# BACTERIAL DISEASES OF FISH

# BACTERIAL DISEASES OF FISH

EDITED BY

## VALERIE INGLIS

*BSc, PhD*
*Head of Bacteriology,*
*Institute of Aquaculture, University of Stirling*

## RONALD J. ROBERTS

*BVMS, PhD, FRCPath, FRCVS, FIBiol, FRSE*
*Director and Professor of Aquatic Pathobiology,*
*Institute of Aquaculture, University of Stirling*

## NIALL R. BROMAGE

*BSc, PhD*
*Senior Lecturer in Reproduction, Genetics and Biotechnology*
*Institute of Aquaculture, University of Stirling*

 INSTITUTE OF AQUACULTURE

Halsted Press: an Imprint of JOHN WILEY & SONS, INC.
NEW YORK    TORONTO

Published in N. America by Halsted Press,
an Imprint of John Wiley & Sons, Inc., New York

Copyright © Blackwell Scientific Publications 1993

Library of Congress Cataloging-in-Publication Data

Bacterial diseases of fish/edited by Valerie Inglis,
  Ronald J. Roberts, Niall R. Bromage.
        p.        cm.
  Includes bibliographical references
  and index.
  ISBN 0470−22120−8
  1. Bacterial diseases in fishes.
I. Inglis, Valerie.  II. Roberts, Ronald J.
III. Bromage, Niall R.
SH177.B3B33   1993
639.3 − dc20                        92−32506
                            CIP

First published in Great Britain in 1993 by
Blackwell Scientific Publications
Osney Mead, Oxford OX2 0EL

Printed in Great Britain

# Contents

# Contributors

**N.R. Bromage**: Institute of Aquaculture, University of Stirling, Stirling, Scotland.

**T.P.T. Evelyn**: Department of Fisheries & Oceans, Biological Sciences Branch, Pacific Biological Station, Nanaimo, BC, Canada.

**Debbie Flett**: Department of Microbiology, College of Biological Science, University of Guelph, Ontario, Canada.

**G.N. Frerichs**: Institute of Aquaculture, University of Stirling, Stirling, Scotland.

**J.L. Fryer**: Department of Microbiology, Oregon State University, Corvallis, Oregon, USA.

**T.S. Hastings**: Scottish Office Agriculture & Fisheries Department, Marine Laboratory, Aberdeen, Scotland.

**Margaret S. Hendrie**: Formerly at Torry Research Station, Aberdeen, Scotland.

**Britt Hjeltnes**: Marine Fisheries Research Institute, Nordnes, Bergen, Norway.

**R.A. Holt**: Department of Microbiology, Oregon State University, Corvallis, Oregon, USA.

**Valerie Inglis**: Institute of Aquaculture, University of Stirling, Stirling, Scotland.

**T. Kitao**: Department of Fisheries, Faculty of Agriculture, Miyazaki University, Miyazaki, Japan.

**A.L.S. Munro**: Scottish Office Agriculture & Fisheries Department, Marine Laboratory, Aberdeen, Scotland.

**J.A. Plumb**: Department of Fisheries & Allied Aquacultures and Alabama Agricultural Experiment Station, Auburn University, Auburn, Alabama, USA.

**Bonnie T. Raymond**: Department of Microbiology, College of Biological Science, University of Guelph, Ontario, Canada.

**R.H. Richards**: Institute of Aquaculture, University of Stirling, Stirling, Scotland.

**J.S. Rohovec**: Department of Microbiology, Oregon State University, Corvallis, Oregon, USA.

**R.J. Roberts**: Institute of Aquaculture, University of Stirling, Stirling, Scotland.

**Rosalynn Stevenson**: Department of Microbiology, College of Biological Science, University of Guelph, Ontario, Canada.

**J.F. Turnbull**: Institute of Aquaculture, University of Stirling, Stirling, Scotland.

**H. Wakabayashi**: Department of Fisheries, Faculty of Agriculture, University of Tokyo, Tokyo, Japan.

**K.N. Woodward**: Veterinary Medicines Directorate, Woodhouse Lane, New Haw, Weybridge, Surrey, England.

# Colour Plates

**Plate 1**  Classic peduncle lesion.

**Plate 2**  Early cold water disease lesion on tail of coho salmon (*Oncorhynchus kisutch*).

**Plate 3**  Severe extensive *Flexibacter psychropila* infection in coho salmon (*Oncorhynchus kisutch*).

**Plate 4**  Columnaris in goldfish (*Carassius auratus*).

**Plate 5**  Swarm of *Flexibacter columnaris* cells forming the characteristic columns.

**Plate 6**  Black patch necrosis in cultured sole (*Solea solea*).

**Plate 7**  Normal dorsal fin on healthy young Atlantic salmon (*Salmo salar*).

**Plate 8**  Typical thickened and eroded dorsal fin of young Atlantic salmon (*Salmo salar*) associated with the condition 'dorsal fin rot'.

**Plate 9**  Peripheral fin rot in plaice (*Pleuronectes platessa*).

**Plate 10**  Japanese eel *Anguilla japonica* infected with *Edwardsiella tarda*.

**Plate 11**  Large white area of depigmentation with central haemorrhagic ulcer on flank of channel catfish (*Ictalurus punctatus*) infected with *E. tarda*.

**Plate 12**  Petechial haemorrhagic ulcers over the surface of channel catfish (*Ictalurus punctatus*) infected with *E. ictaluri*.

**Plate 13**  Ventral reddening and haemorrhage, between opercula in naturally infected young rainbow trout (*Oncorhynchus mykiss*) with redmouth (ERM).

**Plate 14**  *Proteus rettgeri* infection in silver carp (*Hypopthalmichys molitrix*) from ponds fertilized with chicken manure.

**Plate 15**  Oral ulceration in albino plaice (*Pleuronectes platessa*) infected with chronic vibriosis.

**Plate 16**  Deep seated *Vibrio anguillarum* lesion in Atlantic salmon (*Salmo salar*).

**Plate 32**  Direct impression smear from brain of diseased yellowtail (*Seriola quinqueradiata*), showing the arrangement of *Streptococcus* microorganisms.

**Plate 33**  *Streptococcus* spp. showing Gram-positive staining reaction and characteristic chain formation.

**Plate 34**  Tubercle from the liver of a guppy (*Poecilia reticulata*) showing an array of acid fast (red) *Mycobacterium* bacilli in a stroma of caseous necrotic tissue.

**Plate 35**  Epitheliocystis colony between the secondary lamellae of a gilthead bream (*Sparus aurata*).

**Plate 36**  Skin lesions associated with coho salmon (*Oncorhynchus kisutch*) syndrome attributed to *Piscirickettsia salmonis*.

# Preface

This book arose out of the first of the 'Science in Aquaculture' international conferences held at the University of Stirling. These are arranged by the Institute of Aquaculture with BP Nutrition Aquaculture UK and the Scottish Salmon Growers' Association as principal sponsors. Bacterial diseases was chosen as the subject for this first conference since diseases, particularly those caused by bacterial pathogens, are the most important causes of losses among fish farm stocks and a full understanding of this subject is essential for successful therapy and control.

The book has been written as a standard text and is intended for students in aquaculture, veterinarians and microbiologists whose remit includes involvement with the diagnosis or management of fish diseases and for those fisheries scientists who need to know more about bacterial agents of disease in relation to management of fish stocks or production facilities. It is relevant also to workers in the pharmaceutical industry concerned with the development of products aimed at the fish health market and to monitors of human foodstuffs and public health.

The keynote contributors to the conference were asked to provide the individual chapters for the text based on their papers presented at the conference, but also to include material of a general nature and practical information regarding diagnosis, etc. The chapters have been edited to ensure reasonable homogeneity of the text without detracting from the individual nature of the contributions.

The incidence of bacterial diseases of fish in general, and in aquaculture in particular, varies greatly around the world and so it is valuable to have contributions from international authorities directly involved with their management. Chapters on some less important conditions, which had not been the subject of major review papers at the conference, have been added to ensure that the volume is a comprehensive text on fish bacteriology.

The emphasis has been placed on the aetiological agents, their taxonomy, biochemistry, immunology and pathogenicity. Based on an improved scientific understanding of the pathogen and the host-pathogen relationship, control measures are considered. A chapter on the isolation and identification of fish bacterial pathogens is followed by a consideration of their effect on human health both directly and as a result of treatment measures.

The editors hope that this volume will not only prove useful to its readers, but also act as a model for further texts to be derived from this innovative new international conference series.

# Introduction

Much has been written about the bacteriology of fishes. This reflects not only the importance of bacterial activity in relation to diseases of farmed and wild stocks, but also the very important role that they play in the spoilage of fish intended for human consumption. A great deal of this literature, however, has been concerned with the isolation, identification and classification of the relevant, and sometimes irrelevant, bacteria which may be obtained from the tissues of such fishes. Studies on the pathogenesis, ecology, epizootiology and management of bacterial fish diseases are only now becoming developed, in line with the increased economic importance of aquaculture.

The ubiquity of bacteria in the aquatic environment, where they play a major role in both synthetic and degradative processes, makes the task of the fish bacteriologist far from straightforward. The lack of more than a very vestigial taxonomic framework, leading to very incomplete understanding of the relationships between the various groups associated with fish diseases or spoilage, makes logical study or classification problematical. A full understanding of cultural requirements, biochemical properties and antigenic and genetic characteristics is being developed only gradually.

The study of the bacterial diseases of fish is hindered by our less than adequate understanding of the ecological processes, involving interactions between bacteria and their hosts in the aquatic ecosystem. The very different, and often ill-understood physiological features of fishes, characterized particularly by their poikilothermy, contrast with the much better understood physiology of homoiothermic animals. It is from these homoiotherms rather than poikilotherms that virtually all of our present knowledge of epidemiology, immune mechanisms and pathological processes, in relation to bacteria, has been derived. There are often striking differences to be observed when similar processes are studied in poikilotherms (Roberts 1989).

Almost all fish bacterial pathogens are capable of independent existence outside the fish. There is only a very small number of obligatory pathogens. Even these, however, are capable of living for a considerable period within the tissues of their host without any deleterious effect. Usually it is only some major change in the physiology of the host, whether internally driven as, for example, in the case of diseases associated with spawning or due to an external stressor, which allows clinical infections and disease to take place.

Thus it is clear that an understanding of bacterial diseases of fish has to be derived from an appreciation not only of the invading microorganisms but also of their relationship with their environment and their host. Snieszko (1972) was the first to enunciate this when he pointed out that communicable diseases of fish can occur only when susceptible host and virulent pathogen meet in proper environmental conditions requisite for disease induction. The principal bacterial pathogens of fish and associated diseases are given in Table 1. Some are

**Table 1**  Principal bacterial pathogens of fish

**Gram negative gliding bacteria**
    Cytophagaceae:
        *Flexibacter psychrophilus*
        syn: *Cytophaga psychrophila*  cold water disease
        *Flexibacter columnaris*
        syn: *Cytophaga columnaris*    columnaris disease
        *Flexibacter maritimus*        saltwater columnaris
**Cytophaga-like bacteria**    : **Yellow pigmented bacteria**
  (formerly Myxobacteria)    bacterial gill disease and
                     may be associated with fin rot
**Flavobacteriaceae**
  *Flavobacterium branchiophila* bacterial gill disease and
                           may be associated with fin rot
**Gram-negative facultatively anaerobic rods**
    Enterobacteriaceae:
        *Edwardsiella tarda*     edwardsiella septicaemia
        *Edwardsiella ictaluri*  enteric septicaemia of catfish
        *Yersinia ruckeri*       enteric redmouth : ERM
        *Proteus rettgeri*       septicaemia
        *Serratia liquefaciens*  septicaemia
        *Serratia plymuthica*    possible secondary infection
        *Citrobacter freundii*   possible secondary infection
    Vibrionaceae
        *Vibrio alginolyticus*        vibriosis
        *Vibrio anguillarum*          vibriosis
        *Vibrio ordalii*              vibriosis
        *Vibrio salmonicida*          Hitra disease
        *Vibrio vulnificus*           vibriosis

        *Aeromonas salmonicida*        furunculosis
        *Aeromonas hydrophila*         septicaemia
        *Aeromonas caviae*             septicaemia
        *Aeromonas sobria*             septicaemia
    Pasteurellaceae
        *Pasteurella piscicida*        pasteurellosis
**Gram-negative aerobic rods**
    Pseudomonadaceae
        *Pseudomonas fluorescens*       septicaemia
        *Pseudomonas anguilliseptica*  Sekiten-byo
        *Pseudomonas chlororaphus*      not defined
    No family
        *Alteromonas* spp
**Gram-positive aerobic rods**
    No family
        *Renibacterium salmoninarum*   bacterial kidney disease
        *Carnobacterium piscicola*: *Lactococcus piscium*: *Vagococcus salmoninarum*:
        morphologically similar opportunistic pathogens
**Gram-positive facultatively anaerobic cocci**
    No family
        *Streptococcus iniae* septicaemia
        *Streptococcus* spp.
**Gram-positive anaerobic rods**
    Endospore-forming bacteria *Clostridium botulinum* type E botulism
    Irregular non-sporing rods *Eubacterium tarantellus* incriminated in neurological disease

**Table 1** *Continued.*

**Acid fast rods and filaments**
    Mycobacteriaceae:
        *Mycobacterium marinum*   mycobacteriosis
        *Mycobacterium fortuitum*
        *Mycobacterium chelonae*
    Nocardiaceae:
        *Nocardia asteroides*   nocardiosis
        *Nocardia kampachi*
**Rickettsias: Chlamydias: Obligate intracellular parasites**
        *Piscirickettsia salmonis*   salmonid rickettsiosis
        Epitheliocystis organism

important primary pathogens such as *Vibrio anguillarum* and *Aeromonas salmonicida* while others infect more significantly compromised fish. Those present in the environment or as commensals and which are not directly associated with disease have not been included. The nomenclature and classification used here and throughout the text has been based directly on that in Bergey's Manual of Systematic Classification, 8th Edition (Krieg & Holt 1984).

Recently there has been a greater understanding of the need to study bacteria in the context of their environment and their host's physiology and this has led to the conclusion that bacterial diseases of fish are almost invariably 'stress' related. The definition of stress is largely dependent on the user. In relation to fish diseases, however, Brett's (1958) definition is probably the most useful, namely 'Stress is a stage produced by an environmental or other factor(s) which extends the adaptive responses of the individual beyond the normal range, such that its chances of survival are significantly reduced'. When a fish or a population of fish is 'stressed' by almost any form of stressor, the ubiquity of bacteria of pathogenic potential in the environment and even within carrier fish themselves, is such that the fish is likely to be exposed and possibly to succumb to such infection. The exact changes that take place in the fish which trigger the invasion or multiplication of the bacteria are not known, but probably relate to suppression of the non-specific defences such as the reticulo-endothelial system and alterations in the integrity of mucoid surfaces.

Whatever the mechanism for enhanced susceptibility, if the fish's capacity to resist infection is reduced, microorganisms, already within the tissues as in carrier fish, in the gut or in the external environment, will be able to invade and induce clinical disease.

The capacity for such invasion is a major component of the pathogenicity of a bacterial species. Some strains of *Aeromonas salmonicida* (McCarthy & Roberts 1980) or *Mycobacterium marinum* (Aronson 1926) for example, are primary pathogens capable of inducing infection in fish with only the most limited evidence of stress. Others, such as some strains of *Aeromonas hydrophila* (Thorpe & Roberts 1972) can only invade fish already heavily stressed. A third group, virtually saprophytic in their role, can invade fish tissues only prior or post-mortem. They may be present in large numbers, even in moribund fish. Whilst such saprophytes may play a role in the ultimate demise of the host, unlike the primary and secondary pathogens above, they cannot be considered pathogenic *per se*.

The term primary pathogen is thus applied to a microorganism which is capable of initiating a disease on its own or in only minimally stressed stock. Secondary pathogens are those which are generally of limited invasive capacity. Whilst highly significant in the outcome of a disease, secondary pathogens depend on the presence of a primary infection to enable their invasion. Examples of this include many strains of *Aeromonas hydrophila* which exacerbate infections such as those caused by spring viraemia of carp or *Saprolegnia diclina* of salmonids and myxobacterial infections which supervene on *Ichthyobodo necator* and other protozoan infections of the larval branchial cavity.

Bacteria may be associated with many different pathologies in fishes but three responses are archetypal — the septicaemic response, focal dermomyonecrosis leading to ulceration, and the chronic proliferative response.

The septicaemic response, particularly seen in infections caused by the more aggressive of the Gram-negative bacteria, reflects, in the ease with which it becomes generalized, the lack of lymphoid filtration on the circulation system of fishes. They depend for this function largely on the haemopoietic and splenic fixed macrophages. The teleost liver is also deficient in sinusoidal macrophages such as occur in higher animals, although this is made up to a limited extent, in some species, by having a phagocytic atrial lining (Ellis *et al*. 1976). The principal feature of the septicaemic response is the presence of bacteria in virtually all organs. The lesions induced include hyperaemia of capillaries, inflammatory exudation, focal petechial haemorrhages and a leucocytosis which is generally accompanied by significant levels of circulating pigmented macrophages, derived from the melano-macrophage centres, and exophthalmia associated with periorbital oedema (Roberts 1989).

Focal dermomyonecrosis may be a concomitant of acute bacterial septicaemia but generally it is a feature of the less acute, though no less serious, infections where bacteria lodge in the muscle or the dermis. By elaboration of necrotoxins and proteases, they induce significant focal necroses of the tissues within which they are multiplying. This lesion is a particular feature of furunculosis and vibriosis. Often the deeply seated muscle lesion will ultimately extend through the dermis, to ulcerate and release the congery of bacteria and necrotic tissue which play such an important part in disease transmission. The typical abscess, characteristic of such lesions in higher animals, with its yellow purulent exudate of massed neutrophils, does not occur in fishes, where the monocyte or tissue macrophage appears to play a much more significant role.

Pathogenic bacteria of fish often induce chronic, proliferative lesions. These are particularly common in the haemopoietic tissue and are characterized by the presence of ongoing necrosis occurring at the same time as tissue proliferation and repair. This lesion is characteristic of mycobacteriosis, bacterial kidney disease and many other chronic diseases. The central zone of such lesions, containing the initiating bacteria, is gradually enveloped by an epithelioid investment of altered macrophages surrounded by lymphocytes and, gradually, a collar of fibroblasts and collagenous tissue. It had been reported that giant cells, the characteristic multinucleated fused macrophage cells of chronic bacterial lesions of higher vertebrates, did not occur in fishes. Timur *et al.* (1977), however, have shown that although their appearance and regression was temperature and time dependent, they occurred in chronic lesions in all fish species examined.

These types of pathology may all occur in the course of a bacterial infection, but generally one or other is predominant, dependent on the nature of the pathogen and the circumstances of infection. The outcome may be death, complete recovery, or progression to a more chronic condition, where the fish may be seriously compromised and where further stress may lead to recrudescence. Improvement of environmental circumstances, alteration in the fish's susceptibility by use of vaccines, or modification of bacterial reproductive capacity by use of antibiotics, will all move the balance in favour of the fish.

# References

Aronson, J.D. (1926) Spontaneous tuberculosis in salt water fish. *Journal of Infectious Diseases*, **39**, 312−20.

Brett, J.R. (1958) Implications and assessments of environmental stress in the investigation of fish power problems. H.R. MacMillan Lectures, University of British Columbia.

Ellis, A.E., Munro, A.L.S. & Roberts, R.J. (1976) Defence mechanisms in fish. *Journal of Fish Biology*, **8**, 67−78.

Kreig, N.R. & Holt, J.G. (Eds) (1984) *Bergey's Manual of Systematic Bacteriology*. Williams & Wilkins, Baltimore & London.

McCarthy, D.H. & Roberts, R.J. (1980) Furunculosis of fish. *Advances in Microbiology*, **2**, 293−342.

Roberts, R.J. (1989) The pathophysiology and systematic pathology of teleosts. In *Fish Pathology* (Ed. by R.J. Roberts), pp. 56−134. Baillière Tindall, London.

Snieszko, S.F. (1972) Progress in fish pathology in this century. *Symposium of the Zoological Society of London*, **30**, 1−14.

Thorpe, J.E. & Roberts, R.J. (1972) An aeromonad epidemic in the brown trout (*Salmo trutta* L.). *Journal of Fish Biology*, **4**, 441−51.

Timur, G., Roberts, R.J. & McQueen, A. (1977) The experimental pathogenesis of focal tuberculosis in the plaice (*Pleuronectes platessa* L.). *Journal of Comparative Pathology*, **87**, 83−7.

# Part 1:
# Cytophagaceae

Cytophagaceae include several important pathogens of fish which are usually placed in the genera *Cytophaga* and *Flexibacter*. They are Gram-negative rod-shaped bacteria, often pleomorphic and displaying gliding motility. Growth is best on low-nutrient media. On solid media colonies are often yellow, orange or red. Metabolism is chemo-organotrophic and usually aerobic, although some species are facultatively or obligately anaerobic. They are able to degrade biomacromolecules such as gelatin and chitin. The majority are free living in terrestrial and marine environments and some are pathogenic to man and animals including fish, causing disease in both freshwater and marine species.

# Chapter 1:
# Bacterial Cold-Water Disease

The genus *Flexibacter*, within the family Cytophagaceae, consists of Gram-negative, long, slender bacteria which are capable of gliding motility when in contact with a solid surface. The taxonomy of the gliding bacteria is unclear (Reichenbach & Dworkin 1981) but it is gradually being resolved, revealing three important fish pathogens, *Flexibacter psychrophilus* (Borg 1960, Pacha & Ordal 1970, Bernardet & Grimond 1989) and *F. columnaris* (Becker & Fujihara 1978) in freshwater fish and *F. maritimus* (Masumura & Wakabayashi 1977, Hikida *et al.* 1979, Wakabayashi *et al.* 1984, 1986), in marine species.

    *Flexibacter psychrophilus* (syn *Cytophaga psychrophila*) forms slender rods 0.3–0.5 × 2.0–7.0 µm with rounded ends. Optimum growth is at 15°C with no growth at 30°C. Growth occurs on solid media of low nutrient content and proteins such as gelatin and casein are actively decomposed. The mol % G + C in the DNA is 33–34. It is the causative agent of bacterial cold-water disease, a septicaemic infection of salmonids occurring particularly in north-west USA. Outbreaks among alevins may result in 30–50% mortalities; in older fish losses are 20% or less.

## Introduction and historical background

*Flexibacter psychrophilus* syn *Cytophaga psychrophila*, the agent of bacterial cold-water disease has been the focus of recent extensive investigations (Holt 1988). Bacterial cold-water disease (BCWD) is a serious septicaemic infection of hatchery-reared salmonids, especially young coho salmon (*Oncorhynchus kisutch*) in the Pacific Northwest. This bacterium is one of the fish pathogens most frequently isolated from salmonid hatcheries in this region.

The pathology of BCWD in salmonid fish was first described by Davis (1946) at Leetown, West Virginia, USA. He observed a fatal disease of juvenile rainbow trout (*Oncorhynchus mykiss*) in which a characteristic open lesion occurred on or near the peduncle, and for this reason referred to the malady as peduncle disease (Plate 1).

This disease was next observed by Borg (1948) who isolated a bacterium from the kidney and external lesions of diseased juvenile coho salmon in the State of Washington, USA. Signs were similar to those described by Davis, i.e. many of the fish developed a lesion in the area just anterior to the tail which progressed with sloughing of the tissue until the caudal fin was almost detached (Plate 2). Other fish showed lesions on the isthmus, or over the back just anterior to the dorsal fin. Mortality in excess of 30% was observed at certain locations (Borg 1960). The term low temperature or cold-water disease was applied because epizootics were most prevalent when water temperatures were below 10°C. Borg (1960) also successfully infected healthy coho salmon with isolates he obtained from BCWD epizootics.

The aetiological agent described by Borg (1960) was a Gram-negative rod with gliding motility which did not form microcysts or fruiting bodies. Based on the characteristics determined, the bacterium was classified in the genus *Cytophaga* and designated '*Cytophaga psychrophila*' because it failed to grow on culture media when incubated above 25°C. Recently, Bernardet and Grimont (1989) validly published the name *Flexibacter psychrophilus* and designated NCMB 1947 as the type strain. This name will be used for the remainder of this chapter.

## Taxonomy

The taxonomy of *F. psychrophilus* and the entire phylogenetically heterogeneous group of gliding bacteria remains in a state of confusion (Reichenbach & Dworkin 1981). Initially, *F. psychrophilus* was considered a member of the order Myxobacteriales (Borg 1960, Pacha 1968) and was called a myxobacterial fish pathogen. Lewin (1969) concluded that *F. psychrophilus* and a strain of *Cytophaga aurantiaca* isolated from Minnesota, USA garden soil should be considered the same species. He proposed the new name *Flexibacter aurantiacus*. *Bergey's Manual of Determinative Bacteriology*, Eighth Edition (Buchanan & Gibbons, 1974) defined the Order Myxobacteriales as containing only the fruiting myxobacteria with DNA G + C ranging from 67–71%. *Cytophaga* and related genera with much lower %G + C were placed in the Order Cytophagales. Thus, the term myxobacterial fish pathogen is no longer appropriate. *Cytophaga psychrophila* as well as *Flexibacter aurantiacus* were not recognized as a species but were listed as '*Species incertae sedis*' and considered as probable members of the genus *Flexibacter* (Leadbetter 1974). He stated that final classification will depend on the characterization of additional isolates. In the authors' laboratory, *F. aurantiacus* (Lewin 1969) was biochemically and serologically distinct from *F. psychrophilus*. Bernardet and Grimont (1989) further confirmed this by DNA homology.

Christensen (1977) examined the taxonomy of the *Cytophaga* group and recommended that *C. psychrophila* should remain in the genus *Cytophaga* until more work had been done to determine its polysaccharase potential. She also stated, 'the polysaccharase activity of *C. psychrophila* is not fully known and this organism, like *C. columnaris*, may be a *Flexibacter*.' The name *Flexibacter psychrophila* has appeared in the literature (Richards & Roberts 1978, Schneider & Nicholson 1980).

Reichenbach, Behrens & Hirsch (1981) suggested the taxonomy of the cytophagas and related organisms be reconstructed from its very base. There are several roots of the confusion; the group has never been studied on a broad scale; there are many more organisms of this type than previously thought; and all the taxonomic studies published to date are based essentially on morphological and physiological data, not on modern methods of molecular taxonomy (Reichenbach & Dworkin 1981). Reichenbach, Behrens & Hirsch (1981) reported that separation of *Cytophaga* and *Flexibacter* by ability to degrade polysaccharides, as suggested by Leadbetter (1974), was not satisfactory. They proposed to separate *Cytophaga* from *Flexibacter* as follows. *Flexibacter* members have a characteristic cell shape and go through a cyclic change in morphology from long agile thread-like cells (20–30 μm) in young cultures to short nonmotile rods in old ones; all strains contain the flexirubin pigments and the G + C content of DNA is approximately 48%. *Cytophaga*, in contrast, would be divided into two groups; *Cytophaga* (*sensu stricto*), which includes the cellulose decomposers; and *Cytophaga* (*sensu latiore*), which includes short slender rods, with ends often tapering, some containing flexirubin pigments, and with 28–35% G + C content. The *Cytophaga* (*sensu latiore*) group is almost certainly heterogeneous including freshwater and marine organisms, chitin and pectin decomposers, proteolytic strains and fish pathogens from which new genera will most likely result (Reichenbach and Dworkin, 1981).

Reichenbach (1989) listed *C. psychrophila* as one of 20 species in the genus *Cytophaga*. Bernardet and Grimont (1989) compared *F. psychrophilus* strains from France, NCMB 1947 from Dr E.J. Ordal, Washington, and an isolate (SH3–81) from Oregon using phenotypic traits and DNA relatedness. These isolates were compared with type strains of each valid species belonging to the genera *Flexibacter* and *Cytophaga* and with seven *Flavobacterium* species. The *F. psychrophilus* strains formed a tight genomic species whose members were more than 90% related to NCMB 1947. This type strain was only 0 to 5% related to all other *Cytophaga*, *Flexibacter* and *Flavobacterium* species tested. Bernardet and Grimont (1989) followed Leadbetter (1974) in differentiating *Cytophaga* from *Flexibacter* on the basis of polysaccharide degradation and proposed *C. psychrophila* should be in the genus *Flexibacter* as *Flexibacter psychrophilus* pending further reorganization of the whole phylogenetic branch.

## Characteristics of *Flexibacter psychrophilus*

In the authors' laboratory 28 strains of *F. psychrophilus* have been characterized and compared (Holt 1988). These were obtained from widely separated geographical locations in North America and from different pathological and epizootiological situations (Table 1.1). In addition to the work of Borg (1960), other studies have also added to the description of *F. psychrophilus* (Pacha 1968, Pacha & Porter 1968, Bullock 1972, Bernardet & Kerouault 1989).

### Cell morphology

Vegetative cells of *F. psychrophilus* from tryptone-yeast extract (TYE) (Fujihara & Nakatani 1971) or *Cytophaga* broth (Anacker & Ordal 1959) cultures are slender, gram-negative, weakly refractile rods with rounded ends. Cells from a young broth culture (14–24 h) range from 0.3–0.75 μm × 2–7 μm and a few

Table 1.1 *Flexibacter psychrophilus* (*Cytophaga psychrophila*) strains included in a comparative study.

| Designation | Year Isolated | Location | Salmonid Host[a] | Disease, signs or tissue involved |
|---|---|---|---|---|
| SH3–81 | 1981 | Sandy Hatchery, Oregon | juvenile coho salmon | Classical bacterial cold-water disease (BCWD) |
| BC3–81 | 1981 | Big Creek Hatchery, Oregon | juvenile coho salmon | BCWD |
| NN7–81 | 1981 | Nehalem Hatchery, Oregon | juvenile coho salmon | BCWD |
| 84–254[b] | 1984 | Fraser River Hatchery, British Columbia, Canada | juvenile coho salmon | BCWD, including eroded jaw lesion |
| 144a[c] | 1948 | Dungeness Hatchery, Washington | juvenile coho salmon | BCWD |
| NCMB1947 | UNK[d] | Washington | juvenile coho salmon | BCWD |
| MCIK-85 | 1985 | Platte River Hatchery, Michigan | yearling coho salmon | BCWD |
| Ch8-80 | 1980 | Cascade Hatchery, Oregon | yearling coho salmon | BCWD |
| SHSColl-86 | 1986 | Siletz Hatchery, Oregon | juvenile coho salmon | spinal deformed fish |
| BH1–81[e] | 1981 | Bonneville Hatchery, Oregon | juvenile coho salmon | spinal deformed fish |
| SH7–81 | 1981 | Sandy Hatchery, Oregon | juvenile coho salmon | nervous tissue (brain) involvement |
| BFB3–86[f] | 1988 | Butte Falls Hatchery, Oregon | juvenile coho salmon | nervous tissue (brain) involvement |
| BC13S-86 | 1986 | Big Creek Hatchery, Oregon | adult coho salmon | isolated from the spleen |
| SRCo12K-86 | 1986 | Salmon River Hatchery, Oregon | adult coho salmon | isolated from kidney |
| THOF1–86 | 1986 | Trask Hatchery, Oregon | adult coho salmon | isolated from ovarian fluid |
| BCOF19–86 | 1986 | Big Creek Hatchery, Oregon | adult coho salmon | isolated from ovarian fluid |
| THM9–86 | 1986 | Trask Hatchery, Oregon | adult coho salmon | isolated from milt |
| MHChS6–81 | 1981 | McKenzie Hatchery, Oregon | yearling spring chinook | isolated from a white necrotic liver |
| CHChS19–85 | 1985 | Clackamas Hatchery, Oregon | yearling spring chinook | isolated from a white necrotic liver |
| BHURB-86 | 1986 | Bonneville Hatchery, Oregon | yearling fall chinook | mixed infection of BCWD and a blood cell virus |
| SRChF8–81 | 1981 | Salmon River Hatchery, Oregon | yearling fall chinook | anaemic dark pigmented exophthalmic chinook salmon |
| NH67[g] | 1967 | Berlin National Fish Hatchery, New Hampshire | juvenile brook trout | peduncle disease |

| Strain | Year | Location | Host | Disease |
|---|---|---|---|---|
| NB2-79[h] | 1979 | Nootsack Bay, Alaska | juvenile chum salmon | BCWD |
| CCC6-86 | 1986 | Cedar Creek Hatchery, Oregon | juvenile cutthroat trout | BCWD |
| KHRb2-85 | 1985 | Klamath Hatchery, Oregon | juvenile rainbow trout | caudal fin erosion |
| BFRbG3-84[f] | 1984 | Butte Falls Hatchery, Oregon | yearling rainbow trout | eroded gill tissue |
| RbS6-82 | 1982 | Round Butte Hatchery, Oregon | juvenile steelhead trout | BCWD |
| NS3-87 | 1987 | Niagara Springs Hatchery, Idaho | yearling steelhead trout | BCWD |

[a] Cultures were isolated from the kidney except the following strains: NCMB1947 unknown, SHSColl-86 cyst near backbone; SH7-81 and BFB3-86 brain; BC13S-86 spleen; THOF1-86, and BCOF19-86 ovarian fluid, THM9-86 milt; MHChS6-81 liver, and BFRbG3-84 gill lesion.

[b] Isolated by D. Keiser, Nanaimo, British Columbia.

[c] Provided by R.E. Pacha, Ellensburg, Washington.

[d] Unknown.

[e] Isolated by T. Kreps, Clackamas, Oregon.

[f] Isolated by C. Banner, Corvallis, Oregon.

[g] Provided by G.L. Bullock, Leetown, West Virginia.

[h] Isolated by J. Conrad, Clackamas, Oregon.

[i] Isolated by G. Chapman, Eagle, Idaho.

filamentous forms 10−40 μm long are observed. Pleomorphic forms, including cells that are involuted, branched or have thickened ends, appear in older cultures. No microcysts are formed.

Ultrastructure of the outer surface of negatively stained *F. psychrophilus* cells have the granular, crenated, rough appearance reported for other cytophagals (Follett & Webley 1965, Humphrey *et al.* 1979, Strohl & Tait 1978). In addition, vesicular tubular structures similar to those observed on the surfaces of *Cytophaga johnsonii* (Follett & Webley 1965) and *Flexibacter* sp. (Humphrey *et al.* 1979) were evident on the surface of two *F. psychrophilus* strains studied in the authors' laboratory. Based on chemical studies, Humphrey *et al.* (1979) felt these tubular structures were extensions of the outer membrane. No pili were found associated with any of the strains examined. Mesosomes described by Pate & Ordal (1967*a*) in *Flexibacter columnaris* were also observed in negatively stained *F. psychrophilus* cells.

Transmission electron microscopy of sectioned cells (strain 144a) revealed a typical gram-negative cell envelope with a convoluted outer membrane, dense layer (peptidoglycan) and plasma membrane (Fig. 1.1). The convoluted, wavy appearance of the outer membrane is common for the cytophagal bacteria (Follett & Webley 1965, Pate & Orda 1967*b*). Typical colonies of *F. psychrophilus* are shown in Fig. 1.2A and B.

The morphology of *F. psychrophilus* cells in a skin and muscle lesion of a naturally infected juvenile coho salmon was observed by scanning electron microscopy (Fig. 1.3A−C). Figure 1.3A shows an overview of the entire lesion (about 3.5 × 4.5 mm) located laterally just above the pelvic fin. The lesion is typical of most seen with BCWD in which a 'scooped-out' ulcer of skin and muscle occurs. The rough necrotic condition of the surface of the muscle tissue is evident. Within the muscle tissue of the lesion there are massive aggregates or microcolonies of *F. psychrophilus* (Fig. 1.3B and C). Examination of the cells in these microcolonies at 10,000 × magnification reveals no pili but many cells exhibit the rough granular surfaces seen in negatively stained cultured cells. The dimensions of *F. psychrophilus* cells in the lesion of the naturally infected fish are 0.3 × 2.0−2.5 μm. This is smaller than cells grown in culture media.

## Motility

Gliding motility is reported in all studies of *F. psychrophilus*. Bernardet & Kerouault (1989) noted that gliding is slow and difficult to observe. A method that facilitates observation of gliding is to place a coverslip over the peripheral regions of 14−18 h old colonies on a thinly poured moist *Cytophaga* agar (CA) (Anacker & Ordal 1959) plate and to observe microscopically with a wide depth of field oil immersion objective at 1000 × magnification.

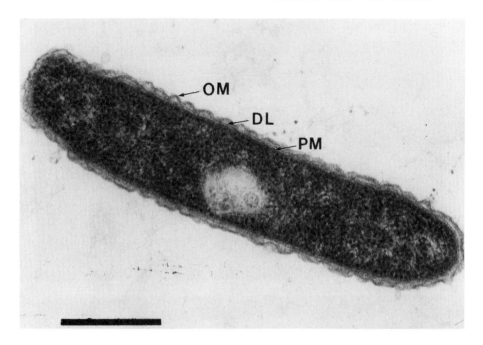

**Fig. 1.1** Electron micrograph of ultrathin section of *Flexibacter psychrophilus* strain 144a. Note wavy convoluted outer membrane (OM), dense layer (DL) and plasma membrane (PM), (Bar = 0.5 μm).

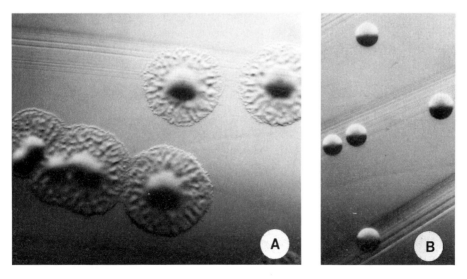

**Fig. 1.2** (A) Photomicrograph demonstrating colony morphology of *Flexibacter psychrophilus* strain SH3−81 showing raised convex centre and thin spreading periphery on *Cytophaga* agar (approx. 8×). (B) Colony morphology of *F. psychrophilus* strain 144a showing the entire colony type on *Cytophaga* agar (approx. 8×).

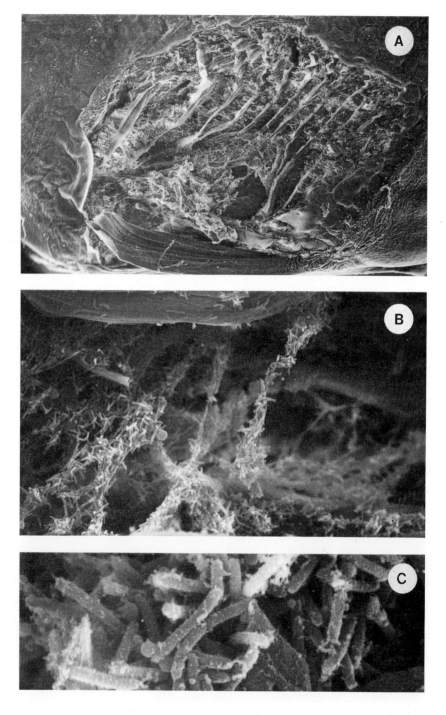

**Fig. 1.3**  (A) Scanning electron micrograph of skin and muscle lesions associated with bacterial cold-water disease. Preparations are from a naturally infected juvenile coho salmon. Overview of entire lesion on lateral-ventral body (× 20). (B) Interior portion of the lesion showing aggregates of cells (× 3000). (C) Microcolony of *F. psychrophilus* cells in the lesion (× 10,000).

**Cultural and environmental characteristics**

*Cytophaga* agar is the most commonly used medium for isolation of *F. psychrophilus* from diseased fish. On this dilute medium after 48−96 h at 15−20°C many strains produce 1−5 mm diameter bright yellow, raised, convex colonies with a thin spreading irregular edge (Fig. 1.2A). Other strains on primary isolation, produce entire, convex, yellow colonies (Fig. 1.2B) or a mixture of the two types.

Investigators have recommended several improved formulations for growth of cytophagals. Shieh (Shieh 1980), modified *Cytophaga* agar (Wakabayashi & Egusa 1974), Hsu-Shotts (Baxa *et al.* 1986) and TYE agar all give good growth. Generally, growth is limited on Tryptic Soy Agar (Difco, Detroit, Michigan) and Lewin's medium (Lewin & Lounsbery 1969).

In liquid media, *F. psychrophilus* grows best in Shieh, modified *Cytophaga* and tryptone yeast extract salts (TYES). TYES is modified TYE and consists of 0.4% tryptone, 0.04% yeast extract, 0.05% $MgSO_4 \cdot 7H_O$, 0.05% $CaCl_2.2H_2O$, and pH 7.2.

*Flexibacter psychrophilus* is strictly aerobic and grows at temperatures between 4 and 23°C (Pacha 1968). Bernardet & Kerouault (1989) examined seven strains and found that all grew well at 10−20°C, but scant growth occurred at 6°C and 25°C; and none at 3°C or above 25°C. In our studies, all 28 *F. psychrophilus* strains grew at 5−23°C, 18 grew slowly at 25°C, and no growth occurred at 30°C (Holt *et al.* 1989). Very slow growth and a generation time of 20−26 h was observed at 3°C. Optimum growth was at 15°C with a generation time of ~2 h.

Several investigators have examined the salt tolerance of this bacterium. Pacha (1968) found that all *F. psychrophilus* strains grew in *Cytophaga* broth with 0.8% NaCl, some with 1.0% and none with 2.0%. Bernardet & Kerouault (1989) observed tolerance to 0.5% NaCl but not to 1.0%. Using TYES broth, all 28 *F. psychrophilus* strains in our study grew in the presence of 0.5 and 1.0% NaCl but none grew in 2.0%.

**Biochemical and physiological properties**

Examination of the nutritional requirements of *F. psychrophilus* has demonstrated little variation among strains (Pacha 1968, Holt 1972, 1988, Otis 1984, Bernardet & Kerouault 1989, Bernardet & Grimont 1989). Minimum variation among strains was noted with the *F. psychrophilus* cultures examined in the authors' laboratory (Table 1.2). They did not utilize simple or complex carbohydrates with the production of acid but were actively proteolytic for casein, gelatin, albumin and collagen. Elastin was degraded by two strains. Pacha (1968) obtained similar results and suggested that this activity may be directly related to the pathogenicity of the bacterium. Otis (1984) did not observe proteolytic activity in five *F. psychrophilus* strains for elastin, and found variable

**Table 1.2**   Biochemical characteristics of the *Flexibacter psychrophilus*[a]

| Characteristic | Results | Characteristic | Results |
|---|---|---|---|
| Degradation of: | | Production of: | |
| Agar | − | Cytochrome oxidase | −[d] |
| Cellulose | − | Indole | − |
| Carboxymethyl cellulose | − | Acetylmethyl carbinol | − |
| Starch | − | | |
| Casein | + | Growth in Broth: | |
| Gelatin | + | 1% Tryptone | + |
| Albumin | + | 1% Casamino acids | − |
| Elastin | +[b] | Koser Citrate | − |
| Collagen | + | | |
| Chitin | − | Other tests: | |
| Tyrosine | +[b] | Methyl red | − |
| Tributyrin | + | Nitrate reduction | − |
| | | Presence of flexirubin | + |
| Carbohydrate utilization: | | | |
| Glucose oxidized | − | Growth on 0.01% | |
| Glucose fermented | − | Sodium lauryl sulfate | − |
| Lactose oxidized | − | | |
| Sucrose oxidized | − | Lysis of dead cells of: | |
| | | *Escherichia coli* | + |
| Production of: | | *Aeromonas hydrophila* | + |
| Ammonia | + | | |
| Hydrogen sulfide | − | | |
| Catalase | +[c] | | |

[a] Twenty eight *F. psychrophilus*
[b] Variable reaction, some strains are positive.
[c] Very slow reaction.
[d] Bernardet & Kerouault (1989) noted positive reaction using a different method.

ability to attack collagen and fibrinogen. All strains degraded chondroitin sulphate and fish muscle. Thus, at least certain strains produced extracellular enzymes that degrade components of fish skin, muscle and cartilage. It appears that the proteolytic nature of *F. psychrophilus* is variable among strains and requires further investigation.

The *F. psychrophilus* strains studied in the authors' laboratory and those reported by Pacha (1968) were catalase positive and cytochrome oxidase negative, and did not produce $H_2S$, indole or acetylmethyl carbinol. Bernardet & Kerouault (1989) reported the presence of cytochrome oxidase but the reaction was weak.

The distribution of flexirubin pigments among yellow pigmented bacteria is considered a useful chemosystematic marker because they are found in most strains of *Flexibacter* and *Cytophaga*-like bacteria isolated from soil and fresh water, in *Sporocytophaga* and in low G + C content flavobacteria (Reichenbach *et al.* 1981). Gram-positive bacteria, flagellated bacteria and most *Cytophaga*-like bacteria isolated from marine environments do not contain these pigments. *Flexibacter psychrophilus* contains flexirubin.

*Flexibacter psychrophilus* strains generally display a homogeneous pattern in susceptibilities to ampicillin, chloramphenicol, erythromycin, oxolinic acid and oxytetracycline. Oxytetracycline incorporated in fish diet is commonly used to control BCWD and two of 28 strains tested were resistant to this antibiotic. Pacha (1968) and Bernardet & Kerouault (1989) also observed homogeneous drug susceptibility patterns. However, some variation in susceptibility to poly-myxin B, kanamycin, nalidixic acid, actinomycin D and sulphonamides was noted.

### DNA studies

The DNA base composition (G + C content) of three strains of *F. psychrophilus* reported by Bernardet & Kerouault (1989) ranged from 32.5 to 33.8 mol% (mean 33.4 mol%). The authors found similar values of 33.2−35.3 mol% with a mean of 34.3% for 13 strains of this bacterium. Relatedness among *F. psychrophilus* strains and with type strains of species in the genera *Flexibacter* and *Cytophaga* was studied by Bernardet & Grimont (1989). Their results were discussed earlier (Taxonomy).

Plasmids have been observed in other bacterial fish pathogens (Toranzo *et al.* 1983) but not in cytophagals from diseased fish. The author found eight of 15 *F. psychrophilus* strains to contain one or two plasmids.

### Serological studies

Pacha (1968) used the slide agglutination method to demonstrate that strains of the bacterium isolated from coho and chinook salmon (*Oncorhynchus tshawytscha*) shared a common antigen. Bullock (1972) found that a strain of *F. psychrophilus* from the western United States shared common antigen(s) with an eastern strain. Pacha & Porter (1968) studied 32 cytophagal strains obtained from the skin of freshwater fish and found none which cross reacted with *F. psychrophilus* rabbit antiserum. They concluded that serological procedures might provide a rapid and useful means for identifying cytophagal fish pathogens.

In the authors' comparison of 28 *F. psychrophilus* strains (Table 1.1) by the slide agglutination method using antiserum prepared with *F. psychrophilus* strain SH3−81 cells, all reacted indicating the presence of common antigen(s). In a serotyping study it was found that *F. psychrophilus* serotypes from New Hampshire, Michigan and Alaska, U.S.A., shared antigen(s) with Oregon strains but were also antigenically different. It is necessary for more strains to be examined before the significance of geographical location and serotype can be determined.

**Diagnostic tests for *Flexibacter psychrophilus***

The following characteristics are important for identification of *F. psychrophilus*:

(1)  Yellow convex colonies on *Cytophaga* agar.
(2)  Thin gram negative rods 0.5−0.75 × 2−7 µm.
(3)  Most rapid growth on dilute media at ∼ 15°C, no growth at 30°C.
(4)  Agglutination with rabbit anti-*F. psychrophilus* serum.
(5)  Actively proteolytic for gelatin and casein.
(6)  No acid production from simple or complex carbohydrates.
(7)  Flexirubin pigments present; colonies turn orange in presence of 20% KOH.
(8)  Weakly catalase positive.
(9)  Scant or no growth on Tryptic Soy Agar or Brain Heart Infusion.
(10) Gliding motility observed, sometimes with difficulty.

## Epizootiology

### Host susceptibility and signs of disease

Cold-water disease probably affects all species of salmonids (Amos 1985) but coho salmon are particularly susceptible. Epizootics of *F. psychrophilus* among coho salmon occur every year at many hatcheries in the north-western United States. The disease usually appears in early spring when water temperatures are between 4−10°C and the severity and specific signs seem to depend on the stage of development of the fry (Wood 1974). When alevins develop the disease, 30−50% mortality may occur and external signs are limited to erosion of the skin covering the yolk. Coagulated-yolk disease often precedes severe BCWD outbreaks. If the epizootic is delayed until the alevins are placed in rearing units and begin feeding, the classic lesion on the peduncle is often observed and losses are usually 20% or less. If BCWD does not occur until several weeks after fish begin to feed, skin and muscle lesions may appear on other areas of the body, i.e. anterior to the dorsal fin, near the vent or on the lower jaw. Morbid fish with no external lesions and dark skin pigmentation are also observed late in epizootics.

A relationship between the severity of BCWD epizootics and the occurrence of deformed juvenile coho salmon when fish are 3−4 months old was reported by Conrad & DeCew (1967). They isolated a bacterium thought to be *F. psychrophilus* from internal organs and this observation was subsequently confirmed by Holt (1972). Wood (1974) reported that this ailment may cause several forms of spinal deformation including compression of the vertebral column, lordosis and scoliosis.

Yearling coho salmon sometimes develop chronic BCWD during the winter months. These fish may exhibit typical lesions of the peduncle muscle (Plate 2), jaw, snout or have no external lesions. They may also be anaemic with haem-orrhagic gills. *Flexibacter psychrophilus* can readily be isolated from internal tissue. Bacterial cold-water disease is sometimes complicated with a red blood cell-associated iridovirus called erythrocytic inclusion body syndrome (EIBS) virus (Leek 1987). This virus may cause anaemia and predispose yearling salmonids to secondary infection with *F. psychrophilus*. The exact role of this virus and *F. psychrophilus* in BCWD of yearling fish has not been determined.

Sockeye (*Oncorhynchus nerka*) and chinook salmon are also susceptible to *F. psychrophilus* infections and exhibit similar disease signs (Rucker *et al.* 1953) to coho salmon. As with yearling coho salmon, certain of the yearling chinook salmon are also infected with the EIBS virus.

Cold-water disease has been reported in rainbow (Davis 1946, Bernardet & Kerouault 1989) and brook trout (*Salvelinus fontinalis*) (Bullock & Snieszko 1970). Schachte (1983) reported that this disease had become a serious problem in cultured fingerling lake trout (*Salvelinus namaycush*) in New York State, USA.

In studies in the authors' laboratory, *F. psychrophilus* isolates have been compared from a variety of different geographic locations, different pathological signs and epizootiological situations. The following was concluded:

(1)  *Flexibacter psychrophilus* probably affects all salmonid species. In our study we have demonstrated that cutthroat trout (*Oncorhynchus clarki*) and chum salmon (*Oncorhynchus keta*) are also susceptible.
(2)  Two identifiable and separate diseases occasionally follow epizootics of BCWD in juvenile coho salmon. The first is the occurrence of fish with spinal deformities. The second is characterized by a nervous spinning behaviour and a dorsal swelling posterior to the skull. Some of the fish have dark pigmentation on one side of their body, possibly indicating affected nervous tissue. *Flexibacter psychrophilus* is readily isolated from brain tissue and less often from internal tissues.
(3)  Strains of *F. psychrophilus* have been isolated from at least two different pathological conditions in yearling chinook salmon. Spring chinook salmon are observed during the winter months with necrotic pale livers and anaemia. Few of these fish have typical BCWD lesions of skin and muscle and most displayed no external skin lesions. Secondly, fall chinook salmon during the summer display anaemia, dark pigmentation of the skin and exophthalmia. A few may also exhibit a swollen, haemorrhagic deep muscle lesion (not open externally) laterally near the vent. In both cases, a mixed infection of *F. psychrophilus* and the EIBS virus is usually noted.
(4)  On rare occasions, *F. psychrophilus* has been isolated from lesions on the gills of yearling rainbow trout.
(5)  *Flexibacter psychrophilus* has been isolated from mature adult coho and chinook salmon tissues including spleen, kidney, ovarian fluid, and milt. Such fish are carriers of the bacterium.

**Histopathology**

Wood & Yasutake (1956) were the first to describe the histopathology of BCWD in naturally infected fish. The disease in coho salmon was found to be an acute bacterial septicaemic infection with the mouth and renal elements of the kidney most affected. The causative agent was found in areas of increased vascularity, including gill secondary lamellar capillaries, kidney, heart and spleen. Bacterial cells were also present in the peritoneum, swim bladder, liver, intestinal muscularis and the pancreas. The cause of death in certain fish was attributed to heart lesions. Wood & Yasutake (1956) noted the characteristic lack of inflammatory response while Borg (1960) observed mild mononuclear infiltration of macrophages. Wolke (1975) reported the histopathology as follows: ulceration of the epidermis and underlying dermis; early lesions having granulocytic infiltration of the dermis and outer muscle masses; as the lesion matures more lymphocytes and then macrophages become apparent; muscle fibres undergo necrosis, leaving empty spaces surrounded by perimysium. Otis (1984) compared the gross and microscopic pathology in steelhead trout (*Oncorhynchus mykiss*) injected intramuscularly, subcutaneously or intraperitoneally with either live *F. psychrophilus* cells or a crude extracellular product preparation from a broth culture. The lesions which developed in both groups were similar and characteristic of cold-water disease, suggesting that extracellular products of *F. psychrophilus* play a significant role in the disease process. Otis (1984) observed internal gross lesions involving widespread systemic haemorrhage of the heart, liver, visceral fat, posterior intestine, air bladder and body wall.

Kent *et al.* (1989) described a spiral swimming behaviour due to cranial and vertebral lesions associated with *F. psychrophilus* infections in salmonid fishes. Histological examination of affected fish revealed subacute to chronic periostitis, osteitis, meningitis and ganglioneuritis. Inflammation and periosteal proliferation of the anterior vertebrae at the junction of the vertebral column with the cranium was a consistent feature of the disease. This condition was observed in populations of fish which had recovered from acute *F. psychrophilus* infections.

**Geographical distribution**

The geographical distribution of *F. psychrophilus* was originally believed to be limited to the North American continent (Anderson & Conroy 1969). Bernardet & Kerouault (1989), however, reported this pathogen in diseased rainbow trout in Europe (France) and it is likely that this bacterium will be identified in fish from most temperate salmonid producing regions of the world.

**Virulence of *Flexibacter psychrophilus***

In the authors' laboratory 19 *F. psychrophilus* strains were compared for their ability to produce disease in yearling coho salmon given subcutaneous injections of viable cells. The percentage mortality caused by the strains varied from 0 to 100% (Holt 1988). This variation in virulence among strains is similar to that reported for *F. columnaris* (Pacha & Ordal 1967).

The experimentally infected fish developed skin necrosis which progressed to open lesions in the musculature (Plate 3). External signs included occasional haemorrhages at the bases of fins or on the opercula and pale gills. Internally, there were petechial haemorrhages of the heart, liver, pyloric caeca, adipose tissue, swim bladder and occasionally the inner body wall. Similar pathology has been observed in naturally infected fish.

## Effect of temperature on progress of the disease

The effect of water temperature on progress of infection in three species, coho and chinook salmon and rainbow trout, has been reported (Holt *et al.* 1989). Fish were held at water temperatures ranging from 3 to 23°C and challenged by subcutaneous injection of a virulent strain of *F. psychrophilus*. Mortality was highest for all three species at temperatures of 3–15°C but decreased progressively up to 23°C. The mean time from infection to death was shortest at 15°C which correlates with the most rapid doubling time for this bacterium in culture medium. Bacterial cold-water disease is in the authors' experience the only infection in which temperatures of 18 and 21°C increased the mean time to death (Holt *et al.* 1989).

## Mode of transmission

The natural reservoirs of *F. psychrophilus* are uncertain. The bacterium does not produce microcysts and apparently maintains itself in a vegetative state throughout the year (Pacha & Ordal 1970). Resident salmonids probably act as carriers (Bullock & Snieszko 1970, Wood 1974). Borg (1960) was not able to demonstrate horizontal transmission unless the mucus and epidermis of the experimental fish were broken. Cytophagal bacteria apparently are part of the aerobic flora of salmonid skin (Pacha & Porter 1968, Horsley 1973) and gills (Trust 1975) but *F. psychrophilus* has not been specifically identified.

*Flexibacter psychrophilus* may be transmitted from sexually mature adult salmonids to eggs and then to susceptible alevins. Borg (1960) reported that *F. psychrophilus* was probably transported on eggs. The first isolation of *F. psychrophilus* from mature adult coho salmon was reported by Holt (1972), who found approximately 50% of the mature adult coho salmon examined to have *F. psychrophilus* in their internal organs and blood. This lends more evidence to the possible association of *F. psychrophilus* with salmon eggs. Studies have demonstrated that cytophagals are the predominant bacterial group on the surface of salmonid eggs (Bell *et al.* 1971, Trust 1972, Yoshimizu *et al.* 1980).

*F. psychrophilus* has been found in skin mucus, kidney and spleen tissue, ovarian fluid and milt of sexually mature male and female chinook and coho salmon. The incidence of the bacterium in female salmon sampled from three fish hatcheries ranged from 20 to 76% and in males from 0 to 66%. In this survey, 110 ovarian fluid samples were collected and *F. psychrophilus* was identified in 38%. There appeared to be fewer *F. psychrophilus* cells in milt. Presence of the bacterium in large numbers in the sexual fluids shows that this bacterium is associated with salmonid eggs and provides a means for vertical transmission (R.A. Holt unpublished observations).

It is not known whether adult salmon carry this bacterium during their salt water phase or became infected on return into fresh water. Adults which have only recently entered fresh water have lower incidences of *F. psychrophilus* than those held for an extended time in fresh water prior to spawning. This suggests that the adults may be infected when they return to fresh water.

## Prevention and control

The most serious outbreaks of BCWD are difficult to treat because they often begin when fish are alevins and incapable of taking medicated food. In coho salmon the pathogen is septicaemic and external bath treatments with surface disinfectants or oxytetracycline are ineffective (Amend 1970). A nitrofuran chemical, nifurpirinol, showed promise for control of BCWD when administered as a bath treatment because it was rapidly absorbed into the tissue of fish (Ross 1972, Wood 1974, Holt *et al.* 1975). However, in the USA at least this nitrofuran is not registered for use in food fish (Schnick & Meyer 1978). Amend *et al.* (1965) tested three sulphonamides incorporated in the fish diet for the control of BCWD in coho salmon. Sulphisoxazole and sulphaethoxy-pyridazine were more effective than sulphamethazine when fish were given a continuous 4 g per 45.4 kg fish per day dosage; however, none of these chemicals completely controlled the disease. Oxytetracycline when incorporated in the diet at 50−75 mg/kg fish/day for 10 days is often more effective than sulphona-mides in controlling BCWD (Snieszko 1964, Wood 1974).

Early infections among trout may be external, and therefore bath treatments with water-soluble oxytetracycline at 10−50 mg/l or quarternary ammonium compounds at 2 mg/l may be beneficial (Bullock & Snieszko 1970, Schachte 1983). Oxytetracycline in the diet is effective for control of BCWD in trout. Schachte (1983) found that the condition in lake trout did not improve with quarternary ammonium compounds or antibiotic therapy when the disease had progressed to the eroded peduncle stage. In this case, a combination of antibiotic and a potassium permanganate flush at 2 mg/l combined with removal of seriously infected fish was required to control mortality.

Wood (1974) reported BCWD to be much less severe in coho salmon alevins kept in shallow rather than deep troughs. Excessive flow through vertical incubators also appears to result in more serious BCWD epizootics. Substrates of various types have been added to incubation trays to reduce alevin movement and mechanical abrasion (Leon & Bonney 1979).

Because there is evidence for *F. psychrophilus* contamination of eggs, Holt (1972) and Schachte (1983) have recommended egg disinfection procedures using organic iodine compounds (Amend 1974). Ross & Smith (1972) demonstrated that 25 mg/l active ingredient of organic iodine effectively killed *F. psychrophilus* in less than 5 minutes. However, recent observations in our laboratory indicate that iodophor treatment of eggs does not prevent BCWD in subsequent fry.

Immunization of fish against *F. psychrophilus* as a means of prevention of BCWD has not been reported and the likelihood of an efficacious bacterin being developed for epizootics in alevins is unlikely. However, because this disease also affects juvenile and yearling age fish, i.e. fish at sizes and ages which have been successfully vaccinated against other fish pathogens (Johnson *et al.* 1982), immunization may be useful.

Protection against *F. psychrophilus* has been demonstrated using a bacterin administered by either injection or immersion (Holt 1988). The injectable bacterin was prepared by mixing equal portions of a formalin killed *F. psychrophilus* cell concentrate and Freund's complete adjuvant. The immersion bacterin was prepared by diluting a cell concentrate with fish pathogen-free well water to obtain a suspension. Replicate groups of coho salmon yearlings were vaccinated, held for 53 days, then challenged with virulent *F. psychrophilus* by subcutaneous injection. We found that intraperitoneal injection of the bacterin provided complete protection of yearling coho salmon compared with 43% loss in control groups. Vaccination by immersion resulted in a reduced level of protection (11%) compared with intraperitoneal exposure.

The occurrence of serologically different strains of *F. psychrophilus* may be important in the development of bacterins. It may be necessary to prepare a polyvalent mixture of the various serotypes and incorporate this into the final bacterin.

# References

Amend, D.F. (1970) Myxobacterial infections of salmonids: prevention and treatment. In *A Symposium on Diseases of Fishes and Shellfishes* (Ed. by S.F. Snieszko), pp. 258−65. Special Publication No. 5, American Fisheries Society, Washington, DC.

Amend, D.F. (1974) Comparative toxicity of two iodophors to rainbow trout eggs. *Transactions of the American Fisheries Society*, **103**, 73−8.

Amend, D.F., Fryer, J.L. & Pilcher, K.S. (1965) Production trials utilizing sulfonamide drugs for the control of 'cold-water' disease in juvenile coho salmon. *Fish Commission of Oregon Research Briefs*, **11**, 14−17.

Amos, K. (Ed.) (1985) *Procedures for the Detection and Identification of Certain Fish Pathogens*, 3rd Edition, pp. 57−8. Fish Health Section, American Fishery Society, Corvallis, Oregon.

Anacker, R.L. & Ordal, E.J. (1959) Studies on the myxobacterium *Chondrococcus columnaris*. I. Serological typing. *Journal of Bacteriology*, **78**, 25−32.

Anderson, J.I.W. & Conroy, D.A (1969) The pathogenic myxobacteria with special reference to fish disease. *Journal of Applied Bacteriology*, **32**, 30−39.

Baxa, D.V., Kawai, K. & Kusuda, R. (1986) Characteristics of gliding bacteria isolated from diseased cultured flounder, *Paralichthys olivaceous*. *Fish Pathology*, **21**, 251−8.

Becker, C.D. & Fujihara, M.F. (1978) *The Bacterial Pathogen* Flexibacter columnaris *and its Epizootiology among Columbia River Fish*. Monograph No. 2, American Fisheries Society,

Washington, DC.

Bell, G.R., Hoskins, G.E. & Hodgkiss, W. (1971) Aspects of the characterization, identification, and ecology of the bacterial flora associated with the surface of stream-incubating Pacific salmon (*Oncorhynchus*) eggs. *Journal of the Fisheries Research Board of Canada*, **28**, 1511−25.

Bernardet, J.F. & Grimont, P.A.D. (1989) Deoxyribonucleic acid relatedness and phenotypic characterization of *Flexibacter columnaris* sp. nov., nom. rev., *Flexibacter maritimus* Wakabayashi, Hikida and Masumura 1986. *International Journal of Systematic Bacteriology*, **39**, 346−54.

Bernardet, J.F. & Kerouault, B. (1989) Phenotypic and genomic studies of 'Cytophaga psychrophila' isolated from diseased rainbow trout (*Oncorhynchus mykiss*) in France. *Applied Environmental Microbiology*, **55**, 1796−800.

Borg, A.F. (1948) Studies on myxobacteria associated with diseases in salmonid fishes. Ph.D. thesis, University of Washington, Seattle.

Borg, A.F. (1960) Studies on myxobacteria associated with diseases in salmonid fishes. *Wildlife Disease*, **8**, 1−85, 2 microcards.

Buchanan, R.E. & Gibbons, N.E. (1974) *Bergey's Manual of Determinative Bacteriology*, 8th edn, pp. 76−119. The Williams and Wilkins Co., Baltimore.

Bullock, G.L. (1972) Studies on selected myxobacteria pathogenic for fishes and bacterial gill disease in hatchery-reared salmonids. Technical Paper No. 60, 30 pp. US Fish and Wildlife Service, Washington, DC.

Bullock, G.L. & Snieszko, S.F. (1970) Fin rot, coldwater disease, and peduncle disease of salmonid fishes. US Department of Interior, Division of Fishery Research, Fishery Leaflet No. 462., Kearneysville, West Virginia.

Christensen, P.J. (1977) The history, biology and taxonomy of the *Cytophaga* group. *Canadian Journal of Microbiology*, **23**, 1599−653.

Conrad, J.F. & DeCew, M. (1967) Observations on deformed juvenile coho salmon. *Fish Commission of Oregon Research Briefs*, **13**, 129.

Davis, H.S. (1946) Care and diseases of trout. US Dept. of the Interior Research Report No. 12, 98 pp. US Government Printing Office, Washington, DC.

Follett, E.A.C. & Webley, D.M. (1965) An electron microscope study of the cell surface of *Cytophaga johnsonii* and some observations on related organisms. *Antonie van Leeuwenhoek Journal*, **31**, 361−82.

Fujihara, M.P. & Nakatani, R.E. (1971) Antibody production and immune responses of rainbow trout and coho salmon to *Chondrococcus columnaris*. *Journal of the Fisheries Research Board of Canada*, **28**, 1253−8.

Hikida, M., Wakabayashi, H., Egusa, S. & Masumura, K. (1979) *Flexibacter* sp., a gliding bacterium pathogenic to some marine fishes in Japan. *Bulletin of the Japanese Society of Scientific Fisheries*, **45**, 421−8.

Holt, R.A. (1972) Characterization and control of *Cytophaga psychrophila* (Borg) the causative agent of low temperature disease in young coho salmon (*Oncorhynchus kisutch*). M.S. Thesis, Oregon State University, Corvallis.

Holt, R.A. (1988) *Cytophaga psychrophila*, the causative agent of bacterial cold-water disease in salmonid fish. Ph.D. Thesis, Oregon State University, Corvallis.

Holt, R.A., Conrad, J.F. & Fryer, J.L. (1975) Furanace for control of *Cytophaga psychrophila*: the causative agent of cold-water disease in coho salmon. *Progressive Fish-Culturist*, **37**, 137−9.

Holt, R.A., Amandi, A., Rohovec, J.S. & Fryer, J.L. (1989) Relation of water temperature to bacterial cold-water disease in coho salmon, chinook salmon, and rainbow trout. *Journal of Aquatic Animal Health*, **1**, 97−101.

Horsley, R.W. (1973) The bacterial flora of the Atlantic salmon (*Salmo salar* L.) in relation to its environment. *Journal of Applied Bacteriology*, **36**, 377−86.

Humphrey, B.A., Dickson, M.R. & Marshall, K.C. (1979) Physicochemical and *in situ* observations on the adhesion of gliding bacteria to surfaces. *Archive für Microbiologie*, **120**, 231−8.

Johnson, K.A., Flynn, J.K. & Amend, D.F. (1982) Onset of immunity in salmonid fry vaccinated by direct immersion in *Vibrio anguillarum* and *Yersinia ruckeri* bacterins. *Journal of Fish Diseases*, **5**, 197−205.

Kent, M.L., Groff, J.M., Morrison, J.K., Yasutake, W.T. & Holt, R.A. (1989) Spiral swimming behavior due to cranial and vertebral lesions associated with *Cytophaga psychrophila* infections in salmonid fishes. *Diseases of Aquatic Organisms*, **6**, 11–16.

Leadbetter, E.R. (1974) The genus *Flexibacter*. In *Bergey's Manual of Determinative Bacteriology*, 8th edn (Ed. by R.E. Buchanan and N.E. Gibbons), pp. 105–7. The Williams and Wilkins Co., Baltimore.

Leek, S.L. (1987) Viral erythrocytic inclusion body syndrome (EIBS) occurring in juvenile spring chinook salmon (*Oncorhynchus tshawytscha*) reared in freshwater. *Canadian Journal of Fisheries and Aquatic Science*, **44**, 685–8.

Leon, K.A. & Bonney, W.A. (1979) Atlantic salmon embryos and fry: effects of various incubation and rearing methods on hatchery survival and growth. *Progressive Fish-Culturist*, **41**, 20–5.

Lewin, R.A. (1969) A classification of flexibacteria. *Journal of General Microbiology*, **58**, 189–206.

Lewin, R.A. & Lounsbery, D.M. (1969) Isolation, cultivation and characterization of flexibacteria. *Journal of General Microbiology*, **58**, 145–70.

Masumura, K. & Wakabayashi, H. (1977) An outbreak of gliding bacterial disease in hatchery-born red sea bream (*Pagrus major*) and gilthead (*Acanthopagrus schlegeli*) fry in Hiroshima. *Fish Pathology*, **112**, 171–7.

Otis, E.J. (1984) Lesions of coldwater disease in steelhead trout (*Salmo gairdneri*): the role of *Cytophaga psychrophila* extracellular products. M.S. Thesis, University of Rhode Island, Kingston.

Pacha, R.E. (1968) Characteristics of *Cytophaga psychrophila* (Borg) isolated during outbreaks of bacterial cold-water disease. *Applied Microbiology*, **16**, 97–101.

Pacha, R.E. & Ordal, E.J. (1967) Histopathology of experimental columnaris disease in young salmon. *Journal of Comparative Pathology*, **77**, 419–23.

Pacha, R.E. & Ordal, E.J. (1970) Myxobacterial diseases of salmonids. In *A Symposium on Diseases of Fishes and Shellfishes* (Ed. by S.F. Snieszko). pp. 243–57, Special Publication No. 5, American Fisheries Society, Washington, D.C.

Pacha, R.E. & Porter, S. (1968) Characteristics of myxobacteria isolated from the surface of freshwater fish. *Applied Microbiology*, **16**, 1901–6.

Pate, J.L. & Ordal, E.J. (1967a) The fine structure of *Chondrococcus columnaris*. I. Structure and formation of mesosomes. *Journal of Cell Biology*, **35**, 1–13.

Pate, J.L. & Ordal, E.J. (1967b) The fine structure of *Chondrococcus columnaris*. III. The surface layers of *Chondrococcus columnaris*. *Journal of Cell Biology*, **35**, 37–51.

Reichenbach, H. (1989) Genus 1. *Cytophaga*. In *Bergey's Manual of Systematic Bacteriology*, Vol. 3 (Ed. by J.T. Staley, M.P. Bryant, N. Pfennig & J.G. Holt), pp. 2015–50. The Williams and Wilkins Co., Baltimore.

Reichenbach, H. & Dworkin, M. (1981) Introduction to the gliding bacteria. In *The Prokaryotes* (Ed. by M.P. Starr, H. Stolp, H.G. Trüper, A. Balows & H.G. Schelgel), pp. 315–27. Springer-Verlag, New York.

Reichenbach, H., Kohl, W. & Ackenbach, H. (1981) The flexirubin-type pigments, chemosystematically useful compounds. In *The* Flavobacterium-Cytophaga *group* (Ed. by H. Reichenbach & O.B. Weeks), pp. 101–9. GBF Monograph Series No. 5, Verlag Chemie, Weinnheim.

Reichenbach, H., Behrens, H., Hirsch, I. (1981) The classification of the *Cytophaga*-like bacteria. In *The* Flavobacterium-Cytophaga *group* (Ed. by H. Reichenbach & O.B. Weeks), pp. 7–15. GBF Monograph Series No. 5, Verlag Chemie, Weinnheim.

Richards, R.H. & Roberts, R.J. (1978) The bacteriology of teleosts. In *Fish Pathology* (Ed. by R.J. Roberts), pp. 183–204. Baillière Tindall, London.

Ross, A.J. (1972) *In vitro* studies with nifurpirinol (P-7138) and bacterial fish pathogens. *Progressive Fish-Culturist*, **34**, 18–20.

Ross, A.J. & Smith, C.A. (1972) Effect of two iodophors on bacterial and fungal fish pathogens. *Journal of the Fisheries Research Board of Canada*, **29**, 1359–61.

Rucker, R.R., Earp, B.J. & Ordal, E.J. (1953) Infectious diseases of Pacific salmon. *Transactions of the American Fisheries Society*, **83**, 297–312.

Schachte, J.H. (1983) Coldwater disease. In *A Guide to Integrated Fish Health Management in the Great Lakes Basin* (Ed. by F.P. Meyer, J.W. Warren & T.G. Carey), pp. 193–197. Special Publication No. 83–2, Great Lakes Fishery Commission, Ann Arbor, Michigan.

Schneider, R. & Nicholson, B.L. (1980) Bacteria associated with fin rot disease in hatchery reared Atlantic Salmon (*Salmo salar*). *Canadian Journal of Fisheries & Aquatic Science*, **37**, 1505–13.

Schnick, R.A. & Meyer, F.P. (1978) Registration of thirty-three fishery chemicals: status of research and estimated costs of required contract studies. Investigations in Fish Control, No. 86, US Department of the Interior, Fish and Wildlife Service, LaCrosse, Wisconsin.

Shieh, H.S. (1980) Studies on the nutrition of a fish pathogen, *Flexibacter columnaris*. *Microbios Letters*, **13**, 129–33.

Snieszko, S.F. (1964) Selected topics on bacterial fish diseases. *Canadian Fish-Culturist*, **32**, 19–24.

Strohl, W.R. & Tait, L.R. (1978) *Cytophaga aquatilis* sp. nov., a facultative anaerobe isolated from the gills of freshwater fish. *International Journal of Systematic Bacteriology*, **28**, 293–303.

Toranzo, A.E., Barja, J.L., Colwell, R.R. & Hetrick, F.M. (1983) Characterization of plasmids in bacterial fish pathogens. *Infection and Immunity*, **39**, 184–92.

Trust, T.J. (1972) The bacterial population in vertical flow tray hatcheries during incubation of salmonid eggs. *Journal of the Fisheries Research Board of Canada*, **29**, 567–71.

Trust, T.J. (1975) Bacteria associated with the gills of salmonid fishes in freshwater. *Journal of Applied Bacteriology*, **38**, 225–233.

Wakabayashi, H. & Egusa, S. (1974) Characteristics of myxobacteria associated with some freshwater fish diseases in Japan. *Bulletin of the Japanese Society of Scientific Fisheries*, **40**, 751–757.

Wakabayashi, H., Hikida, M. & Masumura, K. (1984) *Flexibacter* infection in cultured marine fish in Japan. *Helgoländer Meeresuntersuchungen*, **37**, 587–93.

Wakabayashi, H., Hikida, M. & Masumura, K. (1986) *Flexibacter maritimus* sp. nov., a pathogen of marine fishes. *International Journal of Systematic Bacteriology*, **36**, 296–398.

Wolke, R.E. (1975) Pathology of bacterial and fungal diseases affecting fish. In *The Pathology of Fishes* (Ed. by W.E. Ribelin & G. Migaki), pp. 33–116. University of Wisconsin Press, Madison.

Wood, E.M. & Yasutake, W.T. (1956) Histopathology of fish III. Peduncle ('cold-water') disease. *Progressive Fish-Culturist*, **18**, 58–61.

Wood, J.W. (1974) Diseases of Pacific salmon: their prevention and treatment, 2nd edition, pp. 22–24. State of Washington, Department of Fisheries, Hatchery Division, Olympia.

Yoshimizu, M., Kimura, T. & Sakai, M. (1980) Microflora of the embryo and the fry of salmonids. *Bulletin of the Japanese Society for Scientific Fisheries*, **46**, 967–75.

# Chapter 2:
# Columnaris Disease

*Flexibacter columnaris* syn. *Cytophaga columnaris*, the causative agent of columnaris disease, affects many species of freshwater fish and can cause extensive skin and gill damage and ultimately death. The bacteria are long and slender, with gliding motility achieved by flexing movements. They grow well on low nutrient media producing pale yellow rhizoid colonies. Cellulose starch and agar are not hydrolysed but casein and gelatin are broken down. They have been classified by serotyping and on the basis of sensitivity to the lytic colicin-like substances which they produce. The mol % G + C of the DNA has been reported to be from 30 to 43%.

   *Flexibacter maritimus* causes salt water columnaris. It is similar to *F. columnaris* but has an obligate requirement for sea water. Gliding bacteria, other than this and *F. psychrophilus*, have been associated with disease in freshwater and marine fishes but further work is needed to clarify their taxonomy and pathogenicity (Wakabayashi & Egusa 1974, Schneider & Nicholson 1980).

## Columnaris disease

### Introduction

Columnaris disease was first described by Davis (1922), who observed it in warm-water fish from the Mississippi River, USA. Although Davis did not succeed in isolating the pathogen, he named it *Bacillus columnaris* because, when pieces of infected tissues from diseased fish were examined microscopically in wet mount preparations, column-like masses of the bacteria were observed along the periphery of the tissues.

   The aetiological agent was first isolated by Ordal & Rucker (1944) from hatchery reared sockeye salmon (*Oncorhynchus nerka*) in the summer of 1943 and renamed *Chondrococcus columnaris*. At the same time Garnjobst (1945) isolated the organism from some warm water fishes and assigned it to the genus *Cytophaga*.

   The importance of the disease has led to a significant volume of publications, which have been adequately reviewed by various authors (Davis 1953, Snieszko 1958, Amend 1970, Pacha & Ordal 1970, Becker & Fujihara 1978, Austin & Austin 1987). The precise taxonomy of the agent has been the subject of continuing discussion. In the 8th edition of Bergey's Manual of Determinative Bacteriology, the organism was assigned to the genus *Flexibacter* (Leadbetter 1974). In the 9th edition of Bergey's Manual it was replaced in the genus *Cytophaga* (Reichenbach 1989). In this text, however, the term *Flexibacter columnaris* is used for the causative agent of columnaris disease to avoid confusion in a transitional period during which the new designation may or may not be taken up.

**Disease**

Anderson & Conroy (1969) listed 36 species of fish for which columnaris disease had been described. All freshwater fishes are probably susceptible to columnaris under environmental conditions favourable to the bacterium and stressful to the fish. Generally outbreaks occur when water temperatures reach 15°C and above. *F. columnaris* primarily attacks the external tissues, and uninjured tissue also appears to be attacked. The first indication of the infection is generally the appearance of a white spot on some part of the head, gills, fin or body. This is usually surrounded by a zone with a distinct reddish tinge (Fig. 2.1A), leading to under-running of adjacent skin (Fig. 2.1B). Lesions on the gills or fins extend principally from the distal end towards the base, and the tissues are eroded and destroyed (Figs 2.2 & 2.3). Lesions are covered with a yellowish white mucoid exudate consisting largely of swarms of *F. columnaris* (Plate 4). The bacteria are not usually found systemically until a relatively large amount of external skin or gill damage has taken place; thus it would appear that the bacteria enter the blood stream through the external lesions and are probably not directly involved in causing death (Wood 1974).

**Bacterium**

When infected tissue is examined histologically it is seen to contain large numbers of long slender bacteria. In wet preparations the bacteria show a slow gliding movement and gather into characteristic column-like masses which give the disease its name (Fig. 2.4, Plate 5). The filamentous cells on the columns also display an active flexing movement. The cells are Gram-negative, slender and rather long bacilli, $0.3-0.5\,\mu$m wide and $3-8\,\mu$m long.

Cytophaga agar (CA) (Anacker & Ordal 1959a) is the most frequently used medium for cultivation of the organism. It contains tryptone 0.05%, yeast extract 0.05%, sodium acetate 0.02%, beef extract 0.02% and agar 0.9% and is adjusted to pH 7.2−7.4. According to Song, Fryer & Rohovec (1988a), however, growth responses in Chase, Shieh and Liewes media containing small amounts of salts resulted in a shorter incubation time and higher yields than in CA, which contains no salts. *F. columnaris* produces pale yellow colonies on CA which can vary quite markedly in size and shape. The colonies are of a spreading nature with irregular margins and they adhere to the agar. Under the microscope ($\times 40$), the edges of the colonies appeared rhizoid (Fig. 2.5). *F. columnaris* contains flexirubin type pigments, so that the colonies change their colour from yellow to brown when flooded with 20% KOH solution. In static culture in cytophaga broth (CB) the bacteria form clusters or a pellicle of cells on the surface of the broth. When gently agitated, however, they usually grow homogeneously.

Bernardet & Grimont (1989) described the physiological characteristics of eight strains of *F. columnaris* isolated in Europe, USA and Japan as follows.

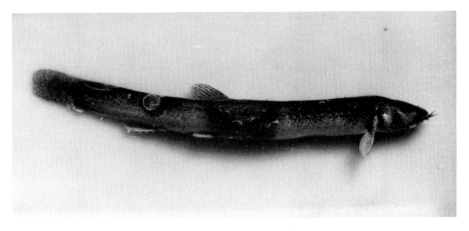

**Fig. 2.1A** Oriental weatherfish, one of the most sensitive hosts to *F. columnaris*. Lesions on the body and fins are surrounded by a hyperaemic zone.

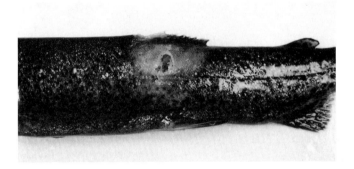

**Fig. 2.1B** Rainbow trout with focal ulcer and associated necrosis below the dorsal fin, a site consistently affected in salmonid columnaris.

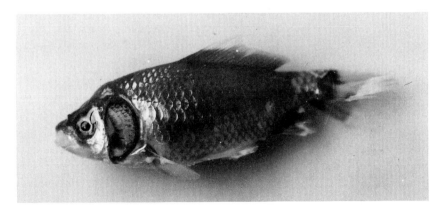

**Fig. 2.2** Goldfish infected with *F. columnaris*. Lesion on the periphery of gills and fins gradually extending towards the body surface.

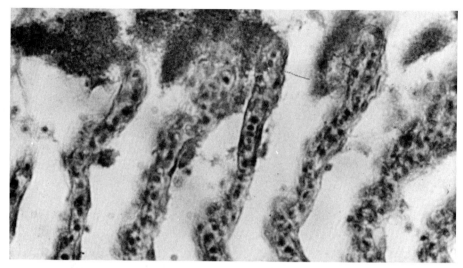

**Fig. 2.3** (above) Cell masses of *F. columnaris* growing on the tips of gill secondary lamellae in the early stages of the infection.

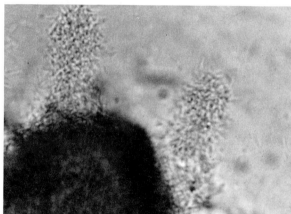

**Fig. 2.4** (left) Columnar formations of *F. columnaris* along the margin of a piece of the tissue.

**Fig. 2.5** (right) A colony of *F. columnaris* growing on cytophaga agar, showing the rhizoid edges to the colony.

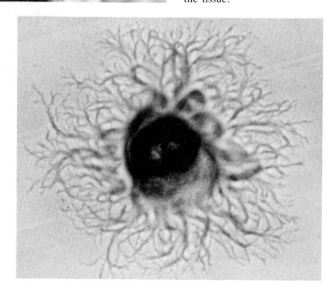

Growth occurs in CB supplemented with 0.1% or 0.5% NaCl and at 10–33°C; strictly aerobic. Catalase and cytochrome oxidase are produced; nitrate is reduced to nitrite; hydrogen sulphide is produced. Cellulose, carboxymethyl cellulose, chitin, starch, aesculin and agar are not hydrolysed. No acid is produced from carbohydrates in ammonium salt-sugar medium. Gelatin, casein (skim milk agar), and tyrosine are hydrolysed. Lysine, arginine and ornithine are not decarboxylated. Tributyrin, lecithin (egg yolk), Tween 20, Tween 80 and DNA are hydrolysed. These characteristics accord with those reported by other workers such as Garnjobst (1945), Wakabayashi *et al.* (1970) and Bootsma & Clerx (1976).

The DNA base composition has been variously defined as between 29.8 and 35.9 mol % G + C (Mitchell *et al.* 1969) or 32.6 and 42.9 mol % G + C (Bootsma & Clerx 1976). According to Bernardet & Grimont (1989) the base compositions of their strains were 32.0–33.2 mol % G + C and the relatedness in DNA-DNA hybridization was more than 76%. Song, Fryer & Rohovec (1988*b*) compared isolates from columnaris diseased fish from Western North America and other areas of the Pacific Rim. They reported that the mol % G + C of the DNA was 29.6–32.5, and that 19 of the 22 strains were 81–98% homologous with their type-species, a USA-Oregon strain of *F. columnaris* isolated from fish in the USA, and it was found that the strains possessed a common species specific antigen and several other antigens (Anacker & Ordal 1959b). On the basis of their antigenic composition, strains were separated into four serotypes and one miscellaneous group. However, no correlation between serotype, geographical origin or species of host-fish and virulence was found.

Many strains of *F. columnaris* were found to produce colicin-like lytic substance and the 134 strains were divided into nine bacteriocin types on the basis of their sensitivity to seven selected bacteriocin preparations (Anacker & Ordal 1959a). Bacteriophage for *F. columnaris* was reported by Anacker & Ordal (1955) and Kingsbury & Ordal (1966). The phage resembled coliphage T2 in shape but infected only *F. columnaris*.

Pacha & Ordal (1963) based their test of virulence of *F. columnaris* on the time required to produce 100% mortality in the experimental fish (yearling sockeye or chinook salmon). The fish were allowed to swim for 2 minutes in standard doses of the organisms and then placed in flowing water at 18.3–20°C. Categories of virulence were determined by the duration of the interval between exposure and 100% mortality of the experimental fish. These were:-

High virulence:            100% killed within 24 h
Moderate virulence:        100% killed within 24–48 h
Intermediate virulence:    100% killed within 48–96 h
Low virulence:             Over 96 h required to kill 100%

There was wide variation in virulence among strains of *F. columnaris* originating from a variety of fish in the waters of the Pacific Northwest.

*Epizootiology*

Geographical distribution
Columnaris has been reported in North America, Asia and Europe and its distribution is probably worldwide (Table 2.1).

Many species have been affected by columnaris disease (Table 2.2), including several of commercial value such as ayu, tilapia and trout.

Water temperature
Columnaris disease attacks fish only at comparatively high temperatures. Davis (1922) first described it as the cause of mortalities among warm water fishes

**Table 2.1**  Geographical distribution of columnaris disease

| | |
|---|---|
| North America | Davis 1922 |
| | Ordal & Rucker 1944 |
| Japan | Wakabayashi & Egusa 1966 |
| | Wakabayashi *et al.* 1970 |
| | Hatai & Hoshina 1971*a,b* |
| Korea | Chun 1975 |
| | Chun *et al.* 1985 |
| Mainland China | Institute of Hydrobiology 1976 |
| Taiwan | Kuo *et al.* 1981 |
| | Chen *et al.* 1982 |
| Netherlands | Bootsma & Clerx 1976 |
| Northern Ireland | Ferguson 1977 |
| Hungary | Farkas & Olah 1986 |
| France | Bernardet 1989 |
| | Bernardet & Grimont 1989 |
| Germany | Alvarado *et al.* 1989 |
| | Bernoth & Korting 1989 |

**Table 2.2**  Species which have been affected by columnaris disease

| | |
|---|---|
| Eels | *Anguilla japonica, A. anguilla* |
| Oriental weatherfish | *Misgurnus anguillicaudatus* |
| Goldfish | *Carassius auratus* |
| Common carp | *Cyprinus carpio* |
| Grass carp | *Ctenopharyngodon idellus* |
| Ayu | *Plecoglossus altivelis* |
| Tilapia | *Oreochromis mossambicus* |
| Pike | *Esox lucius* |
| Tench | *Tinca tinca* |
| Black bullhead | *Ictalurus melas* |
| Sheatfish | *Siluris glanis* |
| Rainbow trout | *Oncorhynchus mykiss* |
| Brook trout | *Salvelinus fontinalis* |

from the Mississippi River which had been transferred to experimental troughs at water temperatures in excess of 21.1°C (70°F). Fish & Rucker (1943) held sockeye salmon fingerlings at different temperatures after exposing them to suspensions of cultured *F. columnaris* for 30 min and demonstrated that *F. columnaris* exerted little effect below 12.8°C. In similar experiments by Ordal & Rucker (1944), 30% of juvenile sockeye salmon held at 16.1°C (61°F) and 100% of those held at 22.2°C (72°F) developed fatal infection. Holt *et al.* (1975) carried out a laboratory experiment on the relationship between water temperature and columnaris disease in steelhead trout (*Oncorhynchus mykiss*), coho (*Oncorhynchus kisutch*) and chinook (*O. tschawytscha*) salmon. No death occurred at temperatures of 9.4°C (49°F) and below. Mortalities varied from 4 to 20% among the three species at 12.2°C (54°F) and increased progressively with increasing temperature to 100% in steelhead trout and coho salmon and 70% in chinook salmon at 20.5°C. The effect of water temperature on columnaris disease in oriental weatherfish was studied by Wakabayashi & Egusa (1972). Fish were infected by the direct contact method whereby a suspension of *F. columnaris* was added to the water at a concentration of about $10^6$ cells/ml, then held at temperatures ranging from 5 to 35°C in 5° intervals. No mortalities occurred in fish held at 5 or 10°C, twenty five per cent of those held at 15°C died and all of the exposed fish held at 20−35°C died. The mean times to death were 7.0, 3.0, 1.8, 1.0 and 1.0 days at 15, 20, 25 and 35°C respectively.

The field studies carried out in the Columbia River system over the period 1955−9 were reviewed by Pacha & Ordal (1970). It was established that the incidence of columnaris disease in salmon, especially sockeye salmon, in the Columbia River Basin, increased with increasing water temperature. Field surveys of Fraser River spawning areas in 1963, 1964 and 1965 revealed that pre-spawning losses of sockeye salmon were associated with high water temperature and columnaris disease (Colgrove & Wood 1966). Pre-spawning losses in 1964 were comparatively very small (less than 5%) owing to the lower temperature prevailing in that year.

The effect of water temperature on the pathogenicity of strains of *F. columnaris* of different levels of virulence was examined by Pacha & Ordal (1970). High-virulence strains were found to infect fish and produce disease at lower water temperature than low-virulence strains. Mortalities were produced at 12.8°C by high-virulence strains whereas low-virulence strains were able to initiate infection only when the temperature was increased to 20°C.

Water quality
Long term survival of the pathogen in environmental water is thought to provide a reservoir of infection. Fijan (1968) indicated that *F. columnaris* could persist for long periods in water of high hardness and organic matter content, but survival time was reduced significantly in water with a pH of 6.0. He suggested that soft water of about 10 ppm $CaCO_3$, especially when acid or of low organic matter content, did not provide a favourable environment for the

organism. Wakabayashi & Egusa (1972) reported that *F. columnaris* could survive for a long time in autoclaved tap water at pH 8.0 which contained $Ca^{++}$ and $Mg^{++}$ at concentrations of 22 and 14 mg/l, respectively. The survival of *F. columnaris* was studied in a variety of waters containing different concentrations of four cations, namely $Na^+$, $K^+$, $Ca^{++}$ and $Mg^{++}$ (Chowdhury & Wakabayashi 1988a). When different categories of water quality were tested it was shown that *F. columnaris* survived for the longest period in water with 0.03% NaCl, 0.01% KCl, 0.002% $CaCl_2$ and 0.004% $MgCl_2.6H_2O$. The formulated water was calculated to be equivalent in hardness to a concentration of $CaCO_3$ of 73.7 mg/l. When the optimal concentrations were diluted 1/10 to 1/100, the survival remained high. In contrast, survival was markedly reduced in the water media containing the salts at a concentration of 10 times optimal or greater. In subsequent experimental work conducted by Chowdhury & Wakabayashi (1988b), experimental infection of weatherfish with *F. columnaris* was also found to vary with different water quality. Infection occurred in every fish at an exposure density of $4-6 \times 10^6$ CFU/ml in both the formulated water and tap water. In contrast, no infection was observed in distilled water and the percentage of infection was low in individual salt solutions.

In a study of the effects of heavy metals on columnaris, MacFarlane *et al.* (1986) showed that arsenic increased the susceptibility of striped bass to *F. columnaris* but copper protected the fish. Hanson & Grizzle (1985) indicated that nitrite at a concentration of 5 ppm enhanced *F. columnaris* infection.

Sugimoto *et al.* (1981) found that *F. columnaris* grew very well on particles of fresh meal derived from the break up of pelleted diets in water. In an experiment, juvenile eels (*Anguilla japonica*) were exposed to a dilute suspension of *F. columnaris* growing on fish meal for 1 h, then placed in aquaria. All fish were dead within 2 days at 26°C. In another experiment, transmission of columnaris disease to healthy fish was enhanced by adding a small quantity of feed pellets to an aquarium containing both diseased and healthy fish. No transmission occurred without addition of the particulate feed matter.

Reservoir host

In field studies carried out in the Columbia River System over the period 1955–9, Pacha & Ordal (1970) found that columnaris disease first appeared in non-salmonid fishes in warm tributaries of the Columbia River. To explore the possibility that such fish served as reservoirs of infection of columnaris disease, six lots of suckers (*Catosformus mersoni*) taken from the river were held in aquaria and the water temperature was slowly raised. Evidence of columnaris disease first appeared at a water temperature of 15°C, followed by outbreaks in all six lots of suckers. It was concluded that fishes such as suckers, carp and white fish could harbour cells of *F. columnaris* and then serve as a source of infection for salmonids when they migrated upstream. Similar experiments were conducted by Colgrove & Wood (1966) in the Fraser River. Suckers captured in the lower Fraser River in April 1965 and held at elevated temperatures in the laboratory developed typical lesions from which *F. columnaris* was isolated. Wakabayashi & Egusa (1967) demonstrated that oriental weatherfish could harbour cells of *F. columnaris*. Apparently healthy fish were purchased from a wholesaler and divided into three groups. Group 1 was placed in running water and group 2 was held in stagnant water. Group 3 was treated with a tetracycline bath at 10 ppm for 24 h, then held in running water. The water temperature ranged from 18 to 24°C during a 17 day period. Columnaris disease first appeared in group 1 on day 10 and subsequently all of 30 fish died by day 14. In contrast, there was no appearance of columnaris disease among groups 2 and 3.

Competitive status with other bacteria
It was reported by Chowdhury & Wakabayashi (1989a) that survival and infectivity of *F. columnaris* declined in the presence of other species of bacteria. The survival of *F. columnaris* was markedly reduced when mixed at a ratio of 1:10 initial density with *Aeromonas hydrophila* or *Citrobacter freundii* in sterile fresh water. In experimental mixed water-borne infection conducted in sterile fresh water, *F. columnaris* failed to invade oriental weatherfish when the initial density of *A. hydrophila* or *C. freundii* was approximately 100 times that of *F. columnaris*. However, *F. columnaris* successfully invaded the fish in the presence of a species of *Streptococcus* or each of two species of *Flavobacterium*, even when the numbers of these bacteria were 1000 times that of *F. columnaris* (Chowdhury & Wakabayashi 1990).

The effect of time-lag between exposures of fish to *F. columnaris* and the competitive bacteria on infections was investigated by Chowdhury & Wakabayashi (1989b). Healthy oriental weatherfish weighing about 10 g were exposed to *F. columnaris* and *C. freundii*. The initial exposure densities of *F. columnaris* and *C. freundii* were $2-4 \times 10^5$ and $2-4 \times 10^7$ CFU/ml, respectively. Fish were not infected by *F. columnaris* and *C. freundii* simultaneously, or when *C. freundii* was added a half hour after exposure to *F. columnaris*. In contrast, when the competitor was added 1 h or later after exposure to *F. columnaris*, the pathogen could successfully invade fish. With such a time-lag, even if the inoculum of *C. freundii* was 1000 times greater than that of *F. columnaris*, *C. freundii* could not prevent the invasion of fish by *F. columnaris*.

Density of fish
A laboratory experiment to show the effect of crowding on susceptibility of juvenile chinook to columnaris disease was carried out by Becker & Fujihara (1978). Experimental fish were held in four troughs (30.5 × 30.5 × 305 cm) with 50, 150, 450 and 900 individuals per trough and exposed to *F. columnaris* from early July until October via incoming Columbia River water (17.5−21°C). No infection or mortality occurred in the 50-fish trough. Crowding hastened infection and mortality in the more crowded troughs, the mortalities in the 150,

450, 900-fish troughs being 1.3, 10.2 and 12.0%, respectively. It seems that crowding not only reduces resistance of fish to *F. columnaris* but also increases chances of the organisms coming into contact with the fish. Effects of crowding fish and exposure density of *F. columnaris* on infection and mortality were studied by Wakabayashi & Egusa (1972). *F. columnaris* suspensions of different densities, namely $\times 10^1$, $\times 10^2$, $\times 10^3$, $\times 10^4$, $\times 10^5$, $\times 10^6$ CFU/ml were prepared in sterile tap water. Oriental weatherfish weighing about 10 g which were previously disinfected by tetracycline baths and well acclimatized, were placed in glass jars containing each bacterial suspension with 1, 5, 10 and 20 individuals per jar. The control groups for each concentration of fish were held in waters containing no bacteria. The water was aerated and the temperature ranged from 22–26°C. Results suggested that the higher the initial density of *F. columnaris* or the concentration of fish, the more certainly infection occurred and the earlier mortalities started to occur.

### Control

Environmental control along with good rearing practice might provide a means of controlling columnaris disease. Auxiliary cold water, if available, is extremely beneficial even if it cools the water by only a few degrees (Wood 1972). Reduction of wild fish in the water supply, possibly by blocking their migration, reduces the number of organisms to which cultured fish are exposed (Wood 1974). The incidence of *F. columnaris* in fish might even be reduced by adding significant numbers of competitive bacteria like *C. freundii* to susceptible fish ponds before *F. columnaris* became established on the fish body (Chowdhury & Wakabayashi 1989*b*).

An excellent review on chemotherapeutics and compounds which have been commonly used for treating columnaris disease was provided by Amend (1970). Since *F. columnaris* primarily affects external surfaces of fish, chemicals are often added directly to the water as a dip, flush, bath or indefinitely prolonged treatment. Heavy metals such as copper sulphate, PMA (pyridylmercuricacetate) etc. were used for many years, but the use of them as therapeutants is now restricted in most countries including UK, Japan and USA because they accumulate in the tissues of treated fish. Benzalkonium chloride (Roccal, Cyncal and Hyamine) or Diquat (6,7-dihydrodipyrido 1,2-a: 2′, 1′-c pyrazidinium dibromide) have been used extensively for treating columnaris disease in the USA. In Japan, nitrofurans such as nifurpyrinol were extensively used for treatment of external infections including columnaris disease until it was suspected of being carcinogenic. For systemic infections, sulphonamides or antibiotics are added to the food. Sulphamerazine and oxytetracycline are administered therapeutically in feed in a two-stage regime, 220 mg/kg/day for 10 days followed by 50 to 75 mg/kg/day for 10 days (Amend 1970).

Fujihara & Nakatani (1971) reported establishment of active immunity to columnaris disease in 3-month-old coho salmon (*Oncorhynchus kisutch*) by oral vaccination with heat killed cells incorporated into fish feed. Studies on oral, parenteral and immersion vaccination of channel catfish (*Ictalurus punctatus*) against *F. columnaris* have been carried out but results were inconclusive (Schachte & Mora 1973). Moore *et al.* (1990) demonstrated the feasibility of immunizing channel catfish against columnaris disease by immersion vaccination with formalin-inactivated bacterins.

## Salt water columnaris disease

### Introduction

*F. columnaris* invades fish only in the freshwater environment. However, marine fish also suffer from columnaris-like disease (Borg 1960, Wood 1968, Anderson & Conroy 1969, Sawyer 1976). Masumura & Wakabayashi (1977) described an outbreak of gliding bacterial disease in hatchery-born Red Sea bream (*Pagrus major*) and Black Sea bream (*Acanthopagrus schlegeli*) fry maintained in net cages in sea water in Japan. The diseased fish were similar in appearance to those with columnaris disease and large numbers of gliding bacteria were observed in scrapings from the lesions. An organism was isolated on cytophaga agar prepared with sea water. The isolate had an obligate requirement for sea water for growth and this could not be replaced by NaCl alone (Hikida *et al.* 1979). Wakabayashi *et al.* (1986) proposed the name *Flexibacter maritimus* for the organism. Subsequently *F. maritimus* infection was reported in Japanese flounder (*Paralichthys olivaceus*) reared in marine hatcheries in Japan (Baxa *et al.* 1986, 1987a). More recent investigation carried out by Bernardet & Grimont (1989) revealed that a strain of a '*Flexibacter columnaris-like*' bacterium deposited in the National Collection of Marine Bacteria (strain NCMB 2158) was synonymous with *F. maritimus*. This strain was originally reported as the aetiological agent of 'black patch necrosis' (BPN) in Dover sole (*Solea solea*) by Campbell & Buswell (1982).

### Disease

Salt water columnaris (*F. maritimus*) was first described as the cause of mortalities among juvenile sea bream cultured in floating net cages in Japan. Japanese flounder reared in hatcheries also often suffer from the disease. Affected fish have eroded mouths, frayed fins and tail rot. In the lesions large numbers of long, slender bacterial rods are observed and give the infected tissue a pale yellow appearance. McVicar & White (1979) described the clinical signs of BPN in Dover sole as slight blistering of the skin surface or darkening of tissue between caudal and marginal fin rays followed by extensive darkening of the area, loss of the epithelial surface and haemorrhage in exposed dermal tissues.

**Bacterium**

*F. maritimus* has an absolute requirement for sea water. No growth occurs on cytophaga medium prepared with the addition of NaCl instead of sea water. At least 30% sea water is required. The bacterium requires KCl as well as NaCl for growth. $Ca^{++}$ enhances growth while $SO_4^{++}$ is slightly inhibitory (Hikida *et al.* 1979).

Colonies on cytophaga agar prepared with sea water are pale yellow, flat and thin with uneven edges and adherent to the agar. The pigment is not flexirubin-type. In unagitated liquid medium, surface growth is in the form of a pellicle.

Bacterial cells from fresh culture are Gram-negative, flexible slender rods. As the cultures age, however, the cells tend to become somewhat shorter and produce round bodies. These spherical cells are not capable of germinating in fresh medium. The organisms have no flagella but exhibit gliding motility on a wet surface. Although columnar formation is not so obvious as in *F. columnaris*, *F. maritimus* also gathers into masses on the periphery of isolated tissues on wet mount preparations (Fig. 2.6).

*F. maritimus* produces catalase, cytochrome oxidase and ammonium and hydrolyses casein, gelatin, tributyrin and tyrosin. It does not produce hydrogen sulphate or indole. Nitrogenous compounds such as tryptone, yeast extract and casamino acids are utilized as sources of carbon and nitrogen for growth. Agar, cellulose, chitin, starch and aesculin are not degraded. Nitrate is reduced to nitrite. Acid is not produced from glucose, galactose, fructose, mannose,

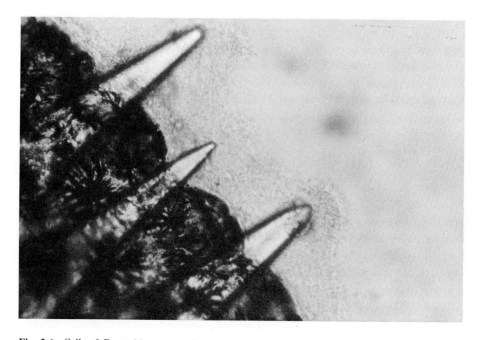

**Fig. 2.6**  Cells of *F. maritimus* swarming on the margin of eroded fin tissues.

lactose, sucrose, sorbose, maltose, cellobiose, trehalose, xylose, rhamnose, raffinose, dextrin, glycogen, inulin, glycorol, adonitol, mannitol, dulcitol, sorbitol, inositol or salicin (Wakabayashi *et al.* 1986).

The DNA base composition of *F. maritimus* has been reported to be 31.3–32.5 mol % G + C (Wakabayashi *et al.* 1986) and 29.0–32.5 mol % G + C (Baxa *et al.* 1987*a*). In DNA-DNA hybridization strain NCMB 2158 isolated from Dover sole in Scotland was 77% related to strain NCMB 2153 isolated from Black Sea bream in Japan (Bernardet & Grimont 1989). Four strains of *F. maritimus* isolated from diseased Japanese flounder were also shown to constitute a tight DNA relatedness group (Baxa *et al.* 1987*a*).

The fact that the Japanese strains examined had a common antigen regardless of source suggests that it may be possible to use a serological test for rapid identification of *F. maritimus* (Wakabayashi *et al.* 1986).

## *Pathogenecity*

*F. maritimus* seems to be less infectious than *F. columnaris*. The ability of *F. maritimus* to produce disease in juvenile Red and Black Sea bream was examined and mortalities among experimental fish varied widely depending on the method of infection (Wakabayashi *et al.* 1984). Fatal infections occurred most frequently when fish were exposed to topical application of the culture on the surface of the mouth or the tail, using an inoculation loop. Infected fish displayed essentially the same clinical signs as naturally infected ones. However, death rarely occurred in experimental fish injected intramuscularly with the bacteria or among those exposed to waterborne organisms. Baxa *et al.* (1987*b*) reported that, although immersion failed to infect Black Sea bream fry with *F. maritimus*, a combination of topical application using a test-tube brush and immersion was effective in producing the disease.

Campbell & Buswell (1982) challenged two groups of 10 Dover sole with a bacterial suspension. The group challenged by scarification showed no signs of the disease, but the group injected subdermally had a 30% mortality after 48 h.

## *Epizootiology*

Salt water columnaris, as it affects sea bream, usually occurs in spring 1 or 2 weeks after transfer from hatchery tanks to inshore net cages and rarely affects fish of more than 60 mm in body length (Wakabayashi *et al.* 1986). Stress imposed by the transfer process is a factor in predisposing hatchery raised fry to *F. maritimus* infection. Although increased water temperature increases the growth of the bacterium, there has been no occurrence of the disease in the summer or autumn. The fact that Red Sea bream is more sensitive to low temperature ($< 15°C$) than Black Sea bream is considered as a possible reason why winter outbreaks have sometimes occurred among Red Sea bream culture in net cages, but not among Black Sea bream.

According to McVicar & White (1979a) BPN in Dover sole occurs in 0-group and 1-group stocks. Clinical signs are generally first observed between 60 and 100 days after hatching and outbreaks are more frequent in summer than in winter. Young fish (0-group) were more seriously affected and death occurred within about 5 days of the first appearance of signs (Plate 6).

*Control*

The standard treatment for salt water columnaris in sea bream and Japanese flounder is to administer antibiotics such as oxytetracycline in the feed. Results, however, are not always satisfactory even though the isolated bacteria are highly sensitive to the drug. Therefore, avoiding overcrowding and overfeeding is recommended, particularly during the expected time of outbreak.

McVicar & White (1979b) reported that a wide range of antibiotics administered orally and as a bath were of little effect in controlling BPN. However, they demonstrated that the addition of a sand substrate to tanks would rapidly cure the disease and remarkably improve hatchery survivals.

# References

Alvarado, V., Stanislawski, D., Boehm, K.H. & Schlotfeldt, H.-J. (1989) First isolation of *Flexibacter columnaris* in eel (*Anguilla anguilla*) in northwest Germany (Lower Saxony). *Bulletin of the European Association of Fish Pathologists*, 9, 96–9.

Amend, D.F. (1970) Myxobacterial infections of salmonids: Prevention and treatment. In *A Symposium on Diseases of Fishes and Shellfishes* (Ed. by S.F. Snieszko), pp. 258–65. American Fisheries Society, Washington, DC.

Anacker, R.L. & Ordal, E.J. (1959a) Studies on the myxobacterium *Chondrococcus columnaris*: II. Bacteriocins. *Journal of Bacteriology*, 78, 33–40.

Anacker, R. & Ordal, E.J. (1959b) Studies on the myxobacterium *Chondrococcus columnaris*: I. Serological typing. *Journal of Bacteriology*, 78, 25–32.

Anacker, R.L. & Ordal, E.J. (1955) Study of a bacteriophage infecting the myxobacterium *Chondrococcus columnaris*. *Journal of Bacteriology*, 70, 738–41.

Anderson, J.I.W. & Conroy, D.A. (1969) The pathogenic myxobacteria with special reference to fish disease. *Journal of Applied Bacteriology*, 32, 30–9.

Austin, B. & Austin, D.A. (1987) Gram-negative pigmented rods. In *Bacterial Fish Pathogens: Disease in Farmed and Wild Fish*, pp. 225–49. Ellis Horwood Ltd, Chichester.

Baxa, D.V., Kawai, K. & Kusuda, R. (1986) Characteristics of gliding bacteria isolated from diseased cultured flounder, *Paralichthys olivaceus*. *Fish Pathology*, 21, 251–8.

Baxa, D.V., Kawai, K. & Kusuda, R. (1987a) Molecular taxonomic classification of gliding bacteria isolated from diseased cultured flounder. *Fish Pathology*, 22, 11–14.

Baxa, D.V., Kawai, K. & Kusuda, R. (1987b) Experimental infection of *Flexibacter maritimus* in Black Sea bream (*Acanthopagrus schlegeli*) fry. *Fish Pathology*, 22, 105–9.

Becker, C.D. & Fujihara, M.P. (1978) The bacterial pathogen *Flexibacter columnaris* and its epizootiology among Columbia River Fish. American Fisheries Society Monograph No. 2, 92pp.

Bernardet, J.F. (1989) *Flexibacter columnaris*: First description in France and comparison with bacterial strains from other origins. *Diseases of Aquatic Organisms*, 6, 37–44.

Bernardet, J.F. & Grimont, P.A.D. (1989) Deoxyribonucleic acid relatedness and phenotypic characterization of *Flexibacter columnaris* sp. nov., nom. rev., *Flexibacter psychrophilus* sp. nov., nom. rev., and *Flexibacter maritimus* Wakabayashi, Hikida & Masumura, 1986. *International Journal of Systematic Bacteriology*, 39(3), 346–354.

Bernoth, E.M. & Korting, W. (1989) First report on *Flexibacter columnaris* in tench (*Tinca tinca*, L.) in Germany. *Bulletin of the European Association of Fish Pathologists*, **9**, 125−7.

Bootsma, R. & Clerx, J.P.M. (1976) Columnaris disease of cultured carp, *Cyprinus carpio* L.: Characteristics of the causative agent. *Aquaculture*, **7**, 371−84.

Borg, A.F. (1960) Studies on myxobacteria associated with diseases of salmonid fishes. *Journal of Wildlife Diseases*, **8**, 1−85.

Campbell, A.C. & Buswell, J.A. (1982) An investigation into the bacterial aetiology of 'black patch necrosis' in Dover sole (*Solea solea* L.). *Journal of Fish Diseases*, **5**, 495−508.

Chen, C.R., Chung, Y.Y. & Kou, G.H. (1982) Studies on the pathogenicity of *Flexibacter columnaris* to eel (*Anguilla japonica*). CAPD Fisheries Series No. 8, *Reports on Fish Disease Research*, **4**, 57−61.

Chowdhury, M.B.R. & Wakabayashi, H. (1988a) Effects of sodium, potassium, calcium and magnesium ions on the survival of *Flexibacter columnaris* in water. *Fish Pathology*, **23**, 231−5.

Chowdhury, M.B.R. & Wakabayashi, H. (1988b) Effects of sodium, potassium, calcium and magnesium ions on *Flexibacter columnaris* infection in fish. *Fish Pathology*, **23**, 237−41.

Chowdhury, M.B.R. & Wakabayashi, H. (1989a) A study on the mechanism of the bacterial competitive effects on *Flexibacter columnaris* infection: Effects of the time-lag between the exposure of fish to *F. columnaris* and its competitor. *Fish Pathology*, **24**, 105−10.

Chowdhury, M.B.R. & Wakabayashi, H. (1989b) Effects of competitive bacteria on the survival and infectivity of *Flexibacter columnaris*. *Fish Pathology*, **24**, 9−15.

Chowdhury, M.B.R. & Wakabayashi, H. (1990) Effects of co-existing bacteria on *Flexibacter columnaris* infection in loach *Misgurnus anguillicaudatus*. In *The 2nd Asian Fisheries Forum* (Ed. by R. Hirano & I. Hanyu), pp. 651−4. Asian Fisheries Society.

Chun, S.K. (1975) The pathogenicity of myxobacteria isolated from infected fish. *Bulletin of National Fisheries University of Busan*, **15**, 31−42.

Chun, S.K., Park, C.Y. & Lee, S.K. (1985) Characteristics of *Flexibacter columnaris* isolated from tilapia (*Tilapia* sp.) *Bulletin of Korean Fisheries Society*, **18**, 369−73.

Colgrove, D.J. & Wood, J.W. (1966) Occurrence and control of *Chondrococcus columnaris* as related to Fraser River sockeye salmon. Progress Report of International Pacific Salmon Fisheries Commission No. 15, 51pp.

Davis, H.S. (1922) A new bacterial disease of freshwater fishes. *Bulletin of US Bureau of Fisheries*, **38**, 261−80.

Davis, H.S. (1953) *Culture and Diseases of Game Fishes*. University of California Press, Berkeley.

Farkas, J. & Olah, J. (1986) Gill necrosis − a complex disease of carp. *Aquaculture*, **58**, 17−26.

Ferguson, H.W. (1977) Columnaris disease in rainbow trout (*Salmo gairdneri*) in Northern Ireland. *Veterinary Record*, **101**, 55−6.

Fijan, N.N. (1968) The survival of *Chondrococcus columnaris* in waters of different quality. *Bulletin de l'Office International des Epizootics*, **69**, 1158−66.

Fish, F.F. & Rucker, R.R. (1943) Infectious disease of Pacific salmon. *Transactions of the American Fisheries Society*, **83**, 297−312.

Fujihara, M.P. & Nakatani, R.E. (1971) Antibody production and immune responses of rainbow trout and coho salmon to *Chondrococcus columnaris*. *Journal of the Fisheries Research Board of Canada*, **28**, 1253−8.

Garnjobst, L. (1945) *Cytophaga columnaris* (Davis) in pure culture: a myxobacterium pathogenic to fish. *Journal of Bacteriology*, **49**, 113−28.

Hanson, L.A. & Grizzle, J.M. (1985) Nitrite-induced predisposition of channel catfish to *Flexibacter columnaris* infection. *Progressive Fish-Culturist*, **47**, 98−101.

Hatai, K. & Hoshina, R. (1971a) Studies on pathogenic myxobacteria − I. Isolation of the organisms and experimental infections. *Fish Pathology*, **5**, 100−6.

Hatai, K. & Hoshina, R. (1971b) Studies on pathogenic myxobacteria − II. Biological and biochemical characteristics. *Fish Pathology*, **6**, 30−6.

Hikida, M., Wakabayashi, H., Egusa, S. & Musumara, K. (1979) *Flexibacter* sp., a gliding bacterium pathogenic to some marine fishes in Japan. *Bulletin of the Japanese Society of Scientific Fisheries*, **45**, 421−8.

Holt, R.A., Sanders, J.E., Zinn, J.L., Fryer, J.L. & Pilcher, K.S. (1975) Relation of water temperature to *Flexibacter columnaris* infection in steelhead trout (*Salmo gairdneri*), coho (*Oncorhynchus kisutch*) and chinook (*O. tschawytscha*) salmon. *Journal of the Fisheries*

*Research Board of Canada*, **32**, 1553−9.

Institute of Hydrobiology (1976) Studies on the white head-mouth disease of grass carp (*Cteno-pharyngodon idellus*). *Acta Hydrobiologica Sinica*, **6**, 53−65.

Kingsbury, D.T. & Ordal, E.J. (1966) Bacteriophage infecting the myxobacterium *Chondrococcus columnaris*. *Journal of Bacteriology*, **91**, 1327−32.

Kuo, S.C., Chung, H.Y. & Kou, G.H. (1981) Studies on artificial infection of the gliding bacteria in cultured fishes. *Fish Pathology*, **15**, 309−14.

Leadbetter, E.R. (1974) Genus II. *Flexibacter* Soriano 1945, 92, Levin 1969, 192 emend. mut. char. In *Bergey's Manual of Determinative Bacteriology*, 8th edn (Ed. by R.E. Buchanan & N.E. Gibbons), pp. 105−7. The Williams & Wilkins Co., Baltimore.

MacFarlane, R.D., Bullock, G.L. & McLaughlin, J.J.A. (1986) Effects of five metals on suscepti-bility of striped bass to *Flexibacter columnaris*. *Transactions of the American Fisheries Society*, **115**, 227−31.

McVicar, A.H. & White, P.G. (1979a) Fin and skin necrosis of cultivated Dover sole *Solea solea* (L.) *Journal of Fish Disease*, **2**, 557−62.

McVicar, A.H. & White, P.G. (1979b) The prevention and cure of an infectious disease in cultivated juvenile Dover sole, *Solea solea* (L.) *Aquaculture*, **26**, 213−22.

Masumura, K. & Wakabayashi, H. (1977) An outbreak of gliding bacterial disease in hatchery-born red sea bream (*Pagrus major*) and gilthead (*Achanthopagrus schlegeli*) fry in Hiroshima. *Fish Pathology*, **12**, 171−7.

Mitchell, T.G., Hendrie, M.S. & Shewan, J.M. (1969) The taxonomy, differentiation and identi-fication of Cytophaga species. *Journal of Applied Bacteriology*, **32**, 40−50.

Moore, A.A., Eimers, M.E. & Cardell, M.A. (1990) Attempts to control *Flexibacter columnaris* epizootics in pond-reared channel catfish by vaccination. *Journal of Aquatic Animal Health*, **2**, 109−11.

Ordal, E.J. & Rucker, R.R. (1944) Pathogenic myxobacteria. *Proceedings of the Society of Experimental Biology and Medicine*, **56**, 15−18.

Pacha, R.E. & Ordal, E.J. (1963) Epidemiology of columnaris disease in salmon. *Bacteriological Proceedings*, **63**, 3−4.

Pacha, R.E. & Ordal, E.J. (1970) Myxobacterial diseases of salmonids. In *A Symposium on Diseases of Fishes and Shellfishes* (Ed. by S.F. Snieszko), pp. 243−7. The American Fisheries Society, Special Publications (5). Washington, DC.

Reichenbach, H. (1989) Genus I. *Cytophaga* Winogradsky 1929, 577, emend. In *Bergey's Manual of Systematic Bacteriology*, Volume 3 (Ed. by J.T. Staley, M.P. Bryant, N. Pfennig & J.G. Holt), pp. 2015−50. The Williams & Wilkins Co., Baltimore.

Sawyer, E.S. (1976) An outbreak of myxobacterial disease in coho salmon (*Oncorhynchus kisutsch*) reared in a marine estuary. *Journal of Wildlife Diseases*, **12**, 575−8.

Schachte, J.H. & Mora, E.C. (1973) Production of agglutinating antibodies in channel catfish (*Ictalurus punctatus*) against *Chondrococcus columnaris*. *Journal of the Fisheries Research Board of Canada*, **30**, 116−18.

Schneider, R. & Nicholson, B.L. (1980) Bacteria associated with fin rot disease in hatchery-reared Atlantic salmon (*Salmo salar*) *Canadian Journal of Fisheries and Aquatic Sciences*, 37, 1505−1513.

Snieszko, S.F. (1958) Columnaris disease of fishes. US Department of Interior, Fish and Wildlife Service, Fisheries Leaflet **46**, 1−3.

Song, Y.L., Fryer, J.L. & Rohovec, J.S. (1988a) Comparison of six media for the cultivation of *Flexibacter columnaris*. *Fish Pathology*, **23**, 91−4.

Song, Y.L., Fryer, J.L. & Rohovec, J.S. (1988b) Comparison of gliding bacteria isolated from fish in North America and other areas of Pacific Rim. *Fish Pathology*, **23**, 197−202.

Sugimoto, N., Kashiwaga, S. & Matsuda, T. (1981) Pathogenic relation between columnaris disease in cultured eel and the formula feeds. *Bulletin of the Japanese Society of Scientific Fisheries*, **47**, 716−25.

Wakabayashi, H. & Egusa, S. (1966) Characteristics of a myxobacterium, *Chondrococcus colum-naris*, isolated from diseased loach. *Bulletin of the Japanese Society of Scientific Fisheries*, **32**, 1015−22.

Wakabayashi, H. & Egusa, S. (1967) Columnaris disease of loach, *Misgurnus anguillicaudatus*. *Fish Pathology*, **1**, 20−6.

Wakabayashi, H. & Egusa, S. (1972) Preliminary experiments on environmental factors influencing the prevalence of columnaris disease. *Fish Pathology*, **7**, 58–63.

Wakabayashi, H. & Egusa, S. (1974) Characteristics of myxobacteria associated with some fresh-water fish diseases in Japan. *Bulletin of the Japanese Society of Scientific Fisheries*, **40**, 751–7.

Wakabayashi, H., Kira, K. & Egusa, S. (1970) Studies on columnaris disease of pond-cultured eel — I. Characteristics and pathogenicity of *Chondrococcus columnaris* isolated from pond-cultured eels. *Bulletin of the Japanese Society of Scientific Fisheries*, **36**, 147–55.

Wakabayashi, H., Hikida, M. & Masamura, K. (1984) *Flexibacter* infection in cultured marine fish in Japan. *Helgoländer Meersuntersuchungen*, **37**, 587–593.

Wakabayashi, H., Hikida, M. & Masumura, K. (1986) *Flexibacter maritimus* sp. nov., a pathogen of marine fishes. *International Journal of Systematic Bacteriology*, **36**, 396–8.

Wood, J.W. (1974) *Diseases of Pacific salmon: Their prevention and treatment* (2nd edn), 82 pp. State of Washington Department of Fisheries, Hatchery Division.

# Chapter 3:
# Bacterial Gill Disease and Fin Rot

The principal genera involved in bacterial gill disease are *Cytophaga*, *Flexibacter* and *Flavobacterium*. These and other less well-defined bacteria are referred to as cytophaga-like bacteria (CLB) or yellow-pigmented bacteria, terms replacing the inappropriate name, 'myxobacteria'. The bacteria associated with fin rot include *CLB*, aeromonads, pseudomonads and others.


## Bacterial gill disease

### Introduction

Bacterial gill disease (BGD) is a condition primarily associated with yellow pigmented, filamentous, Gram-negative bacteria of the genera *Cytophaga*, *Flexibacter* and *Flavobacter*. These bacteria have been referred to as Cytophaga-like bacteria of CLB (Reichenbach 1989). Other Gram-negative Eubacteria have been isolated from cases of BGD (Wood & Yasutake 1957) but these are thought not to play a significant role. Some workers have considered *Flexibacter columnaris* infection of the gills as a form of BGD (Foscarini 1989). However, since *F. columnaris* is covered elsewhere it will not be included here.

Environmental conditions are thought to play some role in the aetiology of BGD. However, the relative significance ascribed to environmental and bacterial components has varied between studies. Some have suggested that adverse environmental conditions are essential to the initiation of BGD (Bullock 1972) or the development of clinical disease (Kimura *et al.* 1978, Wakabayashi *et al.* 1980). Other recent studies have proposed a more primarily pathogenic role for bacteria (Ferguson *et al.* 1991). These results do not necessarily imply a contradiction. BGD may well be a condition resulting from the complex interaction of adverse environmental conditions and bacteria of variable pathogenicity. Therefore similar, if not identical, pathology could result from either the presence of a low grade opportunist pathogen in extreme environmental conditions, or the presence of a highly pathogenic bacterium in marginal environmental conditions.

Since its first report in an experimental salmonid hatchery by Davis (1926), most of the literature has concentrated on BGD in intensively reared salmonids. This is probably a reflection of the economic significance of BGD in salmonid culture. The condition has been reported in other species of intensively reared freshwather fish; however, the literature is not necessarily the best guide to the epidemiology of BGD. For example, BGD is said to be a common condition in Europe (Farkas 1985) but is only rarely reported, since it is easily recognised and treated by farmers.

**Disease and clinical signs**

Affected fish become lethargic and anorexic. They tend to remain near the surface or inlet and may be observed flaring their opercula and coughing. Their respiratory rate is elevated and mucus secretion may increase to the point where strands are obvious trailing from the gills (Bullock & Conroy 1971*a*, Ferguson *et al*. 1991).

Gross pathological changes in mild or early stages include hyperaemia, swelling of the primary lamellae and increased mucus secretion, which often traps debris. These changes may progress to extensive fusion and distortion of the primary lamellae. In the later stages secondary fungal infections and/or opercular damage are commonly observed (Ostland *et al*. 1990).

Histopathological changes detectable under the light microscope usually begin at the tips of the distal secondary lamellae (Kudo & Kimura 1983*a*, Speare *et al*. 1991*a*). This is the site of initial bacterial colonisation, which subsequently spreads proximally. Unfortunately, the bacteria are not always detectable histologically since they may be removed during processing. The early cellular changes can be difficult to resolve with conventional histological techniques but may include hydropic degeneration, exfoliation of the epithelial cells with associated spongiosis or attenuation of the epithelium.

As the disease progresses, more obvious signs of epithelial hyperplasia with associated lamellar fusion are detectable. Such fusion may occur either following apposition of the distal lamellae due to oedema or by cellular proliferation 'filling up' the spaces between secondary lamellae (Speare *et al*. 1991*b*, Kudo & Kimura 1983*a*). If the secondary lamellae fuse distally they form a space lined by epithelial, mucus and chloride cells. This space, which is at least partially enclosed, often contains bacteria, sloughed cells, mucus and other debris (Kudo & Kimura 1983*a*, Speare *et al*. 1991*b*).

The bacterial colonisation and pathological changes are not confined to the secondary lamellae but extend to the primary lamellae and branchial cavity. In these regions the pathology is similar, but with epithelial spongiosis and inflammatory cell infiltration becoming more obvious in severe cases (Ostland *et al*. 1990, Speare *et al*. 1991*a*).

If the condition is successfully treated the gills may recover completely, provided that the basement membrane is intact (Kudo & Kimura 1983*a*).

Electron microscopy reveals further details of the pathological changes. The first signs that have been detected precede bacterial colonisation. They include disfigurement of the epithelial microridges by membrane bound electron lucent vesicles (Speare *et al*. 1991*b*). It is not yet clear how these changes relate to the aetiology of the condition. The first stage of true BGD might be taken as the initial attachment of the bacteria to the microridge tips (Fig. 3.1). The bacteria attach by an extensive glycocalyx containing sloughed material and food particles (Speare *et al*. 1991*b*). A similar structure was also mentioned by Kudo & Kimura (1983*a*) (Fig. 3.2).

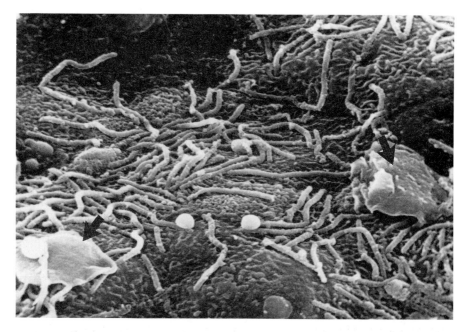

**Fig. 3.1** Gill lamella of rainbow trout showing filamentous bacteria closely adherent to the lamellar surface. Necrotic cells (arrowed) are in the process of exfoliating. SEM × 1600 (Courtesy of Dr D.J. Speare).

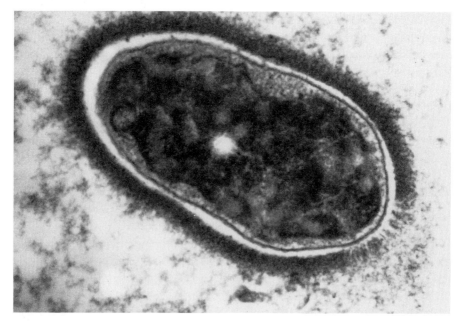

**Fig. 3.2** Continuous and extensive glycocalyx around the bacterial outer cell membrane. TEM × 100,000 (Courtesy of Dr D.J. Speare).

As the numbers of bacteria increase and develop into microcolonies the cellular pathology becomes more obvious. The microridge vesicles fill with cytoplasmic material (Speare *et al.* 1991*a*) and continued superficial vesiculation leads to exfoliation and fusion of adjacent microridges. Both epithelial and chloride cells undergo dilation of the mitochondria, endoplasmic reticulum and cytocavities, indicating hydropic degeneration, and evidence of mucus cell metaplasia has also been reported (Speare *et al.* 1991*a*, Kudo & Kimura 1983*a*).

Thereafter the electron microscopic appearance reflects the histology with extensive proliferation and fusion of the gill epithelium (Fig. 3.3).

The presence of necrosis has been reported by some authors (Ostland *et al.* 1990, Speare *et al.* 1991*b*) but not all (Wakabayashi & Iwado 1985) (See this chapter, Pathogenesis).

## Bacteria

The yellow pigmented, filamentous, Gram-negative bacteria associated with BGD were referred to as 'myxobacteria' in much of the older literature. However it is now agreed that 'myxobacteria' is not an appropriate term for fish pathogens. Most of the organisms are currently thought to belong to the genera *Cytophaga*, *Flexibacter* and *Flavobacter*. Some authors have referred to these organisms as yellow pigmented bacteria (YPB), but for the purpose of this text they will be referred to as Cytophaga-like bacteria (CLB), the

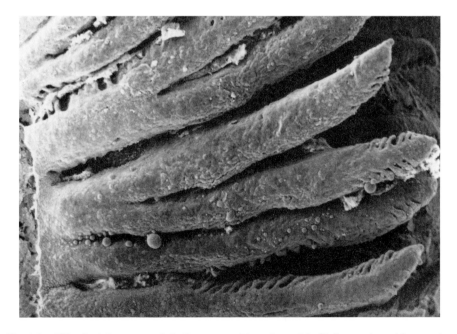

**Fig. 3.3**  Gills of rainbow trout clinically recovered from bacterial gill disease, but with extensive proliferation of lamellar epithelium. SEM × 30 (Courtesy of Dr D.J. Speare).

terminology used in Bergey's Manual of Systematic Bacteriology Volume 3 (See Reichenbach 1989). Probably the most significant bacterium associated with BGD is *Flavobacterium branchiophila*. Wakabayashi *et al.* (1989) proposed that strains from Japan, Ontario and Hungary constituted this new species *F. branchiophila* and deposited strains with the American Type Culture Collection under ATCC35035 and ATCC35036. It would appear that some isolates of this bacteria are highly pathogenic (Ferguson *et al.* 1991).

Whether *F. branchiophila* or other bacteria are involved, it is common to find one strain predominating in any single outbreak, although the strains recovered frequently vary between outbreaks.

The existing information regarding bacteria recovered from BGD is summarised in Table 3.1

## Morphology

The bacteria are characteristically thin rods to filaments found singly or in short chains in broth culture (Wakabayashi *et al.* 1989). Their morphology often varies, depending on environmental conditions and the age of the culture: indeed this is characteristic of *Flexibacter* spp. (Reichenbach 1989). Heo *et al.* (1990*a*) reported the presence of pili approximately 4 nm × 1 μm which appeared to be a common structural component of *F. branchiophila*. Apart from the production of an extensive glycocalyx the bacteria lack other external features.

The bacteria produce yellow/orange cell bound pigments, which in one case was identified as a flexirubin pigment (Ostland *et al.* 1989). Flexirubin pigments are irregularly distributed through the CLB and undergo a characteristic reversible colour change in the presence of potassium hydroxide.

## *Culture*

In common with most CLB the bacteria associated with BGD have a preference for dilute nutrient agar. Cytophaga agar (Anacker & Ordal 1959) is the most commonly used medium. *F. branchiophila* is fastidious and easily overgrown by other bacteria. It produces 0.5−1 mm smooth, round transparent, yellow colonies after 2−5 days. It will grow between 5 and 30°C but not at 37°C.

## *Biochemistry*

This is summarised in Table No. 3.1.

## *DNA studies*

DNA studies have been limited. One study on *Flexibacter* spp. (Pyle & Shotts 1981) demonstrated by DNA homology that they could be separated into four

**Table 3.1** Phenotypic characteristics of bacteria recovered from bacterial gill disease

| Reference | A | B | C | D | E | F | G | H | I | J | K |
|---|---|---|---|---|---|---|---|---|---|---|---|
| **BACTERIA** | | | | | | | | | | | |
| Morphology | M | | | | | | | | | | |
| Size – Diameter | 0.5 × 5–8 | 0.6–0.8 × 4–7 | | | | | | | | | |
| Length | | | | | | | | | | | |
| Flexirubin pigment | – | | +6/11 | | | | | | | | |
| Gliding motility | – | +7/18 | +6/11 | | +16/16 | | | | | | |
| **CULTURE** | | | | | | | | | | | |
| Spreading | – | | +3/11 | | | | | | | | |
| Growth at (°C) 5–30 | + | | +9/11 | | | | ≯25 | | | | |
| 37 | – | | | | | | | + | + | + | ≯25 |
| Growth in >0.1% NaCl | d | | + | + | | | d | d | + | d | d |
| Anaerobic growth | FAC | FAC | – | | | | – | + | – | – | – |
| **BIOCHEMISTRY** | | | | | | | | | | | |
| Cytochrome oxidase | + | + | + | + | + | | + | – | d | d | – |
| Catalase | + | + | + | + | + | | + | + | + | + | + |
| Voges-Proskauer reaction | | | | + | | | | | | | |
| Indole production | – | | – | – | | | – | – | – | – | – |
| H₂S production | + | | – | – | +12/16 | +3/4 | – | d | d | – | – |
| Nitrate reduction | – | | +6/11 | | | | – | d | d | d | d |
| O/F reaction | O | O | O | | | | O/– | | | | |

*continued*

**Table 3.1** *Continued.*

| Reference | A | B | C | D | E | F | G | H | I | J | K |
|---|---|---|---|---|---|---|---|---|---|---|---|
| **HYDROLYSIS/DEGREDATION** | | | | | | | | | | | |
| Aesculin | − | | | | | | d | + | + | + | |
| Casein | + | | + | | | | + | + | + | + | + |
| Cellulose | − | | − | | | | − | − | − | − | − |
| Chitin | − | | | | | | d | + | + | + | |
| Gelatin | + | | + | + | +8/16 | +3/4 | + | + | + | + | + |
| Starch | + | | + | | | | + | + | + | + | + |
| Tributyrin | | | | | | | d | + | + | d | + |
| Tyrosine | | | | | | | + | d | d | d | d |
| **ACID FROM** | | | | | | | | | | | |
| Arabinose | − | | | + | +6/16 | | | | | | |
| Cellobiose | + | | | | | | | | | | |
| Fructose | + | | | | | | | | | | |
| Galactose | − | | | | | | | | | | |
| Glucose | + | | | − | d | +1/4 | − | d | − | − | d |
| Inositol | − | | | | | | | | | | |
| Inulin | + | | | | | | | | | | |
| Lactose | − | | | − | | | − | d | − | − | |
| Maltose | + | | | | | | | d | | | |
| Mannitol | − | | | + | +1/16 | | | | | | |
| Melibiose | + | | | | +6/16 | | | | | | |
| Raffinose | + | | | | | | | | | | |
| Rhaminose | − | | | | | | | | | | |
| Salicin | − | | | | | | | | | | |
| Sucrose | + | | | | +6/16 | | | | | | |
| Sorbitol | − | | | | | | | | | | |
| Trehelose | + | | | | | | | | | | |
| Xylose | − | | | | | | | | | | |

SENSITIVITY TO

| | Penicillin | Nifurprinol |
|---|---|---|
| | S | |
| | S8/18 | |
| | S2/11 | S4/11 |

Key

| | | |
|---|---|---|
| + | = | positive |
| − | = | negative |
| d | = | strain differences |
| FAC | = | Facultative |
| S | = | Sensitive |
| M | = | Microcysts |
| n/n | = | proportion of multiple isolates |
| A | = | *F. branchiophila* references |

Wakabayashi et al. 1980
Farkas 1985
Ototake & Wakabayashi 1985
Austin & Austin 1987
Huh & Wakabayashi 1987
Huh & Wakabayashi 1989
Wakabayashi et al. 1989
Ostland et al. 1989
Heo et al. 1990a
Heo et al. 1990b
Ferguson et al. 1991

| B | = | Ostland et al. 1990 |
| C | = | Ostland et al. 1989 |
| D | = | Acuigrup 1980 |
| E | = | Pyle & Shotts 1981 |
| F | = | Borg 1960 |
| G–J | = | Pacha & Porter 1968 |
| K | = | Bullock 1972 |

groups, one warm water and three cold water, although the clinical conditions from which the bacteria were isolated were not described.

The G + C ratio of *F. branchiophila* was originally reported as 32.9−34 mol% (Wakabayashi *et al.* 1980, Wakabayashi & Iwado 1985), but when the species was formally defined it was stated as 29−30 mol% (Wakabayashi *et al.* 1989).

## *Antigenic studies*

Huh & Wakabayashi (1989) examined the serological characteristics of six strains of *F. branchiophila*. They found common antigens detectable by agglutination and precipitation tests but absorption and precipitation revealed one antigen common to Japanese strains and two common to USA and Hungarian strains.

The extracellular products of *F. branchiophila* include a heat labile haemagglutinin for trout and rabbit and to a lesser extent carp and sheep red blood cells. It also has a non-fimbrial type agglutinin for formalin killed bacterial cells.

Some of the isolates from BGD apparently are phenotypically similar to *F. branchiophila* but do not react with it antigenically (Ostland *et al.* 1989).

## *Diagnostic tests*

The majority of diagnoses are conducted by observation of clinical signs and if necessary fresh smears, histology and bacteriology, although owing to the fastidious nature of *F. branchiophila* confirmation by an immuno fluorescent antibody test is recommended (Huh & Wakabayashi 1987, Heo *et al.* 1990*a*).

## Pathogenesis

Earlier attempts at experimentally infecting fish were either unsuccessful (Rucker *et al.* 1952) or produced only sub-clinical infections (Kimura *et al.* 1978, Wakabayashi *et al.* 1980). However, Bullock (1972) managed to reproduce BGD with a bath challenge in poor water quality, including low dissolved oxygen, high suspended solids and ammonia. This led to the hypothesis that BGD required some form of stress or poor water quality to allow bacterial colonisation. However, recently bacteria have been successfully transmitted in water of controlled quality (Ferguson *et al.* 1991, Speare *et al.* 1991*a*), reproducing clinical disease.

Speare *et al.* (1991*a*) produced a very detailed description of pathology and bacterial colonisation before, during and after a clinical outbreak of BGD. Prior to clinical disease minor changes occur in the microridges, followed by isolated areas of superficial bacterial colonisation (Fig. 3.4). The presence of bacteria immediately precedes degenerative changes in the cells and clinical disease (Fig. 3.5). There is a strong correlation between the number of bacteria and the severity of the histological lesions (Ostland *et al.* 1990). The lesions also heal rapidly following successful removal of the bacteria (Kudo & Kimura

1983*b*,*c*). There is however some dispute regarding some other areas. Kudo & Kimura (1983*b*) and Wakabayashi & Iwado (1985) suggested that the bacteria produce an extracellular hyperplasia inducing factor which can reproduce typical BGD pathology. Ferguson *et al.* (1991) failed to detect any evidence of such a factor although they admitted their study was limited. Speare *et al.* (1991*a*), Ferguson *et al.* (1991), Ostland *et al.* (1989) and Ostland *et al.* (1990) proposed that the hyperplasia was a simple response to the cellular necrosis which they detected. Wakabayashi & Iwado (1985) failed to detect significant necrosis, perhaps owing to different processing techniques.

There is also some disagreement regarding the precise mechanism by which fish are killed. Wood & Yasutake (1957), Snieszko (1981) and Wakabayashi & Iwado (1985) suggested that mortalities were due to the smothering effect of the bacteria on the surface of the gills. Speare *et al.* (1991*b*) maintained that there was insufficient cover of gills by bacteria to produce the observed mortalities. They proposed reduced respiratory diffusion due to spongiosis and damage to the opercular pumps as more probable causes of mortality.

With the exception of Rucker *et al.* (1952) most authors agree that the bacteria are non-invasive (Amend 1970, Ototake & Wakabayashi 1985) or only infiltrate damaged or necrotic cells (Speare *et al.* 1991*b*). This superficial nature may be one of the reasons for the lack of cellular inflammatory response in most cases.

The recovery from BGD which occurs following removal of the bacteria can restore the normal anatomy of the gills, provided that the basement membrane is intact. The predominant process by which recovery takes place is sloughing of the hyperplastic tissue (Kudo & Kimura 1983*a*, and *c*, Ferguson *et al.* 1991) (Fig. 3.6).

**Epizootiology**

BGD has no specific temperature dependencies. There are reports of outbreaks in carp at 5°C (Farkas 1985), in salmonids over 19.7°C (Heo *et al.* 1990*b*) and in eels over 20°C (Funahashi 1980).

Transmission of the associated bacteria is predictably via the water from the environment and other infected fish (Austin & Austin 1987, Ferguson *et al.* 1991), although it can be difficult to isolate *F. branchiophila* in the absence of clinical disease (Heo *et al.* 1990*b*).

**Significance**

As with most conditions in fish pathology, reports of BGD are related more to the location of centres studying the problem than the actual incidence of the disease. Therefore the literature is not necessarily a good guide to the significance and distribution of the disease. Although the majority of the published reports originate from Japan and North America, Snieszko (1981) and Farkas (1985)

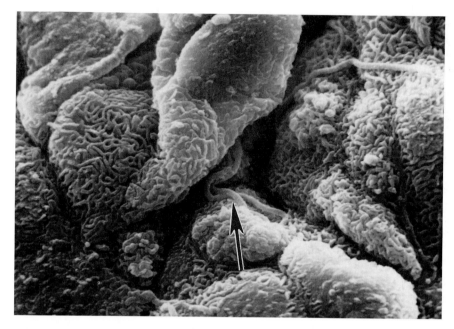

**Fig. 3.4**  Earliest evidence of bacterial colonization (arrow) on gill of rainbow trout. SEM × 2000 (Courtesy of Dr D.J. Speare).

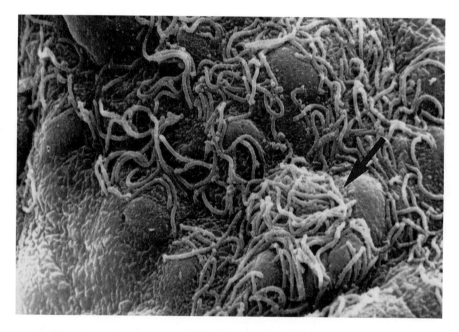

**Fig. 3.5**  Heavy bacterial colonization (arrowed) of area of gill just prior to onset of clinical bacterial gill disease. SEM × 1400 (Courtesy of Dr D.J. Speare).

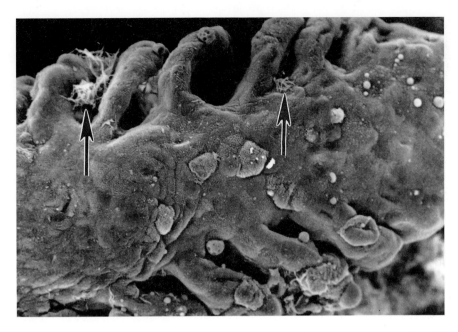

**Fig. 3.6**  Small foci of persistent bacterial colonization (arrowed) on gill of recovered fish. SEM × 280. (Courtesy of Dr D.J. Speare).

indicated that BGD caused significant annual mortalities in many countries. Indeed BGD is said to be common in European salmonid hatcheries but is not reported since it is easy to identify and treat (Bullock & Conroy 1971*a*). Certainly, significant mortalities have been ascribed to BGD, up to 20–25% (Farkas 1985, Ostland *et al.* 1990, Speare *et al.* 1991*a*). Daoust & Ferguson (1983) claimed that it was the most serious problem affecting intensively reared salmonids in Ontario hatcheries.

### Prevention

Preventive measures for a condition with a complex and variable aetiology can be difficult to define. Environmental quality should be maintained by avoiding overcrowding, low dissolved oxygen, suspended solids, and high ammonia levels (Amend 1970, Bullock & Conroy 1971*a*).

At present vaccination does not appear to be a viable proposition. Although Bullock (1972) found evidence of agglutinating antibodies in older trout, Heo *et al.* (1990*b*) found no evidence in younger fish and reported repeated re-infection of populations.

Since the bacteria can spread rapidly through water and there is no evidence of natural resistance, attention to routine hygiene is essential.

**Control**

In common with most fish diseases, control of BGD requires the best possible environmental conditions. Since mortality is assumed to result from asphyxia it is especially important to maintain optimal dissolved oxygen levels. This is also relevant to treatment, since affected fish will be more susceptible to any associated adverse effects.

Many compounds have been employed to treat BGD: initially mercurial compounds such as Lignasan were used (Amend 1970). The compounds are no longer available or appropriate. Quaternary ammonium compounds and chloramine T have been used (Anderson & Conroy 1969, Bullock & Conroy 1971*a*) and some authors also investigated antibiotics for use in BGD (Carlson & Pacha 1968, Amend 1970).

However, since the bacteria are effectively removed by the relatively safe use of 1−5% NaCl for 1−2 min, this must be the treatment of choice.

## Fin rot and miscellaneous CLB infections

Fin rot is a term applied to a wide range of conditions affecting many species (Figs 3.7, 3.8). In addition to the presence of bacteria, fin rot has been linked with traumatic damage, pollution and inappropriate nutrition (Plates 7−9) (reviewed by Turnbull 1992).

Several types of bacteria have been recovered from fin rot, with Cytophaga-like bacteria (CLB) predominating in salmonids (Table 3.2). In most cases the role of the bacteria is still far from clear and varies between different forms of fin rot. Evidence for bacteria as primary pathogens is limited to a study by Oppenheimer (1958), who reproduced fin rot in cod (*Gadus morhua*) by injecting pseudomonads isolated from a clinical case of fin rot. Bullock (1968) proposed that, although the bacteria may be secondary invaders, they might still have a significant effect on the pathogenesis. In yet other cases the bacteria appear to be opportunist secondary invaders, with little effect on the pathology. Dorsal fin rot in freshwater Atlantic salmon was found to be caused by re-peated bite wounds, with bacteria being present for only a short time following such injuries. Their numbers decreased rapidly following re-establishment of epithelial continuity and their presence had little effect on the progression of the disease (Turnbull 1992).

The remaining CLB associated with fish disease are of dubious taxonomic and pathogenic status. Strohl & Tait (1978) recovered 13 isolates from the gills of diseased salmonids and suckers (*Carpoides cyprinus*). These organisms, referred to as *Cytophaga aquatilis*, were similar to those reported by Borg (1960), Pacha & Porter (1968) and Anderson & Conroy (1969). *Cytophaga succinicans* was reported in association with fish disease by Anderson and Ordal (1961), *C. johnsonae* by Christensen (1977) and *C. rosea* by Ross & Smith (1972). Several authors have reported unclassified species of *Flavo-*

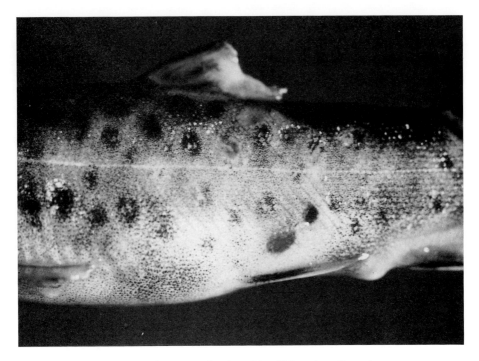

**Fig. 3.7** Dorsal fin rot on salmon parr showing white thickened eroding edge.

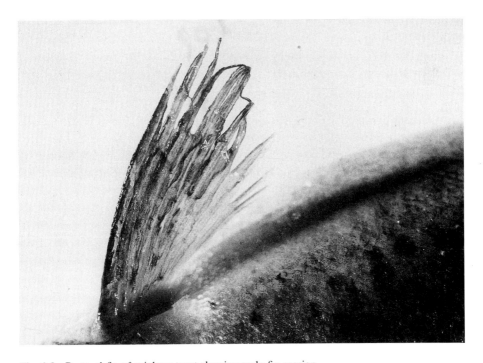

**Fig. 3.8** Pectoral fin of rainbow trout showing early fin erosion.

**Table 3.2**  Bacteria associated with fin rot

| Host species | Bacteria | Reference |
|---|---|---|
| *Salvelinus fontinalis* (brook trout) | CLB | Bullock 1968 |
| Salmonids | CLB | Amend 1970 |
| Salmonids | CLB | Bullock and Snieszko 1970 |
| *Salmo salar* (Atlantic salmon) | CLB | Johansson 1970 |
| Salmonids | CLB, aeromonads & pseudomonads | Bullock & Conroy 1971*b* |
| *S. salar* | *Flexibacter* spp | Schneider & Nicholson 1980 |
| *S. salar* | CLB and others | Turnbull 1992 |
| *Carassius auratus* (gold fish) | aeromonads & pseudomonads | Conroy 1961, 1963, 1964 |
| *Mollienisia sphenops* (black molly) | aeromonads & pseudomonads | Schäperclaus 1950 |
| *Clupea harengus* (herring) | aeromonads & pseudomonads | Sindermann & Rosenfield 1954 |
| *Gadus morhua* (cod) | pseudomonads | Oppenheimer 1958, Khan *et al.* 1981 |
| *Solea solea* (sole) | pseudomonads | Flüchter 1979 |
| *Pomatomus saltatrix* (bluefish) *Paralichthys dentatus* (summer flounder) *Pseudopleuronectes americanus* (winter flounder) *Cynoscion regalis* (weakfish) | aeromonads, pseudomonads & vibrios | Mahoney *et al.* 1973 |
| *P. dentatus* *P. americanus* | unspecified | Murchelano 1975, Murchelano & Ziskowski 1977 |
| Un-specified | aeromonads, pseudomonads vibrios & CLB | Anderson & Conroy 1969 |

*bacterium* in connection with diseased fish, for example Brisou *et al.* (1964), Richards & Roberts (1978), Acuigrup (1980) and Farkas (1985).

Finally organisms were recovered from the surface of a marine salmonid by Wood (1968) and classified as Sporocytophaga following the report of microcysts by Pacha & Ordal (1970).

# References

Acuigrup (1980) Flavobacteriosis in coho salmon (*Oncorhynchus kisutch*). In *Fish Diseases*, Third COPRAQ — Session (Ed. by W. Ahen), pp. 212–7. Springer-Verlag, Berlin.

Amend, D.F. (1970) Myxobacterial infections of salmonids: prevention and treatment. In *A Symposium on Diseases of Fishes and Shellfishes* (Ed. by S.F. Snieszko), pp. 258–65. American Fisheries Society, Washington, DC.

Anacker, R.L. & Ordal, E.J. (1959) Studies on the myxobacterium *Chondrococcus columnaris* I. Serological typing. *Journal of Bacteriology*, **78**, 25–32.

Anderson, J.I.W. & Conroy, D.A. (1969) The pathogenic myxobacteria with special reference to fish disease. *Journal of Applied Bacteriology*, **32**, 30–9.

Anderson, R.L. & Ordal, E.J. (1961) *Cytophaga succinicans* sp. nov., a facultatively anaerobic myxobacterium. *Journal of Bacteriology*, **81**, 130–8.

Austin, B. & Austin, D.A. (1987) Gram-negative pigmented rods. In *Bacterial Fish Pathogens Disease in Farmed and Wild Fish*, pp. 225–244. Ellis Horwood, Chichester.

Borg, A.F. (1960) Studies on myxobacteria associated with diseases in salmonid fishes. *Wild Life Diseases*, **8**, 1–85.

Brisou, J., Tysset, C. & Vacher, B. (1964) Recherches sur les Pseudomonadaceae. Étude de deux souches de Flavobacterium isolées des poissons d'eau douce. *Annales de L'Institute Pasteur*, **74**, 633–8.

Bullock, G.L. (1968) The bacteriology of brook trout with tail rot. *Progressive Fish Culturist*, **30**, 19–22.

Bullock, G.L. (1972) Studies on bacterial gill disease in hatchery-reared salmonids. Bureau of Sport Fisheries and Wildlife, Technical Paper 60, 20–29.

Bullock, G.L. & Conroy, D.A. (1971*a*) Bacterial gill disease. In *Diseases of Fishes*, Book 2A, *Bacterial Diseases of Fishes*. (Ed. by S.F. Snieszko & H.R. Axelrod), pp. 77–87. TFH Publications Inc, Jersey City.

Bullock, G.L. & Conroy, D.A. (1971*b*) Fin rot and tail rot. In *Diseases of Fishes*, 2A, *Bacterial Diseases of Fishes* (Ed by S.F. Sneiszko & H.R. Axelrod), pp. 88–93. TFH Publications Inc, Jersey City.

Bullock, G.L. & Sneiszko, S.F. (1970) Fin rot, coldwater disease and peduncle disease of salmonid fishes. Fish Disease Leaflet, 25, 1–3. US Bureau of Sport Fisheries and Wildlife, Kearnneysville, West Virginia.

Carlson, R.V. & Pacha, R.E. (1968) Procedure for the isolation and enumeration of myxobacteria from aquatic habitats. *Applied Microbiology*, **16**, 795–6.

Christensen, P.J. (1977) The history, biology and taxonomy of the Cytophaga group. *Canadian Journal of Microbiology*, **23**, 1599–653.

Conroy, D.A. (1961) La production de la putrefaccion de la aleta caudal en los peces por la de *Aeromonas punctata*. Microbiologia Española, **14**, 233–8.

Conroy, D.A. (1963) Otras observaciones sobre la putrefaccion de la aleta caudal en los peces. Microbiologia Española, **16**, 63–6.

Conroy, D.A. (1964) Tail rot in fish. *Nature*, **201**, 732–3.

Daoust, P.Y. & Ferguson, H.W. (1983) Gill disease of cultured salmonids in Ontario. *Canadian Journal of Comparative Medicine*, **47**, 358–62.

Davis, H.S. (1926) A new gill disease of trout. *Transactions of the American Fisheries Society*, **56**, 156–60.

Farkas, J. (1985) Filamentous *Flavobacterium* sp. isolated from fish with gill disease in cold water. *Aquaculture*, **44**, 1–10.

Ferguson, H.W., Ostland, V.E., Byrne, P. & Lumsden, J.S. (1991) Experimental production of bacterial gill diseases in trout by horizontal transmission and by bath challenge. *Journal of Aquatic Animal Health*, **3**, 118–23.

Flücher, J. (1979) Identification and treatment of diseases in the common sole (*Solea solea* L). *Aquaculture*, **16**, 271–4.

Foscarini, R. (1989) Induction and development of bacterial gill disease in the eel (*Anguilla japonica*) experimentally infected with *Flexibacter columnaris*: pathological change in the gill vascular structure and in cardiac performance. *Aquaculture*, **78**, 1–20.

Funahashi, N. (1980) Histopathological studies on gill. I. A bacterial gill disease of cultured eel. *Fish Pathology*, **3**, 107–15.

Heo, G.J., Wakabayashi, H. & Watanabe, S. (1990*a*) Purification and characterisation of pili from *Flavobacterium branchiophila*. *Fish Pathology*, **25**, 21–7.

Heo, G.J., Kasai, K.& Wakabayashi, H. (1990*b*) Occurrence of *Flavobacterium branchiophila* associated with bacterial gill disease at a trout hatchery. *Fish Pathology*, **25**, 99–105.

Huh, G.J. & Wakabayashi, H. (1987) Detection of *Flavobacterium* sp. a pathogen of bacterial gill disease, using indirect fluorescent antibody technique. *Fish Pathology*, **22**, 215–20.

Huh, G.J. & Wakabayashi, H. (1989) Serological characteristics of *Flavobacterium branchiophila* isolated from gill diseases of freshwater fish in Japan and Hungary. *Journal of Aquatic Animal Health*, **1**, 142–7.

Johansson, N. (1970) Bakteriologisk undersökning av Laxungar med stjärtfenrota. Swedish Salmon

Research Institute Report, L F I MEDD., 3, 6pp.

Khan, R.A., Campbell, J. & Lear, H. (1981) Mortality in captive Atlantic cod, *Gadus morhua*, associated with fin rot disease. *Journal of Wildlife Diseases*, **17**, 521–8.

Kimura, N., Wakabayashi, H. & Kudo, S. (1978) Studies on bacterial gill disease in salmonids. I Selection of bacterium transmitting gill disease. *Fish Pathology*, **12**, 233–42.

Kudo, S. & Kimura, N. (1983*a*) Transmission electron microscopic studies on bacterial gill disease in rainbow trout fingerlings. *Japanese Journal of Ichthyology*, **30**, 247–60.

Kudo, S. & Kimura, N. (1983*b*) Extraction of a hyperplasia inducing factor. *Bulletin of the Japanese Society of Scientific Fisheries*, **49**, 1777–82.

Kudo, S. & Kimura, N. (1983*c*) The recovery from hyperplasia in an artificial infection. *Bulletin of the Japanese Society of Scientific Fisheries*, **49**, 1635–41.

Mahoney, J.B., Midlidge, F.H. & Deuel, D.G. (1973) A fin rot disease of marine and euryhaline fishes in the New York bight. *Transactions of the American Fisheries Society*, **102**(3), 596–605.

Murchelano, R.A. (1975) The histopathology of fin rot disease in winter flounder from the New York bight. *Journal of Wildlife Diseases*, **11**, 263–8.

Murchelano, R.A. & Ziskowski, J. (1977) Histopathology of an acute fin lesion in the summer flounder, *Paralichthys dentatus* and some speculation on the etiology of fin rot disease in the New York Bight. *Journal of Wildlife Diseases*, **13**, 103–6.

Oppenheimer, C. (1958) Bacterium causing tail rot in the Norwegian codfish. *Publication of the Institute of Marine Science University of Texas*, **5**, 160–4.

Ostland, V.E., Ferguson, H.W. & Stevenson, R.M.W. (1989) Case report: bacterial gill disease in goldfish *Carrasius auratus*. *Diseases of Aquatic Organisms*, **6**, 179–84.

Ostland, V.E., Ferguson, H.W., Prescott, J.F., Stevenson, R.M.W. & Barker, I.K. (1990) Bacterial gill disease of salmonids; relationship between the severity of gill lesions and bacterial recovery. *Diseases of Aquatic Organisms*, **9**, 5–14.

Ototake, M. & Wakabayashi, H. (1985) Characteristics of extracellular products of *Flavobacterium* sp., a pathogen of bacterial gill diseases. *Fish Pathology*, **20**, 167–71.

Pacha, R.E. & Ordal, E.J. (1970) Myxobacterial disease of salmonids. In *A Symposium on Diseases of Fishes and Shellfishes* (Ed. by S.F. Snieszko), pp. 243–257. Special Publication No. 5, American Fisheries Society, Washington, DC.

Pacha, R.E. & Porter, S. (1968) Characteristics of myxobacteria isolated from the surface of freshwater fish. *Applied Microbiology*, **16**, 1901–6.

Pyle, S.W. & Shotts, E.B. (1981) DNA homology studies of selected flexibacteria associated with fish disease. *Canadian Journal of Fisheries and Aquatic Sciences*, **38**, 146–51.

Reichenbach, H. (1989) Order 1. Cytophagales. In *Bergey's Manual of Systematic Bacteriology*, Vol. 3 (Ed. by J.T. Staley, M.P. Bryant, N. Pfennig & J.G. Holt), pp. 2011–15. The Williams and Wilkins Co., Baltimore.

Richards, R.H. & Roberts, R.J. (1978) The Bacteriology of Teleosts. In *Fish Pathology* (Ed. by R.J. Roberts), pp. 183–204. Baillière Tindall, London.

Roberts, R.J. (1989) (Ed.) *Fish Pathology*, 2nd Edn. Baillière Tindall, London.

Ross, A.J. & Smith, C.A. (1972) Effect of two iodophors on bacterial and fungal fish pathogens. *Journal of the Fisheries Research Board of Canada*, **29**, 1359–61.

Rucker, R.R., Johnson, H.E. & Kaydas, G.M. (1952) An interim report on gill disease. *Progressive Fish Culturist*, **14**, 10–14.

Schäperclaus, W. (1950) Uber einen fall von flossenflavle beim schwarzen molly. *Zeitschrift für Fischerei und deren Hilfswissenschaften*, **44**, 13–27.

Schneider, R. & Nicholson, B.L. (1980) Bacteria associated with fin rot disease in hatchery reared Atlantic salmon (*Salmo salar*). *Canadian Journal of Fisheries and Aquatic Sciences*, **37**, 1505–13.

Sindermann, C. & Rosenfeld, A. (1954) Diseases of the fishes of the western north Atlantic I. Diseases of the sea herring (*Clupea harengus*). Research Bulletin Department of Sea Shore Fisheries, 18, 23pp.

Snieszko, S.F. (1981) Bacterial gill disease of freshwater fishes. United States Fish and Wildlife Service, Fish Disease Leaflet, 62. Washington.

Speare, D.J., Ferguson, H.W., Beamish, F.W.M., Yager, J.A. & Yamashiro, S. (1991*a*) Pathology of bacterial gill disease: ultrastructure of branchial lesions. *Journal of Fish Diseases*, **14**, 1–20.

Speare, D.J., Ferguson, H.W., Beamish, F.W.M., Yager, J.A. & Yamashiro, S. (1991*b*) Pathology of bacterial gill disease: sequential development of lesions during natural outbreaks of disease. *Journal of Fish Diseases*, **14**, 21–32.

Strohl, W.R. & Tait, L.R. (1978) *Cytophaga aquatilus* sp. nov. a facultative anaerobe isolated from the gills of freshwater fish. *International Journal of Systematic Bacteriology*, **28**, 293–303.

Turnbull, J.F. (1992) Studies on dorsal fin rot in farmed Atlantic salmon (*Salmo salar* L) parr. Ph.D. Thesis, University of Stirling.

Wakabayashi, H. & Iwado, T. (1985) Effects of a bacterial gill disease on the respiratory function of juvenile rainbow trout. In *Fish and Shellfish Pathology* (Ed. by A.E. Ellis), pp. 153–160. Academic Press, London.

Wakabayashi, H., Egusa, S. & Fryer, J.L. (1980) Characteristics of filamentous bacteria isolated from a gill disease of salmonids. *Canadian Journal of Fisheries and Aquatic Sciences*, **37**, 1499–504.

Wakabayashi, H., Huh, G.J. & Kimura, N. (1989) *Flavobacterium branchiophila*, sp. nov. a causative agent of bacterial gill disease of freshwater fishes. *International Journal of Systematic Bacteriology*, **39**, 213–16.

Wood, E.M. & Yasutake, W.Y. (1957) Histopathology of fish. V. Gill Disease. *Progressive Fish Culturist*, **19**, 7–17.

Wood, J.W. (1968) *Diseases of Pacific Salmon: their Prevention and Treatment*. State of Washington Department of Fisheries, Hatchery Division manual.

# Part 2:
# Enterobacteriaceae

Enterobacteriaceae are a very large family of some 20 genera and more than 100 species of facultatively anaerobic Gram-negative rods (0.3−1.2 × 1.0−6.03 μm. Members are motile by peritrichous flagella, or non-motile, non-sporing and chemo-organotrophic with respiratory and fermentative metabolism. They are cytochrome oxidase-negative and catalase-positive. All but one contain a common enterobacterial antigen.

Enterobacteria are widely disseminated in soil, water, plants and animals. Some, especially *Salmonella* and *Shigella* species, are important pathogens of man and animals, while *Edwardsiella* and *Yersinia* contain species pathogenic for fish. *Proteus rettgeri* and two *Serratia* species also have been implicated in fish disease.

Mol % G + C content of the DNA is 36−60.

# Chapter 4:
## *Edwardsiella* Septicaemia

The genus *Edwardsiella* was first reported by Sakazaki (1962) in Japan and described by Ewing *et al.* (1965). Members exhibit typical characteristics of the *Enterobacteriaceae*. They are Gram-negative small straight rods, $1\,\mu m \times 2-3\,\mu m$, non-spore-forming and motile with peritrichous flagella. Facultatively anaerobic, catalase-positive and oxidase-negative; they ferment D-glucose and a few other compounds but are relatively inactive compared with other taxa in this family. They have been isolated frequently from freshwater and cold-blooded animals. The mol % G + C of the DNA is $55-59$.

Two members of *Edwardsiella* infect fish: *Edwardsiella tarda* (Hoshinae 1962, Ewing *et al.* 1965) and *Edwardsiella ictaluri* (Hawke 1979, Hawke *et al.* 1981). These micro-organisms cause two distinct diseases that differ greatly in their occurrence, clinical signs, pathogenesis and severity. However, each represents a significant problem in relation to fish culture in fresh water.

*Edwardsiella tarda* is the causative agent of septicaemia of warm water fish, particularly catfish and eels, occurring in the United States and Asia. It is disseminated widely in aquatic animals, pond water and muds, providing opportunity for reinfection of cultured fish. Infected fish processed for human consumption is a source of gastroenteritis and, more rarely, other disease of man.

*Edwardsiella ictaluri* causes enteric septicaemia in catfish. It is a highly contagious disease seriously affecting commercial catfish culture in the Southern United States and causing epizootics with mortality rates of $10-50\%$.

## Septicaemia of warm water fish

Edwardsiella septicaemia is a mild to severe systemic disease of primarily warm water fishes in the United States and Asia. The causative agent is *Edwardsiella tarda*. Edwardsiella septicaemia is the currently accepted name for the disease caused by this pathogen, but other names are fish gangrene, emphysematous putrefactive disease of catfish (Meyer & Bullock 1973) and red disease of eels (Egusa 1976). Although channel catfish (*Ictalurus punctatus*) and Japanese eel (*Anguilla japonica*) are the most commonly infected species, *E. tarda* has been isolated from a variety of fish species, both freshwater and marine (Table 4.1). As previously noted, the most serious epizootics related to *E. tarda* infections of fish have been reported from North America and Japan, but disease also occurs in Taiwan, Thailand and Africa. The bacterium probably occurs, however, in other geographical areas as suggested by Wyatt *et al.* (1979).

### Aetiological agent

The first isolation of *E. tarda* was in Japan, where Hoshinae (1962) named the organism *Paracolabacterium anguillimortiferum*. However, Ewing *et al.* (1965), in their description of the genus, designated the microorganism *Edwardsiella tarda*, a name that is now accepted world-wide. Although Wakabayashi &

**Table 4.1**  Species of fish reported to be naturally susceptible to the bacteria *Edwardsiella tarda* and *Edwardsiella ictaluri*

| Common name | Scientific name | Reference |
|---|---|---|
| *Edwardsiella tarda* | | |
| Channel catfish | *Ictalurus punctatus* | Meyer & Bullock 1973) |
| Chinook salmon | *Oncorhynchus tshawytscha* | (Amandi *et al.* 1982) |
| Common carp | *Cyprinus carpio* | (Sae-Oui *et al.* 1984) |
| Crimson seabream | *Evynnis japonicus* | (Kusuda *et al.* 1977) |
| Japanese flounder | *Paralichthys olivaceus* | (Nakatsugawa 1983) |
| Japanese eel | *Anguilla japonica* | (Egusa 1976) |
| Largemouth bass | *Micropterus salmoides* | (White *et al.* 1973) |
| Mullet | *Mugil cephalus* | (Kusuda *et al.* 1976) |
| Red seabream | *Chrysophrys major* | (Yasunaga *et al.* 1982) |
| Striped bass | *Morone saxatilis* | (Herman & Bullock 1986) |
| Tilapia | *Tilapia nilotica* | (Miyashito 1984) |
| Yellowtail | *Seriola gaingu eradiata* | (Yasunaga *et al.* 1982) |

| Common name | Scientific name | Reference |
|---|---|---|
| *Edwardsiella ictaluri* | | |
| Channel catfish | *Ictalurus punctatus* | (Hawke 1979) |
| Brown bullhead | *I. nebulosus* | (Plumb & Sanchez 1983) |
| Blue catfish | *I. furcatus* | (Unpublished) |
| Danio | *Danio devario* | (Waltman *et al.* 1985) |
| Green knifefish | *Eigemannia virens* | (Kent & Lyons 1982) |
| Walking catfish | *Clarias batrachus* | (Kasornchandra *et al.* 1987) |
| White catfish | *I. catus* | (Plumb & Sanchez 1983) |

Egusa (1973) recognized that *E. tarda* was preferable to *P. anguillimortiferum*, however, opposition to naming the organism *E. tarda* rather than *P. anguillimortiferum* occurred as late as 1978 (Sakazaki & Tamura 1978).

Biochemically, *E. tarda* is a typical enteric bacterium (Wakabayashi & Egusa 1973). In addition to being a Gram-negative, motile rod, it ferments carbohydrates and produces gas, grows on media with 3% NaCl and grows at 40°C (Table 4.2). *E. tarda* can be separated from *E. ictaluri* by the former's salt tolerance, indole production, $H_2S$ production on triple sugar iron agar and higher temperature tolerance (Table 4.3). Waltman *et al.* (1986a) compared 116 isolates of *E. tarda* and found little variation in their biochemical and biophysical characteristics, although isolates from Taiwan differed slightly from United States isolates. Positive identification can be made by specific serum agglutination or fluorescent antibody tests. There is no serological similarity between *E. tarda* and *E. ictaluri* (Rogers 1981).

Park *et al.* (1983) identified four *E. tarda* serotypes (A, B, C and D) among 445 isolates from infected eels and environmental sources. Although environmental isolates included similar numbers of all four serotypes, 72% of the

**Table 4.2** Biochemical characteristics not essential to differentiate between *Edwardsiella tarda* and *Edwardsiella ictaluri* (Wakabayashi & Egusa 1973, Hawke *et al.* 1981, Farmer & McWhorter 1984, Waltman *et al.* 1986a,b, Plumb & Vinitnantharat 1989)

| Characteristic | *E. tarda*[1] | *E. ictaluri* | Characteristic | *E. tarda*[1] | *E. ictaluri* |
|---|---|---|---|---|---|
| Voges-Proskauer | − | − | Urea | − | − |
| Phenylalanine | − | − | Cytochrome oxidase | − | − |
| deaminase | | | Catalase | + | + |
| Lysine decarboxylase | + | + | Arginine dihydrolase | − | − |
| Ornithine | + | + | Gelatin hydrolysis | − | − |
| decarboxylase | | | KEN, growth on | − | − |
| Malonate utilization | − | − | d-tartrate | − | − |
| Urease | − | − | Glycerol | + | − |
| Salicin | − | − | Tartrate | − | − |
| Acetate utilization | − | − | Nitrate reduced to | + | + |
| Deoxyribonuclease | − | − | nitrite | | |
| Lipase | − | − | β-Galactosidase | − | − |
| Pectate hydrolysis | − | − | (OIXPG) | | |
| | | | | | |
| Acid from | | | | | |
| Glucose | + | + | Maltose | + | + |
| Lactose | − | − | Sucrose | − | − |
| Mannitol | − | − | Dulcitol | − | − |
| Salicin | − | − | Adonitol | − | − |
| Inositol | − | − | Sorbitol | − | − |
| Arabinose | − | − | Ruffinose | − | − |
| Rhamnose | − | − | Xylose | − | − |
| Trehalose | − | − | Cellubiose | − | − |
| Erythritol | − | − | Esculin | − | − |
| Mannose | + | + | | | |
| | | | | | |
| Triple sugar iron agar | K/AG[2] | K/AG | | | |

[1] + indicates over 90% of isolates are positive for the characteristic and
− indicates over 90% are negative
[2] K represents alkaline or no reaction, A represents acid production and G represents gas production

isolates from fish were serotype A, indicating that this serotype may predominate in disease causation. Also, serotype A was more virulent for fish, especially eels. The bacterium is easily isolated from muscle and internal organs of clinically diseased fish on most general purpose media, such as tryptic soy agar (TSA) or brain heart infusion agar (BHIA). Small punctate colonies develop in 24–48 h on inoculated media incubated at 30°C. Growth of *E. tarda* is more rapid than that of *E. ictaluri*.

## Clinical signs

Clinical signs differ slightly from region to region and from fish species to species. In the United States, where channel catfish is the most commonly

**Table 4.3**  Biochemical and biophysical characteristics that separate *Edwardsiella tarda* from *Edwardsiella ictaluri* (Wyatt *et al.* 1979, Farmer & McWhorter 1984, Waltman *et al.* 1986*a*,*b*, Plumb & Vinitnantharat 1989)

| Characteristic | *E. tarda* | *E. ictaluri* |
|---|---|---|
| Motility | | |
| 25°C | + | + |
| 35°C | + | − |
| Indole production | + | − |
| Methyl red | + | − |
| | | |
| Citrate | | |
| Simmons | − | − |
| Christensen's | + | − |
| H₂S production | | |
| Triple-sugar iron | + | − |
| Peptone iron agar | + | − |
| Tolerance to NaCl | | |
| 1.5% | + | + |
| 3% | + | − |
| Mol 0% G + C of DNA | 55−58 | 53 |

infected species, *E. tarda* infection manifests itself by the presence of small, 3−5 mm, cutaneous lesions located dorso-laterally on the body (Meyer & Bullock 1973). These small lesions progress into abscesses within the flank muscles or caudal peduncle where they develop obvious convex swollen areas and the skin loses pigmentation (Fig. 4.1). When the skin is incised, a foul-smelling gas is emitted and the lesion contains large amounts of necrotized tissue. As infection progresses, the affected fish lose mobility of the caudal portion of the body. Internally, a generalized hyperaemia similar to other bacterial septicaemia is evident. The kidney in particular is enlarged.

In Japan and Taiwan eels with acute infection develop severe hyperaemia with bloody congestion of all fins with echymotic or petechial haemorrhage on various surfaces of the body, as well as gas-filled pockets in the skin. The anal region is swollen and hyperaemic. Internally, there is a general hyperaemia of the peritoneum and the liver is mottled, oedematous, and has abscessation (Fig. 4.2).

**Epizootiology**

Edwardsiella septicaemia of catfish in the United States occurs most often during the warm, summer months. Optimum water temperature for *E. tarda* infections in catfish is approximately 30°C. However, Liu & Tsai (1980) reported that *E. tarda* infections of eels in Taiwan were most common between January

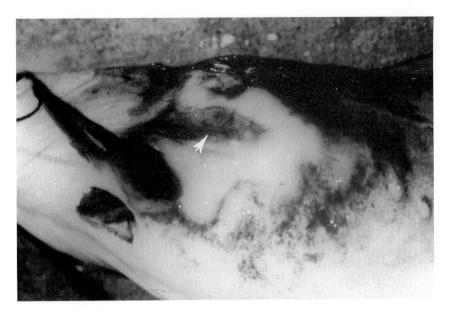

**Fig. 4.1**  *Edwardsiella tarda* infection in channel catfish. Light, depigmented area indicates necrotic muscle underneath with surrounding haemorrhage (arrowed) (Photo by F.P. Meyer).

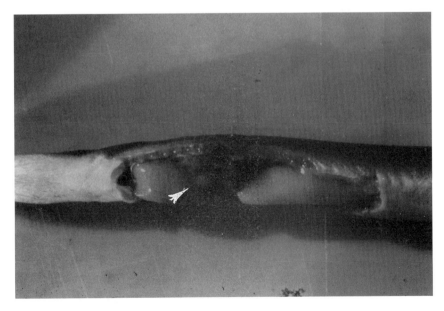

**Fig. 4.2**  *Edwardsiella tarda* infection in Japanese eel with an abscess on the liver (arrowed) (Photo by E.B. Shotts).

and April when water temperatures were 10–18°C. Most of these cases were associated with fluctuating water temperatures. On the other hand, Egusa (1976) stated that *E. tarda* infections of eels in Japan were more prevalent during the warmer summer months. The disease is usually found in larger fish, approximately 0.4 kg catfish and marketable-size eels. However, *E. tarda* also infects elvers and fingerling catfish.

Mortality of channel catfish in ponds is seldom over 5%, however, if the fish are moved into confined holding tanks the rate quickly accelerates to 50% with concomitant mortality. Mortality data are not available for eel populations in Taiwan and Japan. In the United States, *Edwardsiella tarda* was isolated from as many as 88% of dressed domestic catfish (Wyatt *et al.* 1979) and it was found in 30% of imported dressed fish. Additionally, *E. tarda* was isolated from 75% of catfish pond water samples, 64% of catfish pond mud samples and 100% of frogs, turtles and crayfish from catfish ponds. It is apparent that *E. tarda* is a common member of catfish pond microflora and its presence is a constant potentiator of disease.

The source of *E. tarda* is presumably intestinal contents of carrier animals. Fish (catfish and eels) are probably sources of infection, along with carrier amphibians and reptiles. Although environmental stressors are not essential precursors to an *E. tarda* infection, high temperature, poor water quality and crowding probably contribute to the onset and severity of disease. Walters & Plumb (1980) showed that channel catfish fingerlings exposed to low dissolved oxygen, high carbon dioxide and high ammonia concentrations had a higher rate of *E. tarda* infections than those fish that were not environmentally stressed.

*E. tarda* infections are not limited to fish. This organism also causes disease in snakes (Sakazaki 1967), alligators and sea lions (Wallace *et al.* 1966), and *E. tarda* has been implicated in infections in birds (White *et al.* 1969, White *et al.* 1973), cattle (Ewing *et al.* 1965, D'Empaire 1969) and swine (Arambulo *et al.* 1967). In humans, *E. tarda* has been associated with gastroenteritis (King & Adler 1964, Jordan & Hadley 1969, Bockemuhl *et al.* 1971, Van Damme & Vandepitte 1980), abscesses (Fields *et al.* 1967) and meningitis (Sonnenwirth & Kallus 1968, Sachs *et al.* 1974).

**Pathogenesis**

*Edwardsiella tarda* infection of eels spreads from lesions of visceral organs into the musculature and then to the skin, where large lesions develop in the musculature and dermis as previously described (Plate 10) (Egusa 1976). Egusa (1976) further stated that these lesions do not appear to be caused by toxins. However, Ullah & Arai (1983) reported that *E. tarda* does not produce endotoxins as other Gram-negative bacteria do, but that it does produce two exotoxins which could be responsible for the lesions. Pathogenesis in channel catfish appears to be the reverse of that in eels, with initial infection occurring in the dermis, then the musculature and, finally, the pathogen establishes a septicaemia that invades visceral organs (Plate 11). This process has not, however, been well described.

According to Miyazaki and Egusa (1976*a,b,c*) and Miyazaki & Kaige (1985), *E. tarda* in eels causes either nephric or hepatic lesions, with the nephric form of the disease more common. In the nephric form, the kidney is enlarged with various-size abscesses that initially are formed in the sinusoids of hematopoietic tissue of the trunk kidney (Fig. 4.3). Large abscesses are walled off by fibrin, and phagocytic cells contain bacteria (Fig. 4.4). Liquefaction follows, small foci of necrosis are found in other organs and the lateral musculature adjoining the kidney is invaded by the bacteria. In the hepatic form of the disease, livers are usually enlarged with various sized abscesses, some of which leak fluid into the body cavity. Enlarged lesions involve hepatocytes and blood vessels, leading to the formation of emboli and embolic septicaemia.

### Significance

The significance of *E. tarda* depends on fish species and environmental conditions. In Taiwan and Japan, it is one of the most serious bacterial diseases of cultured eels, but in the United States, unless the channel catfish are confined and crowded, it is of little consequence. The greatest problem lies in subclinical infection of catfish when they are being processed. When fish with undetected lesions are skinned, the processing line becomes contaminated, requiring interruption of processing and cleaning and disinfection of equipment.

### Control

The most common treatment for *E. tarda* infections is by application of antibiotic medicated feed. The organism is sensitive to a wide variety of antibiotics and therefore any approved drug can be used (Chen *et al*. 1984, Liu & Wang 1986). In the United States, oxytetracycline at 2.5 g/45 kg of fish is the drug of choice. However, Waltman & Shotts (1986*a*) showed that isolates from Taiwan were generally more resistant to such drugs.

Development of a vaccine has been pursued in Japan and Taiwan. These preparations have involved the use of whole cells, disrupted cells and cell extracts as immunogens (Song & Kou 1979, 1981, Song *et al*. 1982, Salati *et al*. 1983, Salati 1985, Salati & Kusuda 1985*a,b*). All of these preparations are immunogenic, especially by injection, but a practical, commercially available vaccine has not been marketed.

## Enteric septicaemia of catfish

Enteric septicaemia of catfish (ESC) is a highly contagious, systemic disease of cultured catfish that is caused by *Edwardsiella ictaluri*. Enteric septicaemia of catfish is at present the most serious infectious disease affecting the catfish

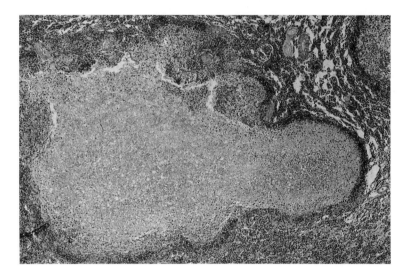

**Fig. 4.3**   Abscess in the kidney of Japanese eel with *Edwardsiella tarda* infection. H&E, × 32 (Photo by T. Miyazaki).

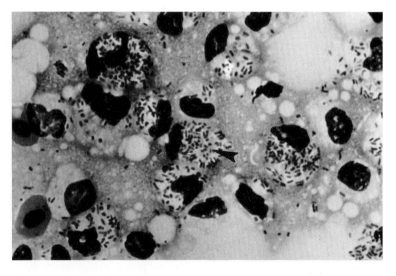

**Fig. 4.4**   Smear of neutrophils from abscess of kidney of Japanese eel. Phagocytic cells are engorged with *Edwardsiella tarda* cells (arrowed). Giemsa, × 1000 (Photo by T. Miyazaki).

industry in the United States. The disease is also called 'hole-in-the-head' owing to the presence of an open lesion appearing in the skull of some chronically ill fish. This name is not, however, an appropriate one, because several other pathogens can cause similar lesions.

*E. ictaluri* has a much more restricted host susceptibility than *E. tarda* (Table 4.1). In addition to channel catfish, it has also been found in blue catfish

(*I. furcatus*), white catfish (*I. melas*) and two aquarium species (Waltman *et al.* 1985) in the United States. The other most notable isolation was from walking catfish (*Clarias batrachus*) in Thailand (Kasornchandra *et al.* 1987). Experimental infections of *E. ictaluri* were established in several non-ictalurids by Plumb & Sanchez (1983), but the most notable were in European catfish (*Silurus glanis*) (Plumb & Hilge 1987), chinook salmon (*Oncorhynchus tshawytscha*) and rainbow trout (*O. mykiss*) (Baxa & Hedrick 1989). Whether or not the non-ictalurid species that are susceptible to *E. ictaluri* can serve as carriers and infect more susceptible species is not known.

ESC occurs primarily across the Southeastern United States where channel catfish are commercially grown, but the disease has also been confirmed in other states, such as Indiana, Idaho, California, Arizona, and New Mexico. With the spread of channel catfish culture to new regions during the past 10 years, it is likely that ESC will eventually be detected in most geographical regions where catfish have been imported.

**Aetiological agent**

ESC was first reported by Hawke (1979) and later the causative agent was named *Edwardsiella ictaluri* (Hawke *et al.* 1981). *E. ictaluri* is a typical member of the Enterobacteriaceae as it is a Gram negative, cytochrome oxidase-negative rod that is weakly motile at 25–30°C but non-motile at higher temperatures (Table 4.2). The organism ferments and oxidizes glucose while producing gas at 20–30°C but not at 37°C, is indole and $H_2S$ negative while producing an acid slant and alkaline butt with gas on TSI agar and is not tolerant of more than 1.5% NaCl. Complete biochemical characteristics were described by Waltmann *et al.* (1986*b*). Plumb & Vinitnantharat (1989) found little biochemical and serological diversity within the species. There are one to three plasmids associated with *E. ictaluri* (Speyerer & Boyle 1987, Newton *et al.* 1988). The function of these plasmids is not yet clear, but they could be important in enhancement of antibiotic resistance. *E. ictaluri* is the most fastidious species of *Edwardsiella*. It grows slowly on culture media, requiring 36–48 h to form punctate colonies on BHI agar at 28–30°C, and it grows poorly or not at all at 37°C.

For detection of ESC, it is essential to observe the primary isolation plates very carefully, because if a more rapidly growing bacterium, such as *Aeromonas* sp., is present, it will over-grow and obscure the more slowly growing *E. ictaluri*. Shotts & Waltman (1990) developed an *E. ictaluri* selective medium, *Edwardsiella ictaluri* agar (EIA), which is excellent for primary isolation and presumptive identification. Identification is by the biochemical characteristics previously outlined, or serologically by specific serum agglutination, fluorescent antibody (FA) (Ainsworth *et al.* 1986), or by enzyme-linked immunosorbant assay (ELISA) (Rogers 1981). Either the FA or ELISA procedures can be used to detect and identify *E. ictaluri* in smears made directly from tissue of infected fish. The importance of an early diagnosis cannot be overemphasized because successful control depends on early diagnosis and immediate application of medicated feed.

## Clinical signs

Some clinical signs of ESC are virtually pathognomonic for the disease. Diseased fish hang listlessly at the surface with a 'head up-tail down' posture, sometimes spinning rapidly in circles, usually followed by death. Externally, petechial haemorrhage or inflammation occurs in the skin under the jaw, on the opercula, and belly. These lesions often become so numerous that the skin is bright red. Inflammation and haemorrhage also occurs at the base of all fins. Small white, depigmented areas (1–3 mm in diameter) appear on the dark skin where they progress into similar size cutaneous ulcers that are inflamed (Fig. 4.5A, Plates 11, 12). In chronically infected fish, an open lesion will develop between the frontal bones of the skull, posterior to or between the eyes (Fig. 4.5B). It is possible to penetrate this lesion with an inoculating loop without cutting the skin or the bone. Also, affected fish have pale gills, exophthalmia, and often an enlarged abdomen.

Internally the body cavity may be filled with a cloudy, bloody or rarely a clear yellow fluid. The kidney and spleen are enlarged and the spleen is dark red. Inflammation occurs in adipose tissue, peritoneum and intestine, and the liver is either pale or mottled with congestion.

## Pathogenesis

*E. ictaluri* can infect fish by two different routes. Water-borne bacteria can invade the olfactory organ via the nasal opening of the fish and migrate into the olfactory nerve and then into the brain (Miyazaki & Plumb 1985, Shotts *et al.* 1986). The infection spreads from meninges to the skull and skin, thus creating the 'hole-in-the-head' condition (Fig. 4.6). *E. ictaluri* can also be ingested and enter the blood through the intestine and result in a septicaemia (Shotts *et al.* 1986). By this route the bacteria apparently colonize capillaries in the dermis causing the necrosis and depigmentation of the skin (Plate 12).

Areechon & Plumb (1983) demonstrated that the most severely affected organs in *E. ictaluri*-infected catfish were the trunk kidney and spleen, both of which were necrotic, while the liver was oedematous and necrotic. Blood characteristics affected included significant decrease in haematocrit, haemoglobin, plasma glucose and plasma protein concentrations. Studies by Jarboe *et al.* (1984), Miyazaki & Plumb (1985) and Shotts *et al.* (1986) demonstrated that interlamellar tissue of the gill proliferated and, where skin epidermis was missing, a mild focal mononuclear infiltration took place in the underlying musculature. Ulcerative lesions of the head showed necrosis and haemorrhage, whereas systemic infection was associated with necrosis of hepatocytes and pancreatic cells. Miyazaki & Plumb (1985) also reported the presence of intact *E. ictaluri* cells in macrophages (Fig. 4.7).

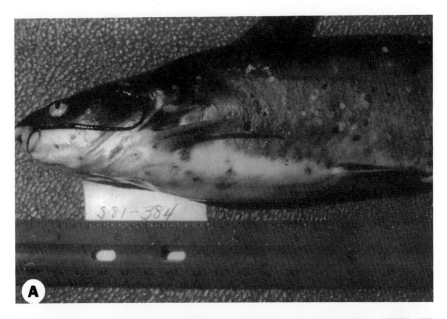

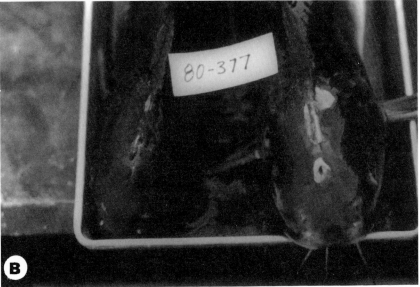

**Fig. 4.5** *Edwardsiella ictaluri* in channel catfish. (A) Depigmented areas precede the haemorrhagic, necrotic ulcers (arrow). (B) Open necrotic lesion in the skull characteristic of chronic *E. ictaluri* infection (Photos by T.E. Schwedler).

Catfish exposed to *E. ictaluri* via oral infection by intubation in the gut developed enteritis, hepatitis, interstitial nephritis and myositis within 2 weeks of infection (Shotts *et al.* 1986). Francis-Floyd *et al.* (1987) described gastro-intestinal lesions, including petechiae or ecchymoses in the mucosa of the gastrointestinal tract, and intestinal distention associated with gas production.

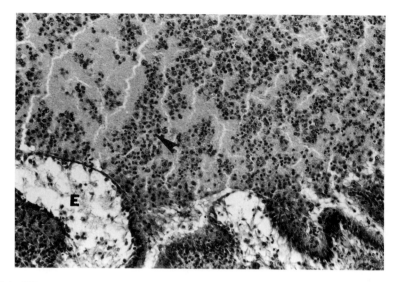

**Fig. 4.6**  Olfactory sac of channel catfish with *Edwardsiella ictaluri* infection. The olfactory sac is packed with neutrophils (arrow) and sensory epithelium (E) is necrotic. H&E, × 110 (Photo by T. Miyazaki).

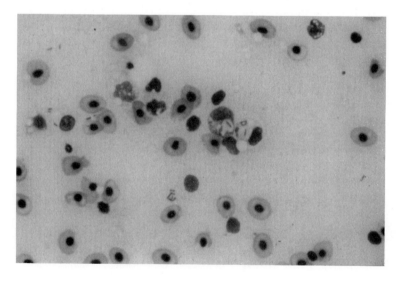

**Fig. 4.7**  Macrophages from *Edwardsiella ictaluri* infected channel catfish. The macrophages contain bacteria. H&E, × 1000 (Photo by T. Miyazaki).

## Epizootiology

When ESC was first described in 1977, it was thought that *E. ictaluri* was an obligate pathogen that would not live for an extended period of time outside of the host (Hawke 1979). However, later work indicated that *E. ictaluri* could survive in pond bottom muds for over 90 days when the temperature was 25°C (Fig. 4.8) (Plumb & Quinlan 1986), a characteristic that could account for recurring epizootics in ponds. The bacterium can probably be carried in the intestines of covertly infected fish. Also *E. ictaluri* has been detected by fluorescent antibody in the lower intestines of fish-eating birds (cormorants and herons). However, it has not been demonstrated that these bacteria are viable (P.W. Taylor, Mississippi Cooperative Extension Service, Personal Communication).

ESC is considered a seasonal disease, occurring primarily in the late spring to early summer and again in the fall (Fig. 4.9). This pattern coincides with air temperatures of 20–27°C. However, the disease has been detected during every month. Francis-Floyd *et al.* (1987) demonstrated that mortalities in experimentally infected channel catfish fingerlings were highest at 25°C, slightly lower at 23°C and 28°C and no deaths due to *E. ictaluri* occurred at 17, 21 or 32°C.

During the first several years following the discovery of ESC, relatively few cases of the disease were detected. However, beginning in the early 1980s, the number of *E. ictaluri* isolates began to climb at an alarming rate (Fig. 4.10). For example, in 1981 47 cases were reported in the Southeastern United States, and in 1985 there were 1042 cases accounting for 28% of all fish diseases in the Southeastern United States. In 1988, there were 1605 cases accounting for 30.4% of all cases of fish disease in the Southeastern United States (A.J. Mitchell, US Fish and Wildlife Service, Personal Communication).

The mortality rates of *E. ictaluri*-infected populations vary from less than 10% to over 50%. The disease occurs in fingerling as well as production-sized fish, and it occurs in all types of cultural conditions, including ponds, race-

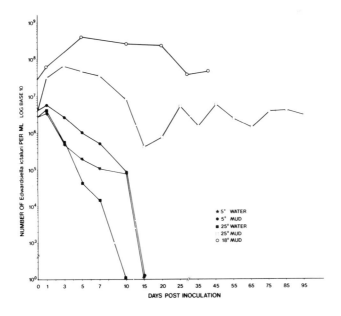

**Fig. 4.8**  Survival of *Edwardsiella ictaluri* in pond water and bottom mud at different temperatures (From Plumb & Quinlan 1986).

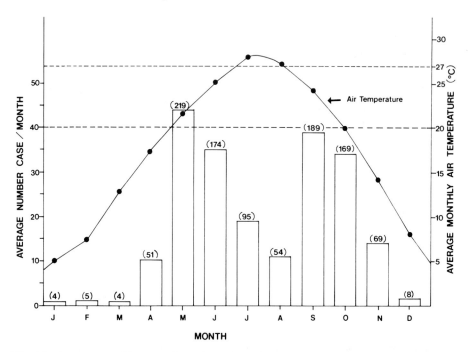

**Fig. 4.9** Average monthly cases of enteric septicaemia of catfish and average monthly air temperature in Alabama from 1985 through 1989 with total number of cases in parentheses (some data from William Hemstreet).

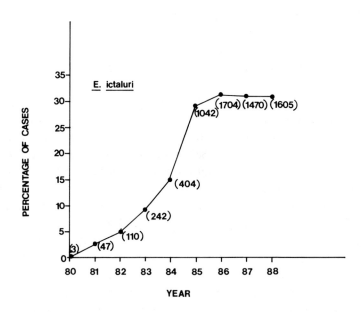

**Fig. 4.10** Yearly increase in percentage of clinical fish disease cases in Southeastern United States that were caused by *Edwardsiella ictaluri* from 1980 through 1988. Total number of *E. ictaluri* cases are in parentheses (Data compiled and supplied by A.J. Mitchell).

ways, recirculating systems and cages. It appears that the higher the fish population density the greater the mortality. Few fish diseases occur without some type of environmental stressor preceding the infection. However, infection of fish due to *E. ictaluri* is one exception. Although the disease is temperature dependent, 20–27°C cannot be considered as stressful for catfish, and ESC occurs under excellent environmental conditions. Nevertheless, poor environmental conditions can increase the severity of infection.

## Significance

During the late 1980s, ESC became the most serious infectious disease of the catfish industry, where it has resulted in losses valued in tens of millions of dollars. ESC can cause a loss of 50% or more of fingerling or food-size populations, and with the disease's widespread nature and an ever expanding catfish culture in the United States and abroad, ESC will continue to be a significant problem in catfish culture.

## Control

The only control of ESC is through the use of antibiotics incorporated into the feed. Oxytetracycline and a potentiated sulphonamide are the only drugs currently in use (Bowser *et al.* 1986, Waltman & Shotts 1986*b*, Plumb *et al.* 1987), but isolates of *E. ictaluri* from clinical cases are showing an increase in the number that are resistant to either or both of these drugs (unpublished data). The major problem in treating ESC with medicated feed is that infected populations quickly become inappetent; therefore, unless medicated feed is given to the fish early in the epizootic, treatment may not be effective. It is extremely important that an early diagnosis be made and medicated feed be applied as soon as possible.

   *E. ictaluri* has a degree of antigenic homogeneity that readily lends itself to successful vaccination as a preventive measure. Although extensive vaccination research has gone and is going on for ESC, no commercial vaccines are currently on the market. Plumb (1988) summarized the immunity and vaccination research for *E. ictaluri*. This bacterium is an excellent antigen and it elicits a strong, rapid immune response when injected into the fish. However, bath exposure to killed bacterins has not resulted in unequivocal protective immunity. Saeed & Plumb (1986) also showed that *E. ictaluri* lipopolysaccharide is immunogenic. Channel catfish immunity to *E. ictaluri* is temperature dependent, whereby the fish will respond at temperatures above 23°C, but not at 12°C, but if the fish are immunized and held at 23°C for 3 days and then placed in 12°C water they will develop an immune response (Plumb *et al.* 1986). These data and results of other researchers indicate the feasibility of vaccine development for *E. ictaluri*. The success depends upon preparation of the antigen and implementation of a delivery technique.

# References

Ainsworth, A.J., Capley, G., Waterstreet, P. & Munson, D. (1986) Use of monoclonal antibodies in the indirect fluorescent antibody technique (IFA) for the diagnosis of *Edwardsiella ictaluri*. *Journal of Fish Diseases*, **9**, 439−44.

Amandi, A., Hiu, S.F., Rohovec, J.S. & Fryer, J.L. (1982) Isolation and characterization of *Edwardsiella tarda* from fall chinook salmon (*Oncorhynchus tsawytscha*). *Applied and Environmental Microbiology*, **43**, 1380−4.

Arambulo, P.V., Westerland, N.E., Sarmiento, R.V. & Abaga, A.S. (1967) Isolation of *Edwardsiella tarda*: a new genus of Enterobacteriaceae from pig bile in the Phillipines. *Far East Medical Journal*, **3**, 385−6.

Areechon, N. & Plumb, J.A. (1983) Pathogenesis of *Edwardsiella ictaluri* in channel catfish, *Ictalurus punctatus*. *Journal of the World Maricultural Society*, **14**, 249−60.

Baxa, D.V. & Hedrick, R.P. (1989) Two more species are susceptible to experimental infections with *Edwardsiella ictaluri*. Fish Health Section/*American Fisheries Society Newsletter*, **17**(1), 4.

Bockemuhl, J., Pan-Urai, R. & Burkhardt, F. (1971) *Edwardsiella tarda* associated with human disease. *Pathogenic Microbiology*, **37**, 393−401.

Bowser, P.R., Munson, A.D., Francis-Floyd, R. & Stiles, F. (1986) Potentiated sulfonamide therapy of *Edwardsiella ictaluri* infection in channel catfish. *Mississippi Agricultural and Forestry Experiment Station Research Report*, **11**, 3.

Chen, S.E., Tung, M.C., Lu, C.F. & Huang, S.T. (1984) Sensitivity *In vitro* of various chemotherapeutic agents to *Edwardsiella tarda* of pond-cultured eels. *CAPD Fisheries Series No. 10, Fish Disease Research*, **6**, 100−6.

Van Damme, L.R. & Vandepitte, J. (1980) Frequent isolation of *Edwardsiella tarda* and *Pleisomonas shigelloides* from healthy Zairese freshwater fish: A possible source of sporadic diarrhoea in the tropics. *Applied and Environmental Microbiology*, **39**(3), 475−9.

Egusa, S. (1976) Some bacterial diseases of freshwater fishes in Japan. *Fish Pathology*, **10**, 103−14.

D'Empaire, M. (1969) Les facteurs de croissance des *Edwardsiella tarda*. *Annales de L'Institut Pasteur*, **116**, 63−8.

Ewing, W.H., McWhorter, A.C., Escobar, M.R. & Lubin, A.H. (1965) *Edwardsiella*, a new genus of Enterbacteriaceae based on a new species, *Edwardsiella tarda*. *International Bulletin of Bacteriological Numerical Taxonomy*, **15**, 33−8.

Farmer, J.J. & McWhorter, A.L. (1984) Genus X *Edwardsiella* Ewing & McWhorter 1965, 37[AL]. In Kreig, N.R. (ed.), *Bergey's Manual of Systematic Bacteriology*, Vol. 1, Baltimore, Williams & Wilkins, 436−491.

Fields, B.N., Uwaydah, M.M., Kunz, L. & Swartz, M.N. (1967) The so-called 'paracolon' bacteria. A bacteriologic and clinical appraisal. *American Journal of Medicine*, **42**, 89−105.

Francis-Floyd, R., Beleau, M.H., Waterstrat, P.R. & Bowser, P.R. (1987) Effect of water temperature on the clinical outcome of infection with *Edwardsiella ictaluri* in channel catfish. *Journal of the American Veterinary Medical Association*, **191**, 1413−16.

Hawke, J.P. (1979) A bacterium associated with disease of pond cultured channel catfish. *Journal of the Fisheries Research Board of Canada*, **36**, 1508−12.

Hawke, J.P., McWhorter, A.C., Steigerwalt, A.G. & Brenner, D.J. (1981) *Edwardsiella ictaluri* sp. nov., the causative agent of enteric septicaemia of catfish. *International Journal of Systematic Bacteriology*, **31**, 396−400.

Herman, R.L. & Bullock, G.L. (1986) *Edwardsiella tarda* as a cause of mortality in striped bass. *Transactions of the American Fisheries Society*, **115**, 232−5.

Hoshinae, T. (1962) On a new bacterium, *Paracolobactrum anguillimortiferum* sp. *Bulletin of the Japanese Society of Scientific Fisheries*, **28**, 162−4.

Jarboe, H.H., Bowser, P.R. & Robinette, H.R. (1984) Pathology associated with a natural *Edwardsiella* infection in channel catfish (*Ictalurus punctatus* Rafinesque). *Journal of Wildlife Diseases*, **20**, 352−4.

Jordan, G.W. and Hadley, W.K. (1969) Human infection with *Edwardsiella tarda*. *Annals of International Medicine*, **70**, 283−8.

Kasornchandra, J., Rogers, W.A. & Plumb, J.A. (1987) *Edwardsiella ictaluri* from walking catfish, *Clarias batrachus* L., in Thailand. *Journal of Fish Diseases*, **10**, 137−8.

Kent, M.L. & Lyons, J.M. (1982) *Edwardsiella ictaluri* in the green knife fish, *Eigemannia virescens*. *Fish Health News*, **11**(1–2), p. ii.

King, B.M. & Adler, D.L. (1964) A previously undescribed group of Enterobacteriaceae. *American Journal of Clinical Pathology*, **41**, 230–2.

Kusuda, R., Toyoshima, T., Iwamura, Y. & Saka, H. (1976) *Edwardsiella tarda* from an epizootic of mullets (*Mugil cephalus*) in Okitsu Bay. *Bulletin of the Japanese Society of Scientific Fisheries*, **42**, 271–5.

Kusuda, R., Itami, T., Mumekiyo, M. & Nakajima, H. (1977) Characteristics of an *Edwardsiella* sp. from an epizootic of cultured crimson sea breams. *Bulletin of the Japanese Society of Scientific Fisheries*, **43**, 129–134.

Liu, C.I. & Tsai, S.S. (1980) Edwardsiellosis in pond-cultured eel in Taiwan. *CAPD Fisheries series No. 3, Reports on Fish Disease Research*, **3**, 109–15.

Liu, E.K. & Wang, J.H. (1986) Drug resistance of fish-pathogenic bacteria-II. Resistance of *Edwardsiella tarda* in aquaculture environment. *EOA Fisheries Series No. 8, Fish Disease Research*, **8**, 56–67.

Meyer, F.P. & Bullock, G.L. (1973) *Edwardsiella tarda*, a new pathogen of channel catfish (*Ictalurus punctatus*). *Applied Microbiology*, **25**, 135–56.

Miyashito, T. (1984) *Pseudomonas fluorescens* and *Edwardsiella tarda* isolated from diseased tilapia. *Fish Pathology*, **19**, 45–50.

Miyazaki, T. & Egusa, S. (1976*a*) Histopathological studies of Edwardsiellosis of the Japanese eel (*Anguilla japonica*) – I. Suppurative interstitial nephritis form. *Fish Pathology*, **11**, 33–43.

Miyazaki, T. & Egusa, S. (1976*b*) Histopathological studies of Edwardsiellosis of the Japanese eel (*Anguilla japonica*) – II. Suppurative hepatitis form. *Fish Pathology*, **11**, 67–75.

Miyazaki, T. & Egusa, S. (1976*c*) Histopathological studies of Edwardsiellosis of the Japanese eel (*Anguilla japonica*) – III. Elvers and anguillettes. *Fish Pathology*, **11**, 127–31.

Miyazaki, T. & Kaige, N. (1985) Comparative histopathology of Edwardsiellosis in fishes. *Fish Pathology*, **20**, 219–27.

Miyazaki, T. & Plumb, J.A. (1985) Histopathology of *Edwardsiella ictaluri* in channel catfish, *Ictalurus punctatus* (Rafinesque). *Journal of Fish Diseases*, **8**, 389–92.

Nakatsugawa, T. (1983) *Edwardsiella tarda* isolated from cultured young flounders. *Fish Pathology*, **18**, 99–101.

Newton, J.C., Bird, R.C., Blevins, W.T., Wilt, G.R. & Wolfe, L.G. (1988) Isolation, characterization, and molecular cloning of cryptic plasmids isolated from *Edwardsiella ictaluri*. *American Journal of Veterinary Research*, **49**, 1856–60.

Park, Soc.-Il, Wakabayashi, H. & Watanabe, Y. (1983) Serotype and virulence of *Edwardsiella tarda* isolated from eel and their environment. *Fish Pathology*, **18**, 85–9.

Plumb, J.A. (1988) Vaccination against *Edwardsiella ictaluri*. In *Fish Vaccination* (Ed. by A.E. Ellis), pp. 152–61. Academic Press, London.

Plumb, J.A. & Hilge, V. (1987) Susceptibility of European catfish (*Silurus glanis*) to *Edwardsiella ictaluri*. *Journal of Applied Ichthyology*, **3**, 45–8.

Plumb, J.A. & Quinlan, E.E. (1986) Survival of *Edwardsiella ictaluri* in pond water and bottom mud. *Progressive Fish-Culturist*, **48**, 212–14.

Plumb, J.A. & Sanchez, D.J. (1983) Susceptibility of five species of fish to *Edwardsiella ictaluri*. *Journal of Fish Diseases*, **6**, 261–6.

Plumb, J.A. & Vinitnantharat, S. (1989) Biochemical, biophysical, and serological homogeneity of *Edwardsiella ictaluri*. *Journal of Aquatic Animal Health*, **1**, 51–6.

Plumb, J.A., Wise, M.L. & Rogers, W.A. (1986) Modulary effects of temperature on antibody response and specific resistance to challenge of channel catfish, *Ictalurus punctatus*, immunized against *Edwardsiella ictaluri*. *Veterinary Immunology and Immunopathology*, **12**, 297–304.

Plumb, J.A., Maestrone, G. & Quinlan, E. (1987) Use of a potentiated sulfonamide to control *Edwardsiella ictaluri* infection in channel catfish (*Ictalurus punctatus*). *Aquaculture*, **62**, 187–94.

Rogers, W.A. (1981) Serological detection of two species of *Edwardsiella ictaluri* infecting catfish. *International Symposium on Fish Biologies: Serodiagnosis and Vaccines. Developments in Biological Standardization*, **49**, 169–72.

Sachs, J.M., Pacin, M. & Counts, G.W. (1974) Sickle hemoglobinopathy and *Edwardsiella tarda* meningitis. *American Journal of Disease of Children*, **128**, 387–8.

Sae-Oui, D., Muroga, K. & Nakai, T. (1984) A case of *Edwardsiella tarda* infection in cultured colored carp *Cyprinus carpio*. *Fish Pathology*, **19**, 197–9.

Saeed, M.O. & Plumb, J.A. (1986) Immune response of channel catfish to lipopolysaccharide and whole cell *Edwardsiella ictaluri* vaccines. *Diseases of Aquatic Organisms*, **2**, 21–5.

Sakazaki, R. (1962) The new group of Enterobacteriaceae, the Asakusa group. *Japanese Journal of Bacteriology*, **17**, 616–17.

Sakazaki, R. (1967) Studies on the Asakusa group of Enterobacteriaceae (*Edwardsiella tarda*). *Japanese Journal of Medical Science and Biology*, **20**, 205–12.

Sakazaki, R. & Tamura, K. (1978) Comment on a proposal of Farmer *et al*. to conserve the specific epithet *tarda* over specific epithet *anguillimortiferum* in the name of the organism known as *Edwardsiella tarda*. *International Journal of Systematic Bacteriology*, **28**, 130–1.

Salati, F. (1985) Immunogenecity of *Edwardsiella tarda* antigens in the eel (*Anguilla japonica*). *Piscicoltura Eittiopatologia*, **20**, 12–26.

Salati, F. & Kusuda, R. (1985*a*) Vaccine preparations used for immunization of eel (*Anguilla japonica*) against *Edwardsiella tarda* infection. *Bulletin of the Japanese Society of Scientific Fisheries*, **51**, 1233–7.

Salati, F. & Kusuda, R. (1985*b*) Chemical composition of the lipopolysaccharide from *Edwardsiella tarda*. *Fish Pathology*, **20**, 187–91.

Salati, F., Kawai, K. & Kusuda, R. (1983) Immunoresponse of eel against *Edwardsiella tarda* antigens. *Fish Pathology*, **18**, 135–41.

Shotts, E.B. & Waltman, W.D. (1990) An isolation medium for *Edwardsiella ictaluri*. *Journal of Wildlife Diseases*, **26**, 214–18.

Shotts, E.B., Blazer, V.S. & Waltman, W.D. (1986) Pathogenesis of experimental *Edwardsiella ictaluri* infections in channel catfish (*Ictalurus punctatus*). *Canadian Journal of Fisheries and Aquatic Sciences*, **43**, 36–42.

Song, Y.L. and Kou, G.H. (1979) Immune response of eels (*Anguilla japonica*) against *Aeromonas hydrophila* and *Edwardsiella anguillimortiferum* (*E. tarda*) infection. Proceedings of the Republic of China – United States Cooperative Science Seminar. National Science Council, Republic of China, Taipei, pp. 107–14.

Song, Y.L. & Kou, G.H. (1981) The immuno-responses of eel (*Anguilla japonica*) against *Edwardsiella anguillimortifera* as studied by the immersion method. *Fish Pathology*, **15**, 249–55.

Song, Y.L., Kou, G.H. & Chen, K.Y. (1982) Vaccination conditions for the eel (*Anguilla japonica*) with *Edwardsiella anguillimortifera* bacterin. *Journal of the Fishery Society of Taiwan*, **4**, 18–25.

Sonnenwirth, A.C. & Kallus, B.A. (1968) Meningitis due to *Edwardsiella tarda*. *American Journal of Clinical Pathology*, **49**, 92–5.

Speyerer, P.D. & Boyle, J.A. (1987) The plasmid profile of *Edwardsiella tarda*. *Journal of Fish Diseases*, **10**, 461–9.

Ullah, A. & Arai, T. (1983) Pathological activities of the naturally occurring strains of *Edwardsiella tarda*. *Fish Pathology*, **18**, 65–70.

Wakabayashi, H. & Egusa, S. (1973) *Edwardsiella tarda* (*Paracolobacterium anguillimortiferam*) associated with pond-cultured eel disease. *Bulletin of the Japanese Society of Scientific Fisheries*, **39**, 931–6.

Wallace, L.J., White, F.H. & Gore, H.L. (1966) Isolation of *Edwardsiella tarda* from a sea lion and two alligators. *Journal of the American Veterinary Medicine Association*, **149**, 881–3.

Walters, G. & Plumb, J.A. (1980) Environmental stress and bacterial infection in channel catfish, *Ictalurus punctatus* Rafinesque. *Journal of Fish Biology*, **17**, 177–85.

Waltman, W.D. & Shotts, E.B. (1986*a*) Antimicrobial susceptibility of *Edwardsiella tarda* from the United States and Taiwan. *Veterinary Microbiology*, **12**, 277–82.

Waltman, W.D. & Shotts, E.B. (1986*b*) Antimicrobial susceptibility of *Edwardsiella ictaluri*. *Journal of Wildlife Disease*, **22**, 173–7.

Waltman, W.D., Shotts, E.B. & Blazer, V.S. (1985) Recovery of *Edwardsiella ictaluri* from Danio (*Danio devario*). *Aquaculture*, **46**, 63–6.

Waltman, W.D., Shotts, E.B. & Hsu, T.C. (1986*a*) Biochemical and enzymatic characterization of *Edwardsiella tarda* from the United States and Taiwan. *Fish Pathology*, **21**, 1–8.

Waltman, W.D., Shotts, E.B. & Hsu, T.C. (1986*b*) Biochemical characteristics of *Edwardsiella ictaluri*. *Applied and Environmental Microbiology*, **51**, 101–4.

White, F.H., Neal, F.E., Simpson, C.F. & Walsh, A.F. (1969) Isolation of *Edwardsiella tarda* from an ostrich and an Australian skink. *Journal of the American Veterinary Medicine Association*, **55**, 1057–8.

White, F.H., Simpson, C.F. & Williams, L.E. Jr. (1973) Isolation of *Edwardsiella tarda* from aquatic animal species and surface waters in Florida. *Journal of Wildlife Diseases*, **9**, 204–8.

Wyatt, L.E., Nickelson, R., II & Vanderzant, C. (1979) *Edwardsiella tarda* in freshwater catfish and their environment. *Applied and Environmental Microbiology*, **38**, 710–14.

Yasunaga, N., Ogawa, S. & Hatai, K. (1982) Characteristics of the fish pathogen *Edwardsiella* isolated from several species of cultured marine fishes. *Bulletin of the Nagasaki Prefecture Institute of Fisheries*, **8**, 57–65.

# Chapter 5:
# Enteric redmouth (ERM) and other enterobacterial infections of fish

The genus *Yersinia*, within the family Enterobacteriaceae consists of Gram-negative small straight rods to coccobacilli $0.5-0.8 \times 1.3\,\mu$m. Endospores are not formed. Species except *Y. pestis* are motile with peritrichous flagella if grown below 30°C although non-motile variants are not uncommon. They are typical of the Enterobacteriaceae but phenotypic characteristics may be temperature dependent with more expressed at 25−29°C than at 35−37°C. The mol % G + C of the DNA is 46−50. *Yersinia* occur widely in live and inanimate habitats and one species, *Y. ruckeri*, is an important primary pathogen of fish. It is the causative agent of enteric redmouth disease affecting rainbow trout primarily and other salmonids and species to a lesser extent. It causes a septicaemic infection in which haemorrhages on the body surface and internal organs commonly occur. The disease is closely stress related and, as such, a problem in intensive culture of rainbow trout. With improved environmental conditions asymptomatic carriers may become established posing a continuing threat. Some species of *Proteus*, *Serratia* and *Citrobacter* have been suggested as potential pathogens of fish. They can be differentiated from other Enterobacteriaceae by specific biochemical tests and by mol % G + C content of their DNA, viz 38−41, 52−60 and 50−52.

## Yersinia

### Introduction

*Yersinia ruckeri*, the causative agent of enteric redmouth (ERM) disease, was first associated with losses in rainbow trout aquaculture in the Hagerman valley of Idaho in the 1950s; hence the previous accusatory name of 'Hagerman redmouth'. Although the disease has predominantly been a problem for rainbow trout in intensive culture, all salmonids and some other fish species can be affected. Losses may be relatively low in chronic infections or can become dramatically higher when water conditions are poor or when fish are exposed to stresses such as handling. As fish become asymptomatic carriers relatively easily, ERM presents a constant threat to salmonid aquaculture.

The organism, *Yersinia ruckeri*, is a member of the Enterobacteriaceae (Ross *et al*. 1966) and the name 'enteric redmouth disease' was used to distinguish it from pseudomonad and aeromonad infections with the same pathological signs. A killed-cell vaccine to protect fish from ERM was already in use (Tebbit *et al*. 1981) before the organism was assigned a formal name. Eventually, taxonomic studies by Ewing *et al*. (1978) assigned it to the genus *Yersinia* on the basis of biochemical and genetic similarities. The species now includes a variety of strains, including six serological varieties.

Recently, disease caused by this organism has been referred to as 'yersiniosis' or 'yersinia septicaemia', as the classic 'redmouth' appearance is not necessarily seen. Overall, the disease is much like other bacterial septicaemias. Haemorrhages on the body surface are common, with reddening at the base of fins and along the lateral line, as well as in the head region. Internally, there can be petechial haemorrhages on the liver, visceral fat and pyloric caeca. The distal part of the intestine and the vent may be inflamed, or fluid may accumulate in the gut. Occasionally, the infection may appear as ulcers, without involvement of internal organs. Chronically-infected fish may appear dark and lethargic, with intermittent reversions to an apparently asymptomatic carrier state.

## The disease

### Pathology

Disease signs can suggest possible mechanisms of pathogenesis. However, there are as yet very few clues to the virulence determinants of *Y. ruckeri*. The gross external changes produced in ERM as first reported by Rucker (1966) in infected rainbow trout were sluggishness and darkening in colour, with reddening around the mouth and operculum, and at the base of the fins (Plate 13). Other pathological signs commonly reported include exophthalmos, reddening around the mouth and local or general darkening of the body (Fig. 5.1) (Fuhrmann *et al.* 1983, Dalsgaard *et al.* 1984, Lesel *et al.* 1983a; Roberts 1983, Giorgetti *et al.* 1985, Bragg *et al.* 1986). Often the characteristic reddened areas around the mouth and operculum are not apparent in more than a very few affected fish, if at all (Frerichs *et al.* 1985, Sparboe *et al.* 1986) and thus absence of classic 'redmouth' does not rule out infection with *Y. ruckeri*.

Internal gross pathological changes are those of a severe haemorrhagic septicaemia and include reddening throughout the peritoneum, in the fat of the body cavity and in the distal portion of the intestine. The stomach may be full

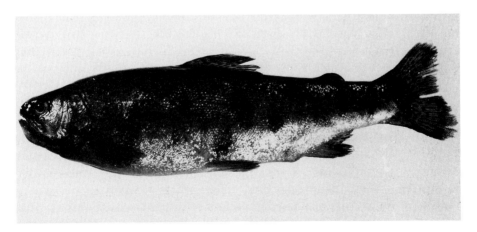

**Fig. 5.1** *Yersinia ruckeri* infected rainbow trout showing generalised ERM signs of reddening under the opercula and focal darkening of skin over affected areas.

of watery fluid, and the intestine may contain yellow fluid. The spleen may be dark and enlarged (Rucker 1966). Wobeser (1973) found petechial haemorrhages in one or more sites in all the fish he examined. The internal gross pathology, characteristic of a haemorrhagic septicaemia (Busch 1978), may be mistaken for furunculosis (Fuhrmann *et al.* 1983). Histopathologically, ERM is characterized by an acute bacteraemia, with low to high concentrations of bacteria observed in virtually all tissues, especially the highly vascularized kidney, spleen, heart, liver and gills (Rucker 1966). Wobeser (1973) observed that infected fish had a severe loss of haematopoietic tissue owing to necrosis in both the anterior and posterior kidney. Normal lymphoid structure in the spleen was lost and changes in cells were observed in the liver. Periocular lesions, with swelling behind the eye (retrobulbar oedema) are also seen (Wobeser 1973).

In a haemorrhagic condition, blood parameters are of obvious interest. Wobeser (1973) found packed red blood cell volume and total blood protein were about 50% of normal values. Quentel & Aldrin (1986) and Lehmann *et al.* (1987) observed decreases in red blood cell counts, haematocrit values, haemoglobin content and leucocyte count in infected rainbow trout. Miller (1983) suggested that the endotoxin of *Y. ruckeri* could affect blood coagulation, ultimately producing thrombosis in the capillaries and haemorrhages.

### Stress effects

ERM disease was first recognized in hatchery-reared rainbow trout in the Hagerman Valley of Idaho in the early 1950s (Busch 1982), a region noted for intensive aquaculture (Busch, 1978). The environment for these fish can be stressful, as crowded conditions result in excess ammonia and metabolic waste products being present in the water. Bullock & Snieszko (1979) suggested that ERM often produces low levels of mortality but large scale epizootics can occur if chronically infected or carrier fish are stressed. Epizootics often follow the weighing and moving of apparently healthy fish (Rucker 1966). Water temperatures (Rucker 1966) and exposure to agents such as copper (Knittel 1981) can act as predisposing factors.

### Host range and vectors

Although ERM disease was first reported in rainbow trout (Ross *et al.* 1966, Rucker 1966), its probable host range appears to include all salmonids (McDaniel 1979). Table 5.1 indicates the isolation sources reported for *Y. ruckeri*, which include salmonids, infected fish of other species and a number of sources that may indicate vectors or casual associations.

The spread of *Y. ruckeri* apparently occurs from fish to fish through water. Cultures of *Y. ruckeri*, or fish that had died from ERM, could induce mortalities when added to a tank containing healthy fish (Rucker 1966). Feral fish (Mitchum

**Table 5.1**   Isolation sources of *Yersinia ruckeri*

|  | Literature reference |
|---|---|
| **Salmonids** | |
| Cutthroat trout (*Salmo clarkii*) | McDaniel (1971) |
| Steelhead trout (*Salmo gairdneri*) | " |
| Silver or coho salmon (*Oncorhynchus kisutch*) | " |
| Chinook salmon (*Oncorhynchus tshawytscha*) | " |
| Brook trout (*Salvelinus fontinalis*) | " |
| Atlantic salmon (*Salmo salar*) | " |
| Brown trout (*Salmo trutta*) | " |
| Sockeye salmon (*Oncorhynchus nerka*) | Dulin *et al.* (1976) |
|  | |
| **Diseased fish** | |
| Emerald shiners (*Notemigonus atherinoides*) | (Mitchum 1981) |
| Minnow (*Pimephales promelas*) | (Michel *et al.* 1986) |
| Cisco (*Coregonus artedii*) | (Stevenson & Daly 1982) |
| Whitefish (*Coregonus peled*) | (Rintamaki *et al.* 1986) |
| (*Coregonus muksun*) | " |
| Sturgeon (*Acipenser baeri*) | (Vuillaume *et al.* 1987) |
| Turbot (*Scophthalmus maximus*) | (Michel *et al.* 1986) |
|  | |
| **Apparently healthy fish** | |
| Goldfish (*Carassius auratus*) | (McArdle & Dooley-Martyn 1985) |
| Carp (*Cyprinus carpio*) | (Fuhrmann *et al.* 1984) |
| Eel (*Anguilla anguilla*) | " |
| Burbot (*Lota lota*) | (Dwilow *et al.* 1987) |
| Coalfish | (Willumsen 1989) |
| Arctic char | |
|  | |
| **Experimentally transmitted to** | |
| Channel catfish (*Icatlurus punctatus*) | (Lewis 1981) |
| Sole and gilthead | (Michel *et al.* 1986) |
|  | |
| **Other sources** | |
| Muskrat (*Ondatra zibethica*) | (Stevenson & Daly 1982) |
| Kestrel and turkey vulture, faeces | (Bangert *et al.* 1988) |
| Crayfish (?) | (Sullivan 1981) |
| Sea gulls | (Willumsen 1989) |
| Human, clinical specimen | (Farmer *et al.* 1985) |
| Sewage | |
| River water | |

1981, Willumsen 1989), imported baitfish (Michel *et al.* 1986) or even ornamentals (McArdle & Dooley-Martyn 1985) have been suggested as sources of ERM. *Y. ruckeri* has been isolated from bird faeces (Table 5.1), and the series of isolations described by Willumsen (1989) from sea gulls and fish farms supports a role for birds in transmission.

Often in relation to fish diseases there is a tendency to attribute the appearance of new problems to fish movements from outwith the area. ERM disease was first recognized in Idaho in the early 1950s (McDaniel 1971) and through the 1960s and 1970s, North American outbreaks of ERM were considered the result of movements of carrier fish or contaminated eggs from Idaho. For example, the first outbreak in Canada (Wobeser 1973) was preceded by importation of fish from Idaho. As the imported fish appeared healthy, it was suggested that they were asymptomatic carriers. However, isolates of *Y. ruckeri* from West Virginia in 1952 and Australia in 1960 led Bullock *et al.* (1977) to suggest that *Y. ruckeri* was present in other areas at the time of the first recognized outbreaks in Idaho.

Certainly now, the number and geographic range of isolations suggests that the organism may be relatively common in fish and the environment, and presents a problem only when fish are exposed to additional stresses. In Canada *Y. ruckeri* has been isolated from hatchery and wild fish in Ontario, yet ERM disease is not known to occur in Ontario (Stevenson & Daly 1982). Similarly, *Y. ruckeri* has been isolated from apparently healthy burbot from the Northwest Territories where it is unlikely that the organism was introduced by stocking (Dwilow *et al.* 1987).

European ERM outbreaks in 1981 were blamed on importation of *Y. ruckeri* along with baitfish from the United States (Michel *et al.* 1986). However, as early as 1977, mortalities in England were presumed to have been caused by *Y. ruckeri*, with confirmed cases by 1981 (Roberts 1983). The many isolations made in diverse European locations suggests that the greater number of outbreaks may be related to more intensive aquaculture. For example, in Germany, the increase from one case of ERM disease in 1981 to 40 outbreaks in 1984–1985 parallels an increase in the number of fish culture sites (Schlotfeldt *et al.* 1985). In addition, isolations may reflect increased surveillance, wider awareness of the organism, and improvements in detection methods for *Y. ruckeri*.

### The carrier state

The carrier state for ERM was recognized early, as Rucker (1966) isolated *Y. ruckeri* from a surviving fish 2 months after experimental exposure. Busch & Lingg (1975) established an asymptomatic carrier state in rainbow trout, by both the parenteral and immersion routes of exposure. For the first 30–60 days after infection, *Y. ruckeri* was readily recovered from the kidney, lower intestine, spleen and liver, even though many fish showed no signs of disease. By 60–65 days post-infection, the pathogen had localized in the lower intestine of 50–75% of the survivors (Busch & Lingg 1975). During the 102 day experiment there was a regular, 36–40 day cycle of intestinal shedding of the organism by fish that had been intraperitoneally infected. This shedding preceded the reappearance of gross pathological changes and mortality by 3–5 days. As the periodicity of the cycle may be altered by seasonal variations in water temperature, loading factors, handling and other stresses, the significance of the 36–40 day cycle is unclear (Busch & Lingg 1975). However, the cyclic phenomenon is often noted to explain fluctuations in the prevalence of the pathogen in groups of fish tested at intervals (Bruno & Munro 1989).

Carrier fish serve as an important source of infection under stress conditions. When the water temperature was raised to 25°C, carriers transmitted *Y. ruckeri* to healthy fish but unstressed fish did not (Hunter *et al*. 1980). In fish that remained carriers after antibiotic treatment, *Y. ruckeri* was not part of the dominant flora isolated from the organs tested (stomach, pyloric caecum, intestine, kidney, liver, heart and muscle) but, rather, it survived in the kidney where it multiplied and eventually invaded other organs when the fish were stressed (Lesel *et al*. 1983*b*). In other attempts to detect the long-term carrier state, it has been useful to culture the lower intestinal tract, as the bacterium may localize in that region. To a considerable extent, successful detection of carrier fish may reflect the microbiological techniques and methods used.

**Diagnostic methods**

Like most Enterobacteriaceae, *Y. ruckeri* grows fairly rapidly, so diagnosis and detection commonly involves culturing organs or lesions and identifying isolates by standard bacteriological procedures. Detection of *Y. ruckeri* in fish is enhanced by a preliminary enrichment, in which tissue samples are placed in tubes of tryptic soy broth and incubated for 2 days at 18°C before streaking onto plates. In virulence trials described by Flett (1989), for example, the prevalence of infection would have been considerably under-estimated if only direct culture was used (Table 5.2). A combination of broth enrichments and sampling the heart, liver and spleen tissue in addition to kidney make culture methods very effective for detecting this and other pathogens (Daly & Stevenson 1985).

For initial plating, trypticase or tryptic soy agar (TSA) is satisfactory, although blood agar is also used. Attempts have been made to enhance recognition of *Y. ruckeri* in mixed cultures on primary plates by using selective and differential media, either intended for *Y. enterocolitica*, or special formulations for *Y. ruckeri* (Waltman & Shotts 1984). However, these media had little advantage over TSA, and were sometimes less effective than TSA (Rodgers & Hudson 1985, Hastings & Bruno 1985). Colonies for further examination are selected from TSA plates on the basis of colony appearance or by slide-agglutination reactions with antiserum. More difficult to describe in a diagnostic protocol is the ability of experienced technicians to 'smell out' *Y. ruckeri* on plates — without infecting themselves! Pure cultures of isolates are further identified by a combination of morphological, serological and biochemical characteristics.

**The microorganism**

*Morphology and growth*

Cells of *Y. ruckeri* are rod-shaped, with filamentous forms seen in older cultures (Ross *et al*. 1966), or earlier in some strains (Austin *et al*. 1982).

**Table 5.2**  Isolation of *Y. ruckeri* from rainbow trout after immersion challenge[a]

| Sv | Strain | Number of fish tested | Average fish wt (g) | cfu/ml bath | % Mortality | % Infection[b] Direct | Broth |
|----|--------|-----------------------|---------------------|-------------|-------------|-----------------------|-------|
| I | RS  7 | 10 | 15.9 | $2.0 \times 10^8$ | 0 | 0 | 70 |
|   | RS 26 | 10 | 15.6 | $3.5 \times 10^8$ | 60 | 100 | 100 |
|   | RS 88*[c] | 10 | 42.6 | $2.4 \times 10^8$ | 80 | 100 | 100 |
|   | RS 89 | 10 | 17.4 | $3.8 \times 10^8$ | 80 | 100 | 100 |
| II | RS  3 | 10 | 61.8 | $1.5 \times 10^8$ | 0 | 60 | 90 |
|   | RS 91 | 10 | 56.6 | $1.0 \times 10^8$ | 90 | 90 | 90 |
| III | RS 20* | 10 | 31.4 | $2.4 \times 10^8$ | 0 | 0 | 60 |
|   | RS 54* | 10 | 33.2 | $1.6 \times 10^8$ | 0 | 0 | 10 |
|   | RS 77* | 10 | 30.9 | $1.9 \times 10^8$ | 0 | 0 | 90 |
| V | RS 25* | 9 | 23.8 | $2.6 \times 10^8$ | 0 | 0 | 22 |
|   | RS 93* | 11 | 38.2 | $2.6 \times 10^8$ | 0 | 0 | 27 |

[a] Fish were challenged by a 1 h immersion in a 1 in 10 dilution of live *Y. ruckeri* cells that were grown in TSB shake-cultures for 48 h at 18°C. Fish were held in flowing water at 10 ± 2°C and mortalities were removed daily. Control groups were immersed in a 1 in 10 dilution of TSB and showed no mortalities and no infection with *Y. ruckeri*

[b] Direct infection rate determined by streaking kidney tissue directly onto TSA. Broth infection rate determined by inoculating TSB with samples of heart, liver, spleen and kidney tissue, incubating tubes 48 h at 18°C then streaking them onto TSA. All plates were incubated 48 h at 18°C

[c] Asterisk (*) indicates 7 day tests, all other tests were 14 days

*Y. ruckeri* is peritrichously flagellated (Ross *et al.* 1966) though non-motile strains are not uncommon. Six of the 33 strains studied by Ewing *et al.* (1978) and many examined by Davies & Frerichs (1989) were non-motile. O'Leary *et al.* (1979) noted that the flagella were not produced at 37°C. In fact, many serovar I strains are unable to initiate growth from a dilute inoculum at 37°C (De Grandis *et al.* 1988), accounting for early comments about poor growth at this temperature. Other serovars and some serovar I strains do grow at 37°C, although optimum growth is between 22°C and 25°C. In addition, concern for maintaining potential virulence factors suggests routine culture at a cautious 18°C.

As a member of the Enterobacteriaceae, *Y. ruckeri* can be routinely cultured on media such as TSA or nutrient agar, and most strains will also grow well on a minimal glucose-salts medium. A few strains, such as ATCC 29904, require a peptone supplement (De Grandis *et al.* 1988).

### Biochemical characteristics

The biochemical characteristics of strains of *Y. ruckeri* have been reported by Ross *et al.* (1966), Wobeser (1973), Ewing *et al.* (1978), Bullock *et al.* (1978), O'Leary *et al.* (1979) and Stevenson & Daly (1982), with summaries provided by Bercovier & Mollaret (1984) and Ewing (1986). Strains of *Y. ruckeri* are fairly homogeneous in biochemical reactions although strains can vary in the methyl red, Voges-Proskauer, lysine decarboxylase, arginine dihydrolase, and lactose fermentation tests (Ross *et al*. 1966, Busch 1973, Wobeser 1973). Different incubation temperatures and test procedures may be the cause of some of the variations reported. For example, many strains of *Y. ruckeri* can produce gas from glucose fermentation when incubated at 18°C, but do so weakly or not at all at 25°C (De Grandis *et al*. 1988).

The sorbitol fermentation reaction of new isolates has been the most diligently noted biochemical characteristic since O'Leary (1977) suggested that a positive reaction indicated serovar II strains. As a result, 'serovar II' has come to include a fairly heterogeneous mixture of strains, including some which react with antiserum against serovar I strains (Dear 1988, Stevenson & Airdrie 1984*a*). Sorbitol fermentation does vary among authentic members of the species; some 32% of strains ferment it. On the other hand, positive reactions for fermentation of L-arabinose, L-rhamnose or D-xylose can be used as tests to clearly exclude an isolate from the species *Y. ruckeri*. DNA from such isolates does not hybridize with that of *Y. ruckeri* (De Grandis *et al*. 1988).

### Genetics and taxonomy

Genetic criteria have been important in determining the taxonomic position of the ERM bacterium. The early description of a Gram-negative, rod-shaped, oxidase negative, peritrichous, fermentative bacterium placed it in the *Enterobacteriaceae* (Ross *et al*. 1966). Within that family, the biochemical reactions of the ERM bacterium most closely resembled those of *Serratia* and *Yersinia*, and it shared approximately equal DNA sequence similarity (about 30%) with species of these two genera (Ewing *et al*. 1978). Eventually, the organism was designated *Yersinia ruckeri* as the DNA base composition (mol % G + C) was 47.5−48%, disqualifying it from the genus *Serratia* at 52−60% (Ewing *et al*. 1978). Similarly, % G + C values exclude *Y. ruckeri* from *Salmonella arizonae* (50−53%), the proposal of Green & Austin (1983). De Grandis *et al*. (1988) found little DNA−DNA homology between these species.

The % G + C values for *Y. ruckeri* are consistent with those of the yersiniae (46−50%). However, *Y. ruckeri* has been described as a species 'searching for a better genus as a final home' (Farmer *et al*. 1985). Ewing *et al*. (1978) had shown that *Y. ruckeri* cultures were not closely related to other named species of *Yersinia* on the basis of DNA−DNA hybridization. Relatedness among most *Yersinia* species is 44−70% or higher, but *Y. ruckeri* is, at most, 38% related (Bercovier & Mollaret 1984). The DNA and phenotypic differences between *Y. ruckeri* and other yersiniae could justify a new genus (Bercovier & Mollaret 1984), but there was reluctance to create one for what was initially a homogeneous group of isolates.

Based on isoenzyme analysis of the products of 15 chromosomal loci in 47 isolates of *Y. ruckeri*, Schill *et al.* (1984) suggested that little genetic diversity was found in this species. However, some genetic distinctions may be seen between strains of different serovars, based on patterns produced by *Eco*RI restriction enzyme treatment of DNA (our observations).

### Plasmids of Y. ruckeri

Taxonomy allows predictions about organisms, based on knowledge of related organisms. Pathogenic strains of several species of *Yersinia* carry plasmids of about 63 kb which encode specific virulence determinants (Portnoy & Falkow 1981). Of 40 serovar I strains of *Y. ruckeri* tested, 75% did have a large plasmid of approximately 88 kb and a smaller plasmid of 15−21 kb (De Grandis 1987, De Grandis & Stevenson 1982). This large plasmid was also observed in serovar I strains by Toranzo *et al.* (1983) and Stave *et al.* (1987). However, the plasmids of *Y. ruckeri* are not homologous with the virulence plasmids of the other yersiniae (De Grandis 1987, Guilvout *et al.* 1988). Most strains carrying the plasmids do not grow at 37°C, are sensitive to polymyxin B, and show bacteriophage sensitivity patterns different from those of strains without the plasmids (De Grandis & Stevenson 1985). However, we were unable to cure strains of plasmids in order to demonstrate unequivocally that these functions are plasmid-encoded.

Serovar II and V strains had a variety of plasmid profiles, while strains of serovar I' and III had either no plasmids or a single plasmid of approximately 88 kb. The only serovar VI isolate studied had one small plasmid of approximately 6.3 kb. There were also strains within serovar I, II, III and V that carried no plasmids (De Grandis 1987). Two serovar I strains carried a transferable 54 kb plasmid which determined plasmid-mediated resistance to tetracycline and sulphonamides (De Grandis & Stevenson 1985).

### Antigens and serotypes of *Yersinia ruckeri*

#### Whole-cell serotypes

The major sub-divisions of the species are based on serological reactions, with six serovars recognized on the basis of whole-cell serology (Table 5.3) The first isolates of *Y. ruckeri* were uniform in their serological reactions, based on 14 isolates studied by Ross *et al.* (1966) and 44 examined by Busch (1973). Antisera used in diagnostic laboratories are generally prepared against formalin-killed whole cells, which avoids many cross-reactions with other enteric bacteria. For example, heated cells (0-antigens) of the ERM bacterium reacted with antiserum to the 0:26 group of *Arizona* (*Salmonella arizonae*) (Ross *et al.* 1966). Similarly, antisera prepared against heated cells of *Y. ruckeri* gave cross-reactions with several enteric bacteria (Stevenson & Airdrie 1984a).

O'Leary (1977) described a new sorbitol-fermenting serovar of *Y. ruckeri*

**Table 5.3**  Summary of whole-cell serotypes of *Yersinia ruckeri*

| Serovar | Designation | No. of isolates | Representative |
|---------|-------------|-----------------|---------------|
| I   | (Hagerman)[a]             | 95 | RS  4 (11.4)          |
| I'  | (Salmonid Blood Spot)[b]  | 10 | RS 20 (0634)         |
| II  | (Oregon)[c] A             | 25 | RS  3 (Big Creek 74) |
|     | B                         | 13 | RS  2 (Ont 258)      |
| III | (Australian)              | 10 | RS 77 (11.43)        |
| IV  | [excluded by DNA homology] | —  |                      |
| V   | (Colorado)                | 5  | RS 25 (2.88)         |
| VI  | (Ontario)                 | 4  | RS 80 (16A)          |

[a] Cross-reactions occur between strains of serovar I, I', III, and V
[b] Serologically the same as serovar III
[c] Includes at least two major serological sub-divisions

from chinook salmon, serovar II. His serological analysis, using whole-cell antisera and whole-cell antigens, indicated that *Y. ruckeri* strains could be differentiated into two serotypes, by two major antigens. A third minor antigen could produce low titre cross-reactions if present (O'Leary *et al.* 1982). O'Leary (1977) and Bullock *et al.* (1978) initially referred to the sorbitol-fermenting serotype as 'serovar 1' and the earlier strains as 'serotype 2', causing some confusion.

In a postscript to a paper, Bullock *et al.* (1978) designated an Australian isolate as serotype 3 as it did not react with antiserum to either serovar I or II. The Australian Salmonid Blood Spot (SBS) bacterium (Llewellyn 1980) is *Y. ruckeri* (De Grandis *et al.* 1988), and was designated as serovar I-prime (I') on the basis of partial cross-reactions with serovar I strains (Stevenson & Airdrie 1984*a*). Contrary to the initial report (Bullock *et al.* 1978), the Australian isolate did cross-react with serovar I antiserum. It was serologically identical to 'serovar I'', so they were combined as serovar III (De Grandis *et al.* 1988, Flett 1989). An additional serovar III (I') isolate from British Columbia was of particular interest because it fermented sorbitol (Stevenson & Daly *et al.* 1982), previously considered to be indicative of serovar II strains. Other sorbitol-fermenting examples of serovar III occur among Norwegian isolates (Flett 1989).

A second example of sorbitol-fermenting strains that reacted with serovar I antiserum but failed to cross-absorb completely came from diseased rainbow trout in Colorado. Antiserum prepared against this strain reacted only weakly with other isolates, including serovar III strains, and strains representing the other serovars did not remove significant amounts of antibody in cross-absorbence studies. As a result, this strain was designated serovar V (Stevenson & Airdrie 1984*a*). Further isolates have since been found (Daly *et al.* 1986), but they have been relatively rare (Table 5.3).

Recent serological re-examination of sorbitol-fermenting strains shows that serovar II is a more heterogeneous group than previously thought, even when serovar III and V isolates are excluded (Pyle & Schill 1985, Flett 1989). Two major subgroups (Table 5.3) can be distinguished by whole-cell reactions. These distinct reactions may have been overlooked in previous studies because of cross-reactions, particularly with newly isolated cultures. Many of our serovar II isolates were selected on the basis of an agglutination reaction with type I antiserum, lost on sub-culture. Stevenson & Daly (1982) described strains which reacted with antisera against both serovar I and II, with fairly high titres ($\geq 160$). When the cells were heat-treated, the cross-reactions with serovar I antiserum were reduced or absent. This suggested different 0-antigens, in contrast to McCarthy & Johnson's (1982) suggestion that serovar II shared some heat-stable 0-antigens with serovar I strains. Their heat-treatment of 15 minutes may not have been sufficient to destroy all heat-labile cross-reacting antigens.

Serovars IV (Stevenson & Airdrie 1984*a*) and VI (Daly *et al.* 1986) were designations given to two Ontario isolates that did not react with antisera prepared against any of the known serovars. DNA hybridization eliminated the single representative of serovar IV, an arabinose and rhamnose fermenting isolate, but confirmed the identity of the serovar VI representative (De Grandis *et al.* 1988).

### Antigens used in serotyping

Whole-cell serologic typing of genera of the Enterobacteriaceae is based on the combined recognition of a variety of cell-surface associated antigen structures, including 0-antigens, flagellar (H) antigens and K (capsular or envelope) antigens. By virtue of the abundance and cellular location of lipopolysaccharide (LPS), the 0-antigen is the major surface antigen for many Gram-negative bacteria and is the basis for detailed serotyping schemes. The LPS extracted from *Y. ruckeri* and other bacteria can be analysed by comparing silver-stained and immunoblotted patterns after separations by polyacrylamide gel electro-phoresis (SDS-PAGE). Strains with the same LPS antigen should have the same banding patterns. These techniques were used to define six 0-serogroups in *Y. ruckeri* (Flett 1989), summarized in Fig. 5.2 and Table 5.4.

Isolates of the whole-cell serovars I and III all have similar LPS profiles, and

**Table 5.4**  0-Antigen serogroups of *Yersinia ruckeri*

| 0-Antigen serogroup | Whole-cell serovars | Antiserum strain | Number of isolates |
|---|---|---|---|
| 0:1 | I, III | RS  4 (11.4) | 110 |
| 0:2 | IIa | RS  3 (BC 74) | 25 |
| 0:3 | IIb | RS  2 (ONT 258) | 13 |
| 0:4 | IIc | RS  6 (ONT 193) | 2 |
| 0:5 | V | RS 25 (2.88) | 5 |
| 0:6 | VI | RS 80 (16A) | 4 |

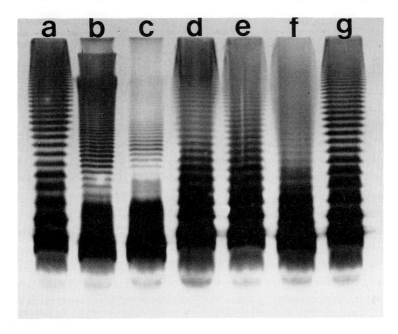

**Fig. 5.2** Comparison by SDS–PAGE and silver staining of LPS preparations from serovars I, II, III, IV and VI strains of *Y. ruckeri*. Proteinase K-digested lysates were added in 5 µl volumes to each well of the 12% PAGE.
Lanes: (a) RS 2 (serovar II), (b) RS 3 (serovar II), (c) RS 6 (serovar II), (d) RS 4 (serovar I),
    (e) RS 77 (serovar III), (f) RS 25 (serovar V), (g) RS 80 (serovar VI).

immunoblots of the LPS patterns with whole-cell antisera against serovar I and serovar III also showed uniform patterns (Flett 1989). This indicates a common LPS or 0-antigen for these strains and accounts for the cross-reactions in whole-cell agglutination reactions. All these strains were assigned to the 0:1 serogroup (the term 'serovar' is used here to refer to whole-cell serology results and the term 'serogroup' for 0-antigen results). As the serovar I and III strains composing the 0:1 serogroup can be distinguished by absorbed sera, there must be other antigens, perhaps outer membrane proteins or flagella, that are not shared by all members of this serogroup. Until those antigens are identified, it is convenient to retain the whole-cell sub-divisions of serovars I and III for this group, as there appears to be some degree of geographic or host specificity in serovar III isolations (Willumsen 1989, and our data). Use of absorbed typing sera on a routine basis in diagnostic laboratories may help resolve this question.

Serovar V strains have similar but not identical LPS patterns to those of the 0:1 group (Fig. 5.2). There are fewer bands overall, especially in the high molecular weight region, and immunoblotting reactions are not completely reciprocal, as type III antiserum did not react with serovar V LPS (Flett 1989). As a result, the serovar V strains have been designated as serogroup 0:5. Their LPS may have some sugars or epitopes in common with that of the 0:1

group, but the arrangements or proportions may differ. As yet the chemical composition is known for only one strain of *Y. ruckeri* (Banoub *et al.* 1988), serovar unknown.

The two major serovar II subgroups could be clearly identified by LPS patterns (Fig. 5.1) and by distinct immunoblots (Flett 1989). The group that includes O'Leary's serovar II strain, Big Creek 74, was designated 0:2, and the other major sub-group, 0:3. Two other minor serogroups, 0:4 and 0:6, were defined by LPS and immunoblot patterns. While the silver-stained LPS patterns of 0:4 strains resembled those of the 0:2 group, they did not interact with type II antiserum in immunoblots. However, heat-treated cells of serogroup 0:4 did agglutinate with this serum. In parallel, the 0:6 group, which is composed of serovar VI strains, has an LPS banding pattern similar to 0:3 (Fig. 5.1), but it did not immunoblot with antiserum prepared against the other representative strains (Flett 1989).

Pyle & Schill (1985) identified four 0-serotypes when they compared the LPS from 17 sorbitol-fermenting isolates of *Y. ruckeri* using similar procedures. However, a direct comparison of the studies is difficult as sorbitol-fermenting strains of serovars III, V or VI may have been included. Based on recognizable strain codes, 0-serotype 2 of Pyle & Schill (1985) is equivalent to our serogroup 0:2 and 0-serotype 4 is equivalent to serogroup 0:3.

Some strains of *Y. ruckeri* autoagglutinate and cannot be serotyped. These strains generally show fewer LPS bands on silver-stained gels than typable strains and may consist of only one or two bands, similar to the situation seen with rough mutants of other enteric bacteria (Hitchcock and Brown 1983).

**Virulence of *Y. ruckeri***

*Distribution of strains*

Strains belonging to serogroup 0:1 accounted for 110 (67%) of 163 strains examined by Flett (1989). This group includes the serovar I strains most often associated with ERM disease (McCarthy & Johnson 1982). Strains of serogroup 0:2, also associated with disease (O'Leary 1977, Cipriano *et al.* 1986), accounted for 25 of 163 strains. The other four serogroups account for only 24 of the 163 strains. Strains of serogroups 0:4, 0:5 and 0:6 have been isolated only in North America, as were the majority of serogroup 0:3 strains (10 of 13).

Most isolates from known fish sources were isolated from rainbow trout (60/110), probably because they are cultured so widely. While most of the large 0:1 serogroup was from rainbow trout, isolates were also made from other fish species. Similarly, isolates of the other serogroups came from both rainbow trout and other species. There is some suggestion of host bias when the serovars isolated from Atlantic salmon and chinook salmon are reviewed. Of 32 isolates from Atlantic salmon culture in Norway, 20 were serogroup 0:1 strains, with 18 isolates belonging to serovar III. Twelve other isolates belonged to serogroup 0:2 (Flett 1989, E. Myhr, unpublished data). Based on the previous Australian serovar III isolates, it was suggested that this serovar was avirulent (Busch 1982). However, the Norwegian serovar III strains were all isolated from diseased fish, suggesting that serovar III strains can be virulent, particularly for Atlantic salmon (Willumsen 1989). Serovar III isolates continue to be isolated from Atlantic salmon in Tazmania and Australia (J. Carson, unpublished data).

Serovar II/ serogroup 0:2 strains have been associated with ERM disease of chinook salmon (O'Leary 1977, Cipriano *et al.* 1986). McCarthy & Johnson (1982) reported serovar II to be avirulent in bath challenges, yet a serovar II strain isolated from an epizootic in chinook salmon produced high mortalities in both brook trout and Atlantic salmon (Cipriano *et al.* 1986). Experimental challenges with serovar II strains did not suggest any difference in the relative virulence of serovar II/0:2 strains for rainbow trout (Table 5.2), chinook salmon (Flett 1989), brook trout (Cipriano *et al.* 1986), and Atlantic salmon (Cipriano *et al.* 1986). Two serovar II strains, RS 3 (BC 74) and RS 91 (11.86), were tested by Cipriano & Ruppenthal (1987) in brook trout, and by Flett (1989) in rainbow trout and chinook salmon. Both strains belong to serogroup 0:2 and were phenotypically similar, but in both studies only RS 91 (11.86) was able to cause mortalities.

### Virulence tests

The results of experimental challenges with *Y. ruckeri* suggest that the virulence of an individual strain cannot be predicted from its serovar or serogroup designation alone. In experiments by Flett (1989) serovar I (RS 26, RS 88) and serovar II (RS 91) strains caused mortalities when administered by injection or immersion (Table 5.2), yet other serovar I (RS 7) and serovar II (RS 3) strains did not cause mortalities. As noted with other pathogens, a strain repeatedly passed on artificial media may lose virulence, although Busch (1982) reported that virulence seemed to be stable and was not lost on subculturing or storage of cultures in frozen, lyophilized, or refrigerated states. Busch & Lingg (1975) reported that maximum virulence of the bacteria could be maintained by four serial passes through rainbow trout.

The results described above and previous virulence data reported in the literature for *Y. ruckeri* show considerable variability (Table 5.5). In addition it is often difficult to compare results from different laboratories as information about the methods used (exposure route, strain of bacteria and growth conditions) and monitoring/standardization of other variables (diet, temperature, water parameters) are not always provided. In addition, while virulence is conveniently quantified as an LD50 value, the dose which is lethal to 50% of the population tested, virulence measured this way only considers the organism's ability to cause deaths. ERM disease, when chronic, can cause low level mortalities over a considerable length of time (Busch 1982). The impact of

**Table 5.5** Results reported for virulence tests on *Y. ruckeri*

| Route and Dose | Species and Weight | Result | Reference |
|---|---|---|---|
| **Injection — Serovar I Strains** | | | |
| subcutaneous 4 × 10³– 4 × 10⁸ cells/ml | Rainbow trout 185 g | LD50 8.5 × 10⁵ bacteria at 5 days | Anderson & Ross 1972 |
| intraperitoneal | Rainbow trout 120 g | LD50 30 bacteria | Busch 1973 |
| intraperitoneal 9.37 × 10⁸– 9.37 cells | Rainbow trout NR[a] | LD5O 9.37 × 10⁸ cells/fish | O'Leary 1977 |
| intraperitoneal 8.0 × 10⁴– 8.0 × 10⁷ cells | Rainbow trout NR | LD50 4.0 × 10⁶ cells/fish | O'Leary 1977 |
| intraperitoneal 5 × 10⁵ cells | Atlantic salmon NR | 100% mortality | Bullock et al. 1976 |
| intraperitoneal 1 × 10⁸ cells/ml | Rainbow trout 200 g | 100% mortality | Dalsgaard et al. 1984 |
| **Injection — Serovar II Strains** | | | |
| intraperitoneal | Rainbow trout NR | LD50 5.95 × 10⁶ | O'Leary 1977 |
| **Bath challenge — Serovar I Strains** | | | |
| 2.75 × 10⁶ bacteria/ml, 1h | Rainbow trout 185 g | 2% mortality at 7 days | Busch & Lingg 1975 |
| 10⁷ cells/ml 30 min | Atlantic salmon NR | 30–50% mortality | Bullock et al. 1976 |

| | | | |
|---|---|---|---|
| $10^8 - 10^9$ cells/ml, 90 s | Rainbow trout 10 g | 65–95% mortality at 15 days | Bullock & Anderson 1984 |
| $1 \times 10^3$ bacteria/ml, 1 h | Steelhead trout NR | LD50 $1.1 \times 10^6$ bacteria/ml | Knittel 1981 |
| $3.5 \times 10^9$ cfu/ml, 60 s | Brook trout 52 g | 90% mortality 14 days | Cipriano et al. 1986 |
| $3.5 \times 10^9$ cfu/ml, 60 s | Atlantic salmon 36 g | 70% mortality 14 days | Cipriano et al. 1986 |

Bath challenge – Serovar II Strains

| | | | |
|---|---|---|---|
| $10^8 - 10^9$ cells/ml, 90 s | Rainbow trout 10 g | 0–20% mortality at 15 days | Bullock & Anderson 1984 |
| $1.4 \times 10^9$ cfu/ml, 60 s | Brook trout 52 g | 70–80% mortality 14 days | Cipriano et al. 1986 |
| $1.4 \times 10^9$ cfu/ml, 60 s | Atlantic salmon 36 g | 100% mortality 14 days | Cipriano et al. 1986 |

Bath challenge – Serovar III Strains

| | | | |
|---|---|---|---|
| $10^8 - 10^9$ cells/ml, 90 s | Rainbow trout 10 g | 0% mortality at 15 days | Busch 1982 |

[a] NR, not reported

chronically infected fish can be significant as they may show decreased growth rates and serve as a source of infection, yet LD50 tests would dismiss such isolates as being of low virulence. For *Y. ruckeri*, both infectivity and mortalities are of interest, particularly as many strains and serovars that do not cause mortalities under the test conditions used by Flett (1989) were still able to establish infection (Table 5.2), potentially significant under stress conditions.

The route of experimental exposure is critical. Injecting bacteria is an artificial situation as it bypasses some of the fish's normal defence mechanisms. Bath challenge may better simulate natural exposure, but results may be inconsistent. For this reason, vaccine trials for ERM are sometimes done using injection challenges (Cossarini-Dunier 1986*a*, Tatner & Horne 1985).

### *Virulence factors*

Differences in the virulence of strains which otherwise appear to be phenotypically similar may help identify the specific virulence factors of *Y. ruckeri*. However, for useful conclusions, the compared strains must be equivalent in other characteristics. For example, the comparison made by Furones *et al.* (1990) was useful in that it restricted comparisons to serovar I isolates. Those results suggested that an unidentified heat-sensitive, lipid-like factor in cell-sonicates explained virulence differences between strains.

Surface antigens of *Y. ruckeri* can affect in the host the ability to establish infection. Some such differences have been noted (Stevenson & Airdrie 1984*b*), but strains do not appear to differ in serum-killing or hydrophobicity tests (our observations). Phagocytosis studies with *Y. ruckeri* have suggested that virulence may be determined, in part, by an ability to circumvent the microbicidal action of fish phagocytes (Stave *et al.* 1987) as serovar I strains elicited a weak chemiluminescent response when compared with serovar II strains. Comparisons across serovars are more difficult to relate to specific virulence factors, and it may be necessary to ask whether the disease produced by virulent *Y. ruckeri* isolates of different serovars is the same pathologic condition. In that regard, there are serovar differences in immunological responses of fish to serovar I and II isolates that may need to be considered.

Overall, the nature of any bacterial factors or characteristics responsible for the pathogenesis of *Y. ruckeri* is not known. Ideally, virulence factors would be demonstrated by comparisons of specific mutations carried by isogenic strains, but with *Y. ruckeri* both the virulence tests and lack of defined virulence characteristics are problems.

### Fish immune responses to *Y. ruckeri*

### *Model antigen*

*Y. ruckeri* has often been used as a test antigen in a broad range of fish immunology studies (Table 5.6). The initial studies of antibody and cellular

**Table 5.6** Examples of immunological tests employing *Y. ruckeri* antigen

| Reaction tested | Literature reference |
|---|---|
| Cellular responses | Anderson *et al.* 1979*a,b,c* |
| Secondary immune response | Anderson & Dixon 1980 |
| | Lamers & van Muiswinkel 1984 |
| | Neumann & Tripp 1986 |
| | Cossarini-Dunier 1986*b* |
| Antigen localization | Lamers & Pilarczyk 1982 |
|   and trapping | Zapata *et al.* 1987 |
| | Herraez & Zapata 1987 |
| Phagocytosis | Griffin 1983 |
| | Stave *et al.* 1987 |
| Immunosuppression | Anderson *et al.* 1982 |
|   by corticosteroids | |
| Thymectomy | Tatner 1987 |
| Gamma irradiation | Chilmonczyk & Oui 1988 |
| Diet and feeding | Blazer & Wolke 1984*a,b* |
| | Henken *et al.* 1987 |
| Toxicant (PCB) effects | Mayer *et al.* 1985 |
| Pesticide effects | Blazer & Wolke 1987*a,b* |
| Manganese ions | Cossarini-Dunier *et al.* 1988 |

immunity and the factors which influence immunity are not generally concerned with the specific antigens and epitopes of the 'model antigen'. However, in some instances the choice of the antigen does affect the responses seen, a consideration in comparing results from different laboratories. For example, the antibody response of fish to serovar I strains of *Y. ruckeri* is significantly lower than to serovar II (BC 74) strains (Flett 1989). Frequently the antigen used in studies has been the serovar II strain, which provided the best response for immunological purposes, yet these responses may not reflect the significant response in infections by serovar I strains or vaccine-induced protection.

### *Vaccination*

The specific antigens of *Y. ruckeri* and the fish response to them are significant from a practical point of view. A bacterin produced using *Y. ruckeri* was the first commercial fish vaccine, and a considerable amount of work in vaccine development and field testing has involved oral, injection and immersion products against ERM, as reviewed by Bullock & Anderson (1984) and Ellis (1988). In 1976, the United States Department of Agriculture issued a product licence for a commercial bacterin against ERM (Tebbit *et al.* 1981). By 1982, Busch (1982) stated that the immunization of fish in production hatcheries against *Y. ruckeri* had become the single most important aspect in the effective management and control of mortality and related losses due to ERM.

In a series of reports based on work carried out over several years, Johnson *et al.* (1982*a,b*, Johnson & Amend 1983 *a,b*) described the parameters of successful vaccination, including information on the size of fish that can be best immunized, the duration of immunity obtained from various protocols, the effects of different delivery systems, and the form of bacterin that should be used for best results. These results, confirmed by Tatner & Horne (1985), provided much of the basic information that needed to be considered for the production and application of fish vaccines.

## Vaccine antigens

Besides the route of exposure used, the potency of bacterins can be influenced by the culture conditions, methods of inactivation, and the strain chosen to produce the bacterin. *Y. ruckeri* used for bacterin production can be grown over a wide pH range (pH 6.5−7.7) and time range (12−96 h) without affecting potency (Amend *et al.* 1983). Inactivation with either chloroform or formalin gives comparable results, and treating the cells with butanol or phenol to extract LPS prior to inactivation does not enhance potency. Lysing the cells by treatment at pH 9.8 did increase the potency (Amend *et al.* 1983). A comparison of four different oral bacterin preparations showed that chloroform-treated cells are more effective in inducing protection than phenol-treated cells and that whole-cells are more effective than sonicated cells (Anderson & Ross 1972). Amend *et al.* (1983) recommended whole-cell vaccines, as opposed to specific antigens such as the 0-antigens used by Anderson *et al.* (1979*a*), because they were adequately potent and less costly to produce.

## Antigen recognition by fish

In the experience of Johnson *et al.* (1982*a*), protective immunity was best demonstrated by challenge with virulent organisms, and antibody level was not a clear indication of the level of protection. The statement that protection against *Y. ruckeri* was not due solely to antibodies was corroborated by Cossarini-Dunier (1986*a*) and Cipriano & Ruppenthal (1987). However, in making such statements about immune responses and protection, it is important to be clear about what, specifically, is being measured. If fish antisera with a high agglutinating titre against serovar I strains is used to immunoblot LPS from serovar I strains, no interaction is seen (Flett 1989, B.T. Raymond, unpublished). In contrast, fish antisera against 0:2/serovar II strains do immunoblot with LPS of those strains. That the LPS of serovar I strains is less immunogenic is also suggested by the results of Anderson & Dixon (1980), who found that 0-antigen prepared from serovar I strains required a dose ten times the dose used for serovar II strains, when using crude LPS preparations to immunize rainbow trout.

Fish do appear capable of recognizing differences in LPS structure similar to those recognized by rabbit antisera, based on the response to serovar II strains (Flett 1989). Immunoblots of the LPS of the serovar I strains with fish sera suggest that this LPS may not be recognized, although rabbit antisera do distinguish it (Flett 1989). Most vaccines are directed only against serovar I strains, since challenges with serovar II strains generally produce poor results (McCarthy & Johnson 1982). In a cross-protection study, Cipriano & Ruppenthal (1987) did show that fish produce circulating antibodies only against the specific serovar (serovar I or II) used for bacterin preparation but that they are protected against experimental challenge with isolates of both serovars. This presents interesting questions in relation to specific and non-specific immune responses. Further studies of both the humoral and cellular immune response of fish to *Y. ruckeri* are required to obtain a complete picture of the fish response to this bacterium. Perhaps the studies can be made more productive by addressing some attention to the specific antigenic components of the cells.

**Future studies**

Studies of *Y. ruckeri* have allowed recognition of the biochemical, phenotypic, genetic and serological diversity of strains in this species. The use of lipopolysaccharide (LPS) profiles and immunoblots to define six 0-serogroups of *Y. ruckeri* begins the necessary thorough analysis of antigens which contribute to whole-cell serological reactions. Strains of serogroup 0 : 1 are the most commonly isolated, with the sub-groups represented by serovar I and III most common in rainbow trout and Atlantic salmon respectively. The 0 : 2 serogroup strains may be more closely associated with disease of chinook salmon, based on isolations. Further work on an antigenic scheme and on analysing other characteristics is required in order to assess the significance of different serological types in fish disease, as it is not yet clear that all infections with all strains of *Y. ruckeri* are identical. Tests of the relative virulence of strains and the relative susceptibility of fish species still give equivocal answers, perhaps because of the strong association of the disease with pre-disposing stress factors. Studies on the nature of the pathogenic activities of *Y. ruckeri* need to be considered in close association with the immune response of fish to specific antigens, both for practical vaccination applications and for interpreting the functions of the fish immune system components.

# Proteus, Serratia, and other enterobacterial pathogens of fish

*Proteus rettgeri* was isolated consistently from the internal organs and lesions of diseased silver carp (*Hypophthalmichthys molitrix*) in Israeli ponds (Bejerano *et al.* 1979). The disease appeared as an acute bacterial septicaemia, with severe mortalities occuring within 3 days when pond water temperatures were 20°C or higher, compared with 8 days at lower temperatures. Some ulceration and muscle degeneration was observed, and there were large, red and often deep ulcerative lesions on the external surface (Plate 14). Intramuscular injection of the isolates of *P. rettgeri*, or exposure of scarified fish to bacteria, produced mortalities and lesions, although with a lower level of mortalities and less severe lesions than in natural infections.

In salmonid fish, two species of *Serratia* have been associated with bacterial septicaemia and mortalities. *S. liquefaciens* was the predominant isolate from dead and dying Atlantic salmon in marine cage sites in Scotland (McIntosh & Austin 1990). The internal organs were affected, particularly the kidney, spleen and liver, but there were few external signs of infection. *S. liquefaciens* was also a common isolate from the organs of lake trout and brook trout from an Ontario fish hatchery with a low but consistent level of mortalities (S. Lord, unpublished observations). In both cases, the results of biochemical tests on the isolates closely resembled those reported for this species of *Serratia* (Grimont & Grimont 1982). However, the Atlantic salmon isolate was difficult to identify initially because its anomalous oxidase reaction and flagella arrangement suggested it was an aeromonad (McIntosh & Austin 1990). When reinjected into Atlantic salmon, the salmon isolate produced damage to muscle tissue at the site of injection and rapid mortalities (72 h for doses of $10^3$ cells). Rainbow trout also showed muscle and internal organ necrosis when injected with high doses of the organism ($10^7$), but mortalities did not occur (McIntosh & Austin 1990). Extensive, spreading muscle necrosis can appear when *S. liquefaciens* is injected subcutaneously into rainbow trout (S. Lord, unpublished observation), perhaps owing to the action of the many exoenzymes produced by this bacterium.

A red-pigmented species, *Serratia plymuthica*, was isolated repeatedly from moribund rainbow trout fingerlings in a hatchery in northwest Spain (Nieto *et al.* 1990). Again there were no external signs of disease, and the organism was detected after bacteriological culture of the organs. A mean lethal dose of $10^5$ cells was reported for intraperitoneal injections into rainbow trout, and again there were signs of tissue damage from the injection challenge.

Based on the above reports, some species of *Serratia* and *Proteus* do appear to be opportunistic pathogens of fish. Not only have they been found as the predominant isolate from diseased animals but they also produce disease in fish experimentally exposed to them. Other species of enteric bacteria, notably *Citrobacter freundii* (Sato *et al.* 1982, Baya *et al.* 1990) and *Enterobacter agglomerans* (Hansen *et al.* 1990) have been suggested as possible pathogens on the basis of isolations from infections and mortalities. However, further evidence is needed to substantiate these species as more than incidental pathogens. As enterobacteria are ubiquitous in the environment, it is not surprising that some should be opportunistic pathogens of fish, reptiles and insects as well as of mammals, birds and plants. They would present a particular risk in warm water ponds that are frequently exposed to faecal material, such as the silver carp ponds regularly fertilized with poultry manure (Bejerano *et al.* 1979).

# References

Amend, D.F., Johnson, K.A., Croy, T.R. & McCarthy, D.H. (1983) Some factors affecting the potency of *Yersinia ruckeri* bacterins. *Journal of Fish Diseases*, **6**, 337–44.
Anderson, D.P. & Dixon, O.W. (1980) Immunological memory in rainbow trout to a fish disease bacterin administered by flush exposure. In *Phylogeny of Immunological Memory* (Ed. by

M.J. Manning), pp. 103—9. Elsevier/North-Holland Biomedical Press.

Anderson, D.P. & Ross, A.J. (1972) Comparative study of Hagerman redmouth disease oral bacterins. *Progressive Fish Culturist*, **34**, 226—8.

Anderson, D.P., Roberson, B.S. & Dixon, O.W. (1979*a*) Plaque-forming cells and humoral antibody in rainbow trout (*Salmo gairdneri*) induced by immersion in a *Yersinia ruckeri* 0-antigen preparation. *Journal of the Fisheries Research Board of Canada*, **36**, 636—9.

Anderson, D.P., Roberson, B.S. & Dixon, O.W. (1979*b*) Cellular immune response in rainbow trout *Salmo gairdneri* Richardson to *Yersinia ruckeri* 0-antigen monitored by the passive haemolytic plaque assay test. *Journal of Fish Diseases*, **2**, 169—78.

Anderson, D.P., Roberson, B.S. & Dixon, O.W. (1979*c*) Induction of antibody-producing cells in rainbow trout, *Salmo gairdneri*; by flush exposure. *Journal of Fish Biology*, **15**, 317—22.

Anderson, D.P., Roberson, B.S. & Dixon, O.W. (1982) Immunosuppression induced by a corticosteroid or an alkylating agent in rainbow trout (*Salmo gairdneri*) administered a *Yersinia ruckeri* bacterin. *Developmental and Comparative Immunology*, Supplement 2, 197—204.

Austin, B., Green, M. & Rodgers, C.J. (1982) Morphological diversity among strains of *Yersinia ruckeri*. *Aquaculture*, **27**, 73—8.

Bangert, R.L., Ward, A.C.S., Stauber, E.H., Cho, B.R. & Widders, P.R. (1988) A survey of the aerobic bacteria in the faeces of captive raptors. *Avian Diseases*, **32**, 53—62.

Banoub, J.H., Nakhla, N.A. & Patel, T.R. (1988) Structural elucidation of the 0-antigen isolated from the lipopolysaccharide of *Yersinia ruckeri*. Canadian Society of Microbiology, Annual Meeting, Abstract MP7, 55.

Baya, A.M., Lupiani, B., Hetrick, F.M. & Toranzo, A.E. (1991) Increasing importance of *Citrobacter freundii* as a fish pathogen. *FHS/AFS Newsletter*, **18**(4), 4.

Bejerano, Y., Sarig, S., Horne, M.T. & Roberts, R.J. (1979) Mass mortalities in silver carp *Hypophthalmichthys molitrix* (Valenciennes) associated with bacterial infection following handling. *Journal of Fish Diseases*, **2**, 49—56.

Bercovier, H. & Mollaret, H.H. (1984) Genus XIV. *Yersinia*. In *Bergey's Manual of Systematic Bacteriology*, Vol. 1 (Ed. by N.R. Krieg), pp. 498—506. Williams and Wilkins, Baltimore.

Blazer, V.S. & Wolke, R.E. (1984*a*) The effects of α-tocopherol on the immune response and non-specific resistance factors of rainbow trout (*Salmo gairdneri* Richardson). *Aquaculture*, **37**, 1—9.

Blazer, V.S. & Wolke, R.E. (1984*b*) Effect of diet on the immune response of rainbow trout (*Salmo gairdneri*). *Canadian Journal of Fisheries and Aquatic Sciences*, **41**, 1244—7.

Bragg, R.R. & Henton, M.M. (1986) Isolation of *Yersinia ruckeri* from rainbow trout in South Africa. *Bulletin of the European Association of Fish Pathologists*, **6**, 5—6.

Bruno, D.W. & Munro, A.L.S. (1989) Immunity in Atlantic salmon, *Salmo salar* L., fry following vaccination against *Yersinia ruckeri*, and the influence of body weight and infectious pancreatic necrosis virus (IPNV) on the detection of carriers. *Aquaculture*, **81**, 205—11.

Bullock, G.L. & Anderson, D.P. (1984) Immunization against *Yersinia ruckeri*, cause of enteric redmouth disease. In *Symposium on Fish Vaccination* (Ed. by P. de Klinkelin), pp. 151—66. Office International des Epizooties, Paris.

Bullock, G.L. & Snieszko, S.F. (1979) Enteric redmouth disease of salmonids. *Fish Disease Leaflet* No. 57. U.S. Fish & Wildlife Service, Washington, D.C.

Bullock, G.L., Stuckey, H.M. & Herman, R.L. (1976) Comparative susceptibility of Atlantic salmon (*Salmo salar*) to the enteric redmouth bacterium and *Aeromonas salmonicida*. *Journal of Wildlife Diseases*, **12**, 376—9.

Bullock, G.L., Stuckey, H.M. & Shotts, E.B., Jr (1977) Early records of North American and Australian outbreaks of enteric redmouth disease. *Fish Health News*, **6**, 96—7.

Bullock, G.L., Stuckey, H.M. & Shotts, E.B., Jr (1978) Enteric redmouth bacterium: comparison of isolates from different geographic areas. *Journal of Fish Diseases*, **1**, 351—6.

Busch, R.A. (1973) The serological surveillance of salmonid populations for presumptive evidence of specific disease association. Ph.D. Thesis, University of Idaho, Moscow, Idaho.

Busch, R.A. (1978) Enteric red mouth disease (Hagerman strain). *Marine Fisheries Review*, **40**, 42—51.

Busch, R.A. (1982) Enteric redmouth disease (*Yersinia ruckeri*). In *Antigens of Fish Pathogens* (Ed. by D.P. Anderson, M. Dorson & Ph. Dubourget), pp. 201—23. Marcel Merieux, Lyon.

Busch, R.A. & Lingg, A.J. (1975) Establishment of an asymptomatic carrier state infection of enteric redmouth disease in rainbow trout (*Salmo gairdneri*). *Journal of the Fisheries Research Board of Canada*, **32**, 2429−32.

Chilmonczyk, S. & Oui, E. (1988) The effects of gamma irradiation on the lymphoid organs of rainbow trout and subsequent susceptibility to fish pathogens. *Veterinary Immunology and Immunopathology*, **18**, 173−80.

Cipriano, R.C. & Ruppenthal, T. (1987) Immunization of salmonids against *Yersinia ruckeri*: significance of humoral immunity and cross protection between serotypes. *Journal of Wildlife Diseases*, **23**, 545−50.

Cipriano, R.C., Schill, W.B., Pyle, S.W. & Horner, R. (1986) An epizootic in chinook salmon (*Oncorhynchus tshawytscha*) caused by a sorbitol-positive serovar II strain of *Yersinia ruckeri*. *Journal of Wildlife Diseases*, **22**, 488−92.

Cossarini-Dunier, M. (1986*a*) Protection against enteric redmouth disease in rainbow trout, *Salmo gairdneri* Richardson, after vaccination with *Yersinia ruckeri* bacterin. *Journal of Fish Diseases*, **9**, 27−33.

Cossarini-Dunier, M. (1986*b*) Secondary response of rainbow trout, *Salmo gairdneri* to DNP-haemocyanin and *Yersinia ruckeri*. *Aquaculture*, **52**, 81−6.

Cossarini-Dunier, M., Demael, A., Lepot, D. & Guerin, V. (1988) Effect of manganese ions on the immune system of carp (*Cyprinus carpio*) against *Yersinia ruckeri*. *Developmental and Comparative Immunology*, **12**, 573−9.

Dalsgaard, I., From, J. & Horlyck, V. (1984) First observation of *Yersinia ruckeri* in Denmark. *Bulletin of the European Association of Fish Pathologists*, **4**, 10.

Daly, J.G. & Stevenson, R.M.W. (1985) Importance of culturing several organs to detect *Aeromonas salmonicida* in salmonid fish. *Transactions of the American Fisheries Society*, **114**, 909−10.

Daly, J.G., Lindvik, B. & Stevenson, R.M.W. (1986) Serological heterogeneity of recent isolates of *Yersinia ruckeri* from Ontario and British Columbia. *Diseases of Aquatic Organisms*, **1**, 151−3.

Davies, R.L. & Freichs, G.N. (1989) Morphological and biochemical differences among isolates of *Yersinia ruckeri* obtained from wide geographical areas. *Journal of Fish Diseases*, **12**, 357−65.

Dear, G. (1988) *Yersinia ruckeri* isolated from Atlantic salmon in Scotland. *Bulletin of the European Association of Fish Pathologists*, **8**, 18−20.

Dulin, M.P., Huddleston, T., Larson, R.E. & Klontz, G.W. (1976) *Enteric Redmouth Disease*. Bulletin No. 6, College of Forestry, Wildlife, & Range Sciences, University of Idaho, Moscow, 15pp.

Dwilow, A.G., Souter, B.W. & Knight, K. (1987) Isolation of *Yersinia ruckeri* from burbot, *Lota lota* (L.), from the Mackenzie River, Canada. *Journal of Fish Diseases*, **10**, 315−17.

Ellis, A.E. (1988) Vaccination against enteric redmouth (ERM). In *Fish Vaccination* (Ed. by A.E. Ellis), pp. 85−92. Academic Press, London.

Ewing, W.H. (1986) *Edwards and Ewing's Identification of Enterobacteriaceae*, 4th edition (Ed. by W.H. Ewing), pp. 472−3. Elsevier Science Publishing Co., Inc., New York.

Ewing, E.W., Ross, A.J., Brenner, D.J. & Fanning, G.R. (1978) *Yersinia ruckeri* sp. nov., the redmouth (RM) bacterium. *International Journal of Systematic Bacteriology*, **28**, 37−44.

Farmer, J.J. III, Davies, B.R., Hickman-Brenner, F.W., McWhorter, A., Huntley-Carter, G.P., Asbury, M.A., Riddle, C., Wathen-Grady, H.G., Elias, C., Fanning, G.R., Steigerwalt, A.G., O'Hara, C.M., Morris, G.K., Smith, P.B. & Brenner, D.J. (1985) Biochemical identification of new species and biogroups of Enterobacteriaceae isolated from clinical specimens. *Journal of Clinical Microbiology*, **21**, 46−76.

Flett, D.E. (1989) 0-Antigen serogroups of *Yersinia ruckeri*. M.Sc. Thesis, University of Guelph.

Frerichs, G.N., Stewart, J.A. & Collins, R.O. (1985) Atypical infection of rainbow trout, *Salmo gairdneri* Richardson, with *Yersinia ruckeri*. *Journal of Fish Diseases*, **8**, 383−7.

Fuhrmann, H., Böhm, K.H. & Schlotfeldt, H.-J. (1983) An outbreak of enteric redmouth disease in West Germany. *Journal of Fish Diseases*, **6**, 309−11.

Fuhrmann, H., Bohm, K.H. & Schlotfeldt, H.-J. (1984) On the importance of enteric bacteria in the bacteriology of freshwater fish. *Bulletin of the European Association of Fish Pathologists*, **4**, 42−6.

Furones, M.D., Gilpin, M.J., Alderman, D.J. & Munn, C.B. (1990) Virulence of *Yersinia ruckeri* serotype I strains is associated with a heat-sensitive factor (HSF) in cell extracts. *FEMS Microbiology Letters*, **66**, 339−44.

Giorgetti, G., Ceshia, G. & Bovo, G. (1985) First isolation of *Yersinia ruckeri* in farmed rainbow trout in Italy. In *Fish and Shellfish Pathology* (Ed. by A.E. Ellis), pp. 161—6. Academic Press, London.

Grandis, S.A. de (1987) The DNA relatedness and plasmid profiles of strains of *Yersinia ruckeri*. Ph.D. Thesis, University of Guelph, Guelph, Ontario.

Grandis, S.A. de & Stevenson, R.M.W. (1982) Variations in plasmid profiles and growth characteristics of *Yersinia ruckeri* strains. *FEMS Microbiology Letters*, **15**, 199—202.

Grandis, S.A. de & Stevenson, R.M.W. (1985) Antimicrobial susceptibility patterns and R plasmid-mediated resistance of the fish pathogen *Yersinia ruckeri*. *Antimicrobial Agents and Chemotherapy*, **27**, 938—42.

Grandis, S.A. de, Krell, P.J., Flett, D.E. & Stevenson, R.M.W. (1988) Deoxyribonucleic acid relatedness of serovars of *Yersinia ruckeri*, the enteric redmouth bacterium. *International Journal of Systematic Bacteriology*, **38**, 49—55.

Green, M. & Austin, B. (1983) The identification of *Yersinia ruckeri* and its relationship to other representatives of the Enterobacteriaceae. *Aquaculture*, **34**, 185—92.

Griffin, B.R. (1983) Opsonic effect of rainbow trout (*Salmo gairdneri*) antibody on phagocytosis of *Yersinia ruckeri* by trout leukocytes. *Developmental and Comparative Immunology*, **7**, 253—9.

Grimont, P.A.D. & Grimont, F. (1984) Genus VIII. *Serratia* Bizio 1823, 288[AL]. In *Bergey's Manual of Systematic Bacteriology*, Vol. 1 (Ed. by N.R. Kreig & J.G. Holt), pp. 477—484. Williams & Wilkins, Baltimore.

Guilvout, I., Quilici, M.L., Rabot, S., Lesel, R. & Mazigh, D. (1988) *Bam*HI restriction endonuclease analysis of *Yersinia ruckeri* plasmids and their relatedness to the genus *Yersinia* 42- to 47-megadalton plasmid. *Applied Environmental Microbiology*, **54**, 2594—7.

Hansen, G.H., Raa, J.K. & Olafsen, J.A. (1990) Isolation of *Enterobacter agglomerans* from dolphin fish, *Coryphaena hippurus* L. *Journal of Fish Diseases*, **13**, 93—6.

Hastings, T.S. & Bruno, D.W. (1985) Enteric redmouth disease: survey in Scotland and evaluation of a new medium, Shotts-Waltman, for differentiating *Yersinia ruckeri*. *Bulletin of the European Association of Fish Pathologists*, **54**, 2594—7.

Henken, A.M., Tigchelaar, A.J. & van Muiswinkel, W.B. (1987) Effects of feeding level on antibody production in African catfish, *Clarias gariepinus* Burchell, after injection of *Yersinia ruckeri* 0-antigen. *Journal of Fish Diseases*, **11**, 85—8.

Herraez, M.P. & Zapata, A. (1987) Trapping of intraperitoneal-injected *Yersinia ruckeri* in the lymphoid organs of *Carassius auratus*: the role of melano-macrophage centres. *Journal of Fish Biology*, **31**(Supplement A), 235—7.

Hitchcock, P.J. & Brown, T.M. (1983) Morphological heterogeneity among *Salmonella* lipopolysaccharide chemotypes in silver-stained polyacrylamide gels. *Journal of Bacteriology*, **154**, 269—77.

Hunter, V.A., Knittel, M.D. & Fryer, J.L. (1980) Stress-induced transmission of *Yersinia ruckeri* infection from carriers to recipient steelhead trout, *Salmo gairdneri* Richardson. *Journal of Fish Diseases*, **3**, 467—72.

Johnson, K.A. & Amend, D.F. (1983*a*) Comparison of efficacy of several delivery methods using *Yersinia ruckeri* bacterin on rainbow trout, *Salmo gairdneri* Richardson. *Journal of Fish Diseases*, **6**, 331—6.

Johnson, K.A. & Amend, D.F. (1983*b*) Efficacy of *Vibrio anguillarum* and *Yersinia ruckeri* bacterins applied by oral and anal intubation of salmonids. *Journal of Fish Diseases*, **6**, 473—6.

Johnson, K.A., Flynn, J.K. & Amend, D.F. (1982*a*) Onset of immunity in salmonid fry vaccinated by direct immersion in *Vibrio anguillarum* and *Yersinia ruckeri* bacterins. *Journal of Fish Diseases*, **5**, 197—205.

Johnson, K.A., Flynn, J.K. & Amend, D.F. (1982*b*) Duration of immunity in salmonids vaccinated by direct immersion with *Yersinia ruckeri* and *Vibrio anguillarum* bacterins. *Journal of Fish Diseases*, **5**, 207—13.

Knittel, M.D. (1981) Susceptibility of steelhead trout, *Salmo gairdneri* Richardson to redmouth infection *Yersinia ruckeri* following exposure to copper. *Journal of Fish Diseases*, **4**, 33—40.

Lamers, C.H.J. & Pilarczyk, A. (1982) Immune response and antigen localization in carp (*Cyprinus carpio*) after administration of *Yersinia ruckeri* 0-antigen. *Developments in Comparative Immunology*, Supplement 2, 107—14.

Lamers, C.H.J. & Muiswinkel, W.B. van. (1984) Primary and secondary immune response in carp (*Cyprinus carpio*) after administration of *Yersinia ruckeri* 0-antigen. In *Fish Diseases*, Fourth

CoPRAQ Session Acuigrup (Ed.), pp. 119–27. ATP, Madrid.

Lehmann, J., Sturenberg, F.-J. & Mock, D. (1987) The changes in haemogram of rainbow trout (*Salmo gairdneri* Richardson) to an artificial and natural challenge with *Yersinia ruckeri*. *Journal of Applied Ichthyology*, **3**, 174–83.

Lesel, R., Lesel, M., Gavini, F. & Vuillaume, A. (1983*a*) Outbreak of enteric redmouth disease in rainbow trout, *Salmo gairdneri* Richardson, in France. *Journal of Fish Diseases*, **6**, 385–7.

Lesel, R., Gavini, F., Lesel, M. & Darroze, S. (1983*b*) Dynamique de la flore bacterienne de la truite arc-en-ciel, lars d'une enterosepticemie a *Yersinia ruckeri*. INSERM Colloque International de Bacteriologie, Lille, May 1983 (poster).

Lewis, D.H. (1981) Immunoenzyme microscopy for differentiating among systemic bacterial pathogens of fish. *Canadian Journal of Fisheries and Aquatic Sciences*, **38**, 463–6.

Llewellyn, L.C. (1980) A bacterium with similarities to the redmouth bacterium and *Serratia liquefaciens* (Grimes and Hennerty) causing mortalities in hatchery reared salmonids in Australia. *Journal of Fish Diseases*, **3**, 29–39.

McArdle, J.F. & Dooley-Martyn, C. (1985) Isolation of *Yersinia ruckeri* type I (Hagerman strain) from goldfish *Carassius auratus* (L.). *Bulletin of the European Association of Fish Pathologists*, **5**, 10–11.

McCarthy, D.H. & Johnson, K.A. (1982) A serotypic survey and cross-protection test of North American field isolates of *Yersinia ruckeri*. *Journal of Fish Diseases*, **5**, 323–8.

McDaniel, D.W. (1971) Hagerman redmouth. *American Fishes U.S. Trout News.*, **15**, 14–28.

McDaniel, D. (Ed.) (1979) *Procedures for the Detection and Identification of Certain Fish Pathogens.* American Fisheries Society/Fish Health Section.

Mayer, K.S., Mayer, F.L. & Witt, A., Jr (1985) Waste transformer oil and PCB toxicity to rainbow trout. *Transactions of the American Fisheries Society*, **114**, 869–86.

McIntosh, D. & Austin, B. (1990) Recovery of an extremely proteolytic form of *Serratia liquefaciens* as a pathogen of Atlantic salmon, *Salmo salar*, in Scotland. *Journal of Fish Diseases*, **36**, 765–72.

Michel, C., Faivre, B. & Kinkelin, P. de (1986) A clinical case of enteric redmouth in minnows (*Pimephales promelas*) imported in Europe as bait-fish. *Bulletin of the European Society of Fish Pathologists*, **6**, 97–9.

Miller, T. (1983) Blood coagulation in ERM infected trout: role of bacterial endotoxin. Proceedings of the Eighth Annual FHS/AFS Workshop, Kearneysville, WV, p. 48.

Mitchum, D.L. (1981). Concurrent infections: ERM and furunculosis found in emerald shiners. *FHS/AFS Fish Health Newsletter*, **9**, 2.

Neuman, D.A. & Tripp, M.R. (1986) Influence of route of administration on humoral immune response of channel catfish (*Ictalurus punctatus*) to *Yersinia ruckeri*. *Veterinary Immunology and Immunopathology*, **12**, 163–74.

Nieto, T.P., Lopez, L.R., Santos, Y., Nunez, S. & Toranzo, A.E. (1990) Isolation of *Serratia plymuthica* as an opportunistic pathogen in rainbow trout, *Salmo gairdneri* Richardson. *Journal of Fish Diseases*, **13**, 175–7.

O'Leary, P.J. (1977) Enteric redmouth bacterium of salmonids: a biochemical and serological comparison of selected isolates. M.Sc. thesis, Oregon State University, Corvallis.

O'Leary, P.J., Rohovec, J.S. & Fryer, J.L. (1979) A further characterization of *Yersinia ruckeri* (enteric redmouth bacterium). *Fish Pathology*, **14**, 71–8.

O'Leary, P.J., Rohovec, J.S., Sanders, J.E. & Fryer, J.L. (1982) Serotypes of *Yersinia ruckeri* and their immunogenic properties. Sea Grant College Program Publication No. ORESU-T-82–001, Oregon State University, Corvallis. 15pp.

Portnoy, D.A. & Falkow, S. (1981) Virulence-associated plasmids from *Yersinia enterocolitica* and *Yersinia pestis*. *Journal of Bacteriology*, **148**, 877–83.

Pyle, S.W. & Schill, W.B. (1985) Rapid serological analysis of bacterial lipopolysaccharides by electrotransfer to nitrocellulose. *Journal of Immunology Methods*, **85**, 371–82.

Quentel, C. & Aldrin, J.F. (1986) Blood changes in catheterized rainbow trout (*Salmo gairdneri*) intraperitoneally inoculated with *Yersinia ruckeri*. *Aquaculture*, **53**, 169–85.

Rintamaki, P., Valtonen, E.T. & Frerichs, G.N. (1986) Occurence of *Yersinia ruckeri* infection in farmed whitefish, *Coregonus peled* Gmelin and *Coregonus muksun* Pallas, and Atlantic salmon *Salmo salar* L., in northern Finland. *Journal of Fish Diseases*, **9**, 137–40.

Roberts, M.S. (1983) A report of an epizootic in hatchery reared rainbow trout, *Salmo gairdneri*

Richardson, at an English trout farm, caused by *Yersinia ruckeri*. *Journal of Fish Diseases*, **6**, 551−2.

Rodgers, C.J. & Hudson, E.B. (1985) A comparison of two methods for isolation of *Yersinia ruckeri* from rainbow trout (*Salmo gairdneri*). *Bulletin of the European Association of Fish Pathologists*, **5**, 92−93.

Ross, A.J., Rucker, R.R. & Ewing, W.H. (1966) Description of a bacterium associated with redmouth disease of rainbow trout (*Salmo gairdneri*). *Canadian Journal of Microbiology*, **12**, 763−70.

Rucker, R.R. (1966) Redmouth disease of rainbow trout (*Salmo gairdneri*). *Bulletin de L'Office International des Epizooties*, **65**, 825−30.

Sato, N., Yamane, N. & Kawamura, T. (1982) Systemic *Citrobacter freundii* infection among sunfish *Mola mola* in Matsushima Aquarium. *Bulletin of the Japanese Society of Scientific Fisheries*, **48**, 1551−7.

Schill, W.B., Phelps, S.R. & Pyle, S.W. (1984) Multilocus electrophoretic assessment of genetic structure and diversity of *Yersinia ruckeri*. *Applied Environmental Microbiology*, **48**, 975−9.

Schlotfeldt, H.-J. von, Böhm, K.H., Pfortmuller, F. & Pfortmuller, K. (1985) Rotmaulseuche/ ERM (Enteric redmouth disease) der Forelle and anderen Nutzfischen in Nordwestdeutschland − Varkommen, Terapie und Vakzinierungsergebnisse. *Tierarztliche Umschau*, **40**, 985−95.

Sparboe, O., Koren, C., Håstein, T., Poppe, T. & Stenwig, H. (1986) The first isolation of *Yersinia ruckeri* from farmed Norwegian salmon. *Bulletin of the European Association of Fish Pathologists*, **6**, 41−2.

Stave, J.W., Cook, T.M. & Roberson, B.S. (1987) Chemiluminescent responses of striped bass, *Morone saxatilis* (Walbaum), phagocytes to strains of *Yersinia ruckeri*. *Journal of Fish Diseases*, **10**, 1−10.

Stevenson, R.M.W. & Airdrie, D.W. (1984a) Serological variation among *Yersinia ruckeri* strains. *Journal of Fish Diseases*, **7**, 247−54.

Stevenson, R.M.W. & Airdrie, D.W. (1984b) Isolation of *Yersinia ruckeri* bacteriophages. *Applied Environmental Microbiology*, **47**, 1201−5.

Stevenson, R.M.W. & Daly, J.D. (1982) Biochemical and serological characteristics of Ontario isolates of *Yersinia ruckeri*. *Canadian Journal of Fisheries and Aquatic Sciences*, **39**, 870−6.

Sullivan, J. (1981) Enteric redmouth. In *Alaskan Wildlife Diseases* (Ed. by R.A. Dieterich), pp. 406−10. University of Alaska, Fairbanks.

Tatner, M.F. (1987) The effect of thymectomy on the vaccine-induced protection to *Yersinia ruckeri* in rainbow trout, *Salmo gairdneri*. *Developmental and Comparative Immunology*, **11**, 427−30.

Tatner, M.F. & Horne, M.T. (1985) The effects of vaccine dilution, length of immersion time, and booster vaccinations on the protection levels induced by direct immersion vaccination of brown trout, *Salmo trutta*, with *Yersinia ruckeri* (ERM) vaccine. *Aquaculture*, **46**, 11−18.

Tebbit, G.L., Erikson, J.D. & Vande Water, R.B. (1981) Development and use of *Yersinia ruckeri* bacterins to control enteric redmouth disease. In *International Symposium on Fish Biologics: Serodiagnostics and Vaccines*. Leetown, WV, *Developments in Biological Standardization*, **49**, 395−401.

Toranzo, A.E., Barja, J.L., Colwell, R.R. & Hetrick, F.M. (1983) Characterization of plasmids in bacterial fish pathogens. *Infection and Immunity*, **39**, 184−92.

Vuillaume, A., Brun, R., Chene, P., Sochon, E. & Lesel, R. (1987) First isolation of *Yersinia ruckeri* from sturgeon, *Acipenser baeri* Brandt, in south west of France. *Bulletin of the European Association of Fish Pathologists*, **7**, 18−19.

Waltman, W.D. & Shotts, E.B., Jr (1984) A medium for the isolation and differentiation of *Yersinia ruckeri*. *Canadian Journal of Fisheries and Aquatic Sciences*, **41**, 804−6.

Willumsen, B. (1989) Birds and wild fish as potential vectors of *Yersinia ruckeri*. *Journal of Fish Diseases*, **12**, 275−7.

Wobeser, G. (1973) An outbreak of redmouth disease in rainbow trout (*Salmo gairdneri*) in Saskatchewan. *Journal of the Fisheries Research Board of Canada*, **30**, 571−5.

Zapata, A.G., Torroba, M., Alvarez, F., Anderson, D.P., Dixon, O.W. & Wisniewski, M. (1987) Electron microscopic examination of antigen uptake by salmonid gill cells after bath immunization with a bacterin. *Journal of Fish Biology*, **31**(Supplement A), 209−17.

# Part 3:
# Vibrionaceae

Vibrionaceae is a family of facultatively anaerobic Gram-negative rods, 0.3–1.0 × 1–3.5 µm, straight or slightly curved and non spore-forming. They are motile by means of polar flagella or non-motile. Metabolism is chemo-organotrophic, with both oxidative and fermentative respiration. Most are oxidase positive. They are found primarily in water and in association with aquatic animals. Several *Vibrio* and *Aeromonas* species are important in diseases of fish.

# Chapter 6:
# Vibriosis

The genus *Vibrio* consists of Gram-negative straight or slightly curved rods 0.5−0.3 μm × 1.4−2.6 μm. They are non spore-forming and motile by monotrichous or multitrichous sheathed polar flagella. All are facultative anaerobes and chemo-organotrophs and most are oxidase positive. Most species grow well in media with a sea water base; sodium ions stimulate the growth of all species and for many are an absolute requirement. They are sensitive to the vibriostat 2,4-diamino − 6,7 − diisopropyl pteridine phosphate (0/129). They are common in aquatic habitats, particularly in marine and estuarine environments and in association with marine animals. Several species are pathogenic for man as well as marine animals. The mol % G + C of the DNA is 38−51.

This genus contains the most significant marine fish bacterial pathogens. As with aeromonads in fresh water, they are ubiquitous, especially where organic loads are high. Only certain species are pathogenic, and while particular strains within a species may be highly pathogenic, others may be innocuous or act only as secondary invaders.

The vibrios *Vibrio alginolyticus*, *V. anguillarum*, *V. ordalii*, *V. salmonicida*, and *V. vulnificus* are marine fish pathogens. All are associated with acute bacterial septicaemias or chronic focal lesions in marine fish. Generally vibriosis in fish accompanies some other stress or physical trauma, but some strains, especially of *V. anguillarum* or *V. salmonicida*, appear to be highly infectious primary pathogens. Infection of Atlantic salmon with *V. salmonicida* is known as cold water vibriosis or Hitra disease.

## Introduction

*Vibrio anguillarum* was the first *Vibrio* to be isolated from fish, from eels in the Mediterranean (Canestrini 1883) and for many years all pathogenic vibrios were ascribed to this taxon. However, with the expansion of international interest in fish culture it became clear that in particular geographical areas and culture systems, other distinct species were playing a role. Thus *V. alginolyticus* was a problem particularly as a secondary invader of traumatized sea bream (*Sparus aurata*) in Israel (Colorni *et al.* 1981), while *V. vulnificus*, a lactose-fermenting, species is generally restricted to eels and largely, though not exclusively, to Japanese waters (Muroga *et al.* 1979, Biosca *et al.* 1991).

It is *Vibrio anguillarum* itself, however, and the two species subsequently designated from closely related strains, viz *V. ordalii* (Schiewe *et al.* 1981) and *V. salmonicida* (Egidius *et al.* 1986) that appear to be the most seriously pathogenic. The last two are principally associated with disease in Pacific and Atlantic salmon respectively. The original *Vibrio anguillarum* taxon, however, still remains rather heterogeneous for a true species (West *et al.* 1983) and it seems likely that as experience with other intensively cultured marine fishes is increased other separate, host-related species may well emerge.

Species differentiation is usually on the basis of biochemical properties, as there is some serological cross-reactivity between species. Within species they are generally serologically homogeneous, although there are at least two sero-logically distinct subspecies of *Vibrio salmonicida* (Schroder *et al.* 1991).

## Biological characteristics of the fish pathogenic vibrios

Marine vibrios, including the fish pathogens, are found in all saline waters. They are more frequent where static water and soft benthos occur in combination with high organic load. Their frequency is greatly reduced in areas where rocky shores or high energy beaches combine with well-aerated waters.

They are characterized by their vibrionic, or comma shape (Fig. 6.1), which may be more or less obvious depending on the medium of growth. Metabolism is aerobic or facultatively anaerobic and carbohydrates are fermented with the production of acid but not gas. They produce 3-butanediol, reduce nitrates and produce a variety of enzymes including catalase, oxidase, β-galactosidase and arginine dihydrolase. Their main characteristic in laboratory culture, however, and the feature which most readily distinguishes them from the aeromonads, is their susceptibility to the pteridine vibriostat 0/129, which inhibits their multi-plication. Table 6.1 gives their principal distinguishing biochemical features.

In culture, good growth of all marine vibrios can generally be obtained on most general purpose media, provided they contain 1−2% sodium chloride.

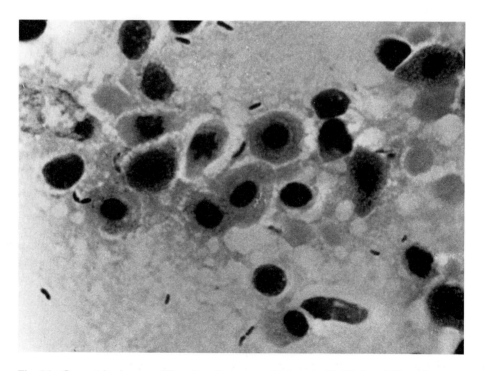

**Fig. 6.1** Gram stained smear of liver from European eel infected with *Vibrio vulnificus* biotype 2. The comma shaped bacteria are well demonstrated by phase contrast (× 1600) (Courtesy of Dr G. Biosca).

**Table 6.1** Biochemical characteristics of fish pathogenic *Vibrio* species. All are Gram-negative, fermentative, oxidase-positive and motile, have a requirement for sodium ions for growth and are sensitive to the vibriostat 0/129 phosphate (150 μg). Some distinguishing features are given

| | *V. alginolyticus* | *V. anguillarum* | *V. ordalii* | *V. salmonicida* | *V. vulnificus* |
|---|---|---|---|---|---|
| Swarming on complex solid media | + | − | − | − | − |
| Arginine dihydrolase | − | + | − | − | − |
| Reduce $NO_3^-$ to $NO_2^-$ | + | + | − | − | + |
| Vosges-Proskauer reaction | + | + | − | − | − |
| Grow at 40°C | + | − | − | − | + |
| Utilize sucrose | + | + | + | − | − |
| Utilize L-arabinose | − | + | − | − | − |
| Utilize D-sorbitol | − | + | − | − | − |

The biochemical activity of *V. salmonicida* has been investigated in detail by Egidius *et al.* (1986), who first proposed it as a separate species. It has a low growth temperature, 1−22°C with an optimum of 15°C. Further, *V. salmonicida* has been distinguished from *V. anguillarum* and *V. ordalii* by DNA hybridization experiments (Wiik & Egidius 1986).

Thiosulphate citrate bile salt agar is a medium which selectively promotes growth of pathogenic vibrios other than *V. ordalii*, while inhibiting other bacteria. Colonies are smooth, convex and grey-white and appear within 48 h at 20°C on non-selective media.

The G + C molar percentage of the DNA of vibrios varies. *V. anguillarum* type I, the archetypal species, has a G + C content of 45.6%, while that of *V. ordalii* is 43−44 moles % (Kiehn & Pacha 1969, Schiewe *et al.* 1979, Schiewe 1981).

## Antigenic structure

*Vibrio anguillarum* is serologically diverse, and up to ten '0' antigen serotypes have been described (Sørensen & Larsen 1966). Originally, three serotypes were associated with salmonid isolates, corresponding to different geographical areas (Pacha & Kiehn 1969). This has now been extended to six by Japanese workers (Kitao *et al*. 1983), who encompassed strains from eel and other marine species such as ayu as well as salmonids in their serological study.

*Vibrio ordalii* was first elevated to species level on biochemical grounds, from strains that had previously been classified as biotypes within *V. anguillarum*. This was done despite the strong antigenic cross-reactivity between the two biotypes. The separation into two species was subsequently fully justified on the basis of DNA/DNA hybridization comparisons and very disparate plasmid profiles, but nevertheless the antigenic links suggest a strong relationship between the two (Schiewe *et al*. 1981).

The protective antigens of *V. anguillarum* and *V. ordalii* are known. The antigens are heat stable lipopolysaccharides in the cell wall, which may also be released into the culture supernatant (Chart & Trust 1984). They are large molecules of 100 kilodaltons (kD) and are able to withstand severe extraction methods. Various proteins in the outer membrane were also found to be antigenic, and two of these, of weaker antigenic potential, also have a molecular weight of 40 kD (Chart & Trust 1984). These are heat labile. The proteins and lipopolysaccharides in the membrane of *V. anguillarum* have been extensively characterized in the six different O serogroups identified among Japanese strains of the bacterium (Aoki *et al*. 1981, Tajima *et al*. 1990). The protein components in the outer membrane were different among the serogroups, with serogroup B lacking the major protein of molecular weight 38−44 kD.

*Vibrio salmonicida* isolates form a homogeneous grouping in relation to their biochemistry (Espelid *et al*. 1988). Two distinct serotypes exist, one of which is more prevalent among non-salmonid species such as cod, but both can be found in the different species. *Vibrio salmonicida* of all serotypes, however, is more pathogenic in salmon than in other fishes (Schroder *et al*. 1991).

The surface layer antigen of *Vibrio salmonicida* has been isolated and characterized by Hjelmeland *et al*. (1988). Called the CS-PI antigen, this cell surface product is a single polypeptide, the monomeric form of which has an apparent molecular weight of 40 kD. There are also oligomeric forms with molecular weight in the range 300−700 kD. The antigen contains 6% carbohydrate and several isomeric forms can be distinguished.

## Toxin production and virulence mechanisms

Little is known of the toxigenicity or virulence mechanisms of the other fish pathogenic vibrios, but in the case of *Vibrio anguillarum* a considerable body of information is available, much of which may also relate to the other species, given the similarities in clinical lesions and pathology with which they are associated.

The outstanding feature of clinical vibriosis is the level of anaemia which results in all but the most acute cases. This is haemolytic in nature (Frerichs & Roberts 1989), and McArdle (1973) was the first to demonstrate that the exotoxin involved was heat labile and protein in nature. Munn (1980) showed subsequently that it was enzymic and occurred only during the stationary phase of growth, possibly explaining why infections have to be well established before severe anaemia occurs. Proteases have also been described (Kodama *et al.* 1984), accounting for the severe focal myonecrosis and liquefaction that occur in principal lesions, usually within the skeletal musculature.

The capacity of the micro-organism to produce haemolytic anaemia, which results in high circulating and melano-macrophage related iron levels in affected fish (Roberts 1975), is related to its high requirement for iron. In support of this, pathogenic strains have a well developed iron sequestering mechanism based on secretion of a siderophore, which induces separation of plasma and tissue iron from its transferrin or ferritin binding proteins. This complexes to the siderophore and attaches to specific complex transporting outer cell membrane proteins for absorption into the bacterial cells (Actis *et al.* 1985).

As with some other highly pathogenic bacteria, such as *Corynebacterium diphtheriae*, the possession of pathogenic capacity, in this case due to the siderophore and iron-complex transporting mechanism, by a strain, is coded for by a plasmid which is only present in highly pathogenic strains (Crosa 1980). When it is experimentally cleansed from such strains they lose their pathogenicity (Crosa *et al.* 1980). Although generally plasmid associated, the specifying codons can on occasion be integrated within the host cell genome rather than in the plasmid DNA (Toranzo *et al.* 1983).

## Diseases associated with fish pathogenic vibrios

Whenever marine fishes are stressed or traumatized, both under farming conditions and in the wild, vibrios are enabled to produce infections which take the form of focal haemorrhagic ulcers on the mouth (Plate 15) or skin surface, or else focal necrotic lesions in the muscle, the orbit or along the edge of the fins. Where the lesion is sub-epidermal, a black overlying area is apparent on the skin, and if this ulcerates, a shallow, but extensive, haemorrhagic ulcer with a white (dermal collagenous) rim and a black pigmentary halo is produced.

Such lesions may be associated with strains of *Vibrio anguillarum* and are also characteristic of the pathology associated with the other vibrios such as *Vibrio vulnificus* in eels (Biosca *et al.* 1991) (Fig. 6.2). In addition to this general chronic necrotizing syndrome, however, *Vibrio anguillarum*, *V. ordalii* and *V. salmonicida* have particular clinico-pathological syndromes associated with them.

### Vibrio anguillarum

*Vibrio anguillarum*, as the name suggests, was first described in eels in the Camachio lagoon area of Italy (Hofer 1904). To this day, whenever high temperatures and high salinities stress the fish there, an acute haemorrhagic

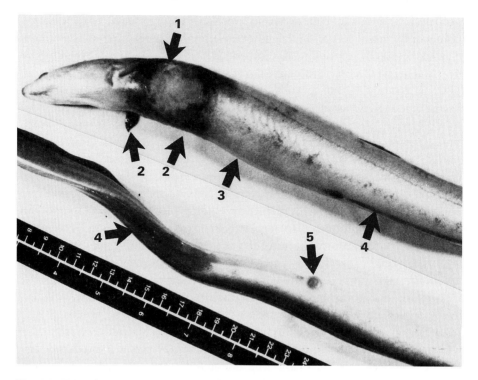

**Fig. 6.2**  Eels suffering from vibriosis caused by *Vibrio vulnificus*, showing (1) a skin ulcer, (2) reddened operculum (3) distended abdomen, (4) haemorrhagic anal fin and (5) protrusion of haemorrhagic rectum (Courtesy of Dr G. Biosca).

condition known as 'red pest' breaks out, and it has been recorded widely in eels elsewhere. It is, however, not dissimilar from acute vibriosis, caused by the same species of *Vibrio* in salmonids and marine flatfish, for both of which more pathological data are available.

Vibriosis usually occurs in warm weather, particularly when stocking densities, whether in farmed or wild fish, are high, and when salinities and organic loads are also high. The occurrence of other stressors such as parasitism or handling trauma may well precipitate the condition, but with many strains inherent pathogenicity is such that often no predisposing cause can be found. Outbreaks have also been recorded in freshwater species, fed (presumptively infected) marine fish offals (Hacking & Budd 1971, Kitao *et al.* 1983). Incubation period varies with strain and temperature.

When an outbreak occurs in young fish, mortalities can be 50% or higher. In older fish, losses may be lower, but infected fish do not feed or grow, and when harvested apparently normal fish may have large focal necrotic lesions in the middle of the muscle mass (Plate 16).

The first signs of the disease are usually anorexia, with darkening either of the whole fish or of particular areas of the dorsum, above developing lesions. The peracute condition, found in young cultured salmon and turbot (Frerichs

& Roberts 1989), results in death without any other clinical signs except occasional periorbital or abdominal oedema. In older fish subsequent acute and chronic stages occur, during each of which there may be heavy losses. In the acute stage fish have dark skin swellings which ulcerate to release a red effusion of necrotic tissue containing very large numbers of infective bacteria. Internal lesions include deep seated muscle lesions and consistent enlargement and liquefactive necrosis of the spleen, which becomes cherry red in colour and loses its sharp edges.

Chronically infected fish generally have large granulating lesions deep in the muscle. Gills are very pale, reflecting the severe anaemia, and fibrinous adhesions may be found between visceral and parietal peritoneum. The eye is often infected, and is suffused with blood beneath a grey corneal opacity which progresses to ulceration.

When sections from affected fish are examined histologically, they show a variety of features depending on the stage of development of the disease. In peracute cases severe cardiac myopathy (Fig. 6.3), renal and splenic necrosis associated particularly with the erythroid haemopoietic tissue (Fig. 6.4), and periorbital oedema may be all that can be observed.

In the acute cases, cardiac lesions are less marked (although in eels small colonies of bacteria are commonly found within cardiac muscle) and it is the skin lesions which are most obvious. These appear to originate in the hypodermis but extend deep into the muscle. There is severe necrosis of muscle (Figs 6.5, 6.6) and collagen of the dermis, with eventual ulceration of the overlying epidermis. In the liver there is severe focal necrosis and, in the spleen and kidney, massive depletion and necrosis of haemopoietic elements (Fig. 6.7).

Chronic cases are characterized by heavy deposition of haemosiderin within melano-macrophage centres, and concurrent organization and necrosis within the large focal lesions found in the muscle.

### *Vibrio ordalii*

*Vibrio ordalii* induces a pathogenesis not particularly different from that of *V. anguillarum*, but generally less severe. Peracute cases rarely occur. Infection may be via ascending infection from the posterior gut, or through the skin, but it is rarely found outside salmonids (Ransom *et al.* 1984). The bacterium does not contain the siderophore plasmid.

### *Vibrio salmonicida*

*Vibrio salmonicida* is specifically responsible for the condition of Atlantic salmon known as cold-water vibriosis or Hitra disease, which has caused heavy losses in Norway since the 1970s. Although the term has tended to be used generically to describe any heavy losses in winter, the specific syndrome associ-

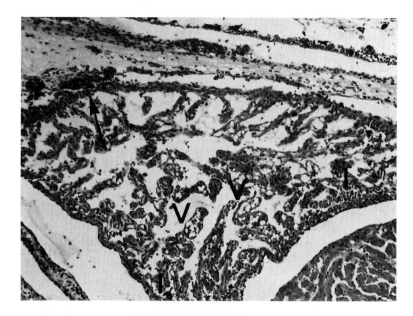

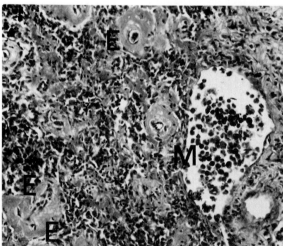

**Fig. 6.3** (above) Atrium of Dover sole with peracute vibriosis. There is extensive vacuolation (V) of the sarcoplasm with small foci of inflammatory cells (I) and hyperaemia of the pericardium (arrowed) (H&E × 400) (Courtesy of Dr G.N. Frerichs).

**Fig. 6.4** (right) Section of spleen with acute vibriosis. There is depletion of haemopoietic tissue, swelling of the wall of the ellipsoid (E) and considerable numbers of pigment containing cells in the splenic vessels (M) (H&E × 200) (Courtesy of Dr T. Hastein).

ated with this homogeneous taxon, serologically distinct from *V. anguillarum* and *V. ordalii*, is now recognized as an entity (Egidius *et al.* 1986).

First clinical signs of Hitra disease are inappetence and disorganized swimming. Fish may, however, die in the peracute phase without any obvious clinical signs. Pathology varies with the stage in the disease process, but common external signs are pallor of the gills, haemorrhage on the fin base, redness and swelling, with occasional prolapse at the rectum, and petechial haemorrhage on the ventral abdominal wall. Haemorrhagic ulceration or dark patches on the operculum and dorsum are common findings.

Internally the fish is pale due to anaemia, and there are ascites and haemor-

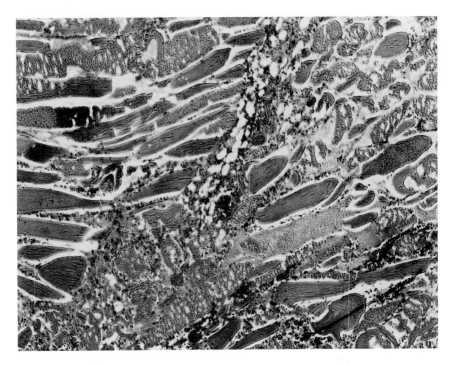

**Fig. 6.5** Section of Atlantic salmon muscle in late stages of vibriosis. There is extensive sacroplasmic necrosis with the inflammatory response extending down the intermyotomal fascia (H&E × 50) (Courtesy of Dr T. Hastein).

rhage on the swimbladder, within the abdominal fat and on the hepatic and other visceral peritoneal surfaces, and a moruloid, pale grey spleen (Plates 17, 18). Liver colour may vary from grey-brown to yellow. Histopathologically the condition resembles that of *Vibrio anguillarum* infections, but often with severe heart and muscle changes. Imprints or touch-smears of spleen or kidney show large numbers of bacteria among the haemopoietic cells when stained appropriately (Fig. 6.8).

The pathogenesis does not appear to depend on a plasmid mediated iron sequestering system and virulence is not associated with specific plasmid profiles (Wiik *et al*. 1989).

## Control

Control of vibriosis, as with other bacterial septicaemias, is best achieved by maintenance of water quality, good husbandry and low stocking densities. This is not, however, always possible, and where outbreaks occur, treatment with an oral antibiotic is the only option. Its value is limited, however, since clinically affected fish do not eat and therefore cannot be treated, and so once a diagnosis has been made immediate treatment is of the essence, before too many fish go off their food.

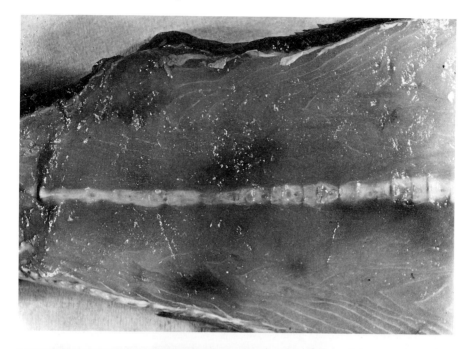

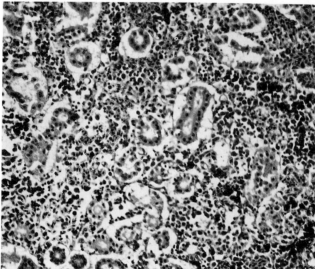

**Fig. 6.6**  (above) Longitudinal section of salmon muscle showing deep seated necrotic muscle lesions caused by *Vibrio anguillarum* (Courtesy Dr T. Hastein).

**Fig. 6.7**  (left) Section of mid-kidney of salmon with acute vibriosis. There is tubular necrosis as well as haemopoietic depletion and necrosis. (H&E × 150) (Courtesy of Dr T. Hastein).

As with other bacterial pathogens, resistance to antibiotics is a serious problem with the vibrios. Not only are many strains of both *V. anguillarum* and *V. salmonicida* now resistant to the commonly used oxytetracycline, but multi-resistance to oxytetracycline, sulphonamides and even oxolinic acid is growing in areas where salmon culture is intensive (Hjeltnes *et al.* 1987, Olsen & Skiewe 1988).

Because of its importance in salmonid culture, vibriosis was the first disease to which major efforts at vaccination were applied and these met with consider-able success. Killed vaccines against *Vibrio anguillarum*, which confer protec-tion by virtue of the presence of heat stable lipopolysaccharides derived from the cell walls, have been available since 1980. All of the licensed vaccines available are highly effective against *Vibrio* diseases, which in the Northern hemisphere include both *V. anguillarum* and *V. ordalii* infection. In Norway, a *Vibrio anguillarum* and *Vibrio salmonicida* combined vaccine is also available.

The success of these vaccines was largely due to the early identification of the protective antigens during the vaccine development stage. These are lipo-polysaccharides in the cell wall (they may also be released into the culture supernatant). They are very heat stable, can withstand severe extraction methods, and are excellent immunogens in most fish species. They do not require booster doses to maintain vaccinal immunity and are very effective at stimulating both the humoral and cell mediated, immune defence mechanisms in fish. They work well without adjuvants and are consistently found to provide high levels of protective immunity. No advantage was found in trying to improve on the simple foundations of the early vaccines (inactivated cultures of whole cells and their extracellular products), and even more importantly, the *Vibrio* vaccines were found to work well by all the delivery methods being tested in the early stages of fish vaccine research, i.e. by injection (Hayashi *et al.* 1964), orally (Fryer *et al.* 1978) and by immersion (Egidius & Anderson 1979).

*Vibrio* vaccines have proved effective for other farmed species, such as cod and eels, with little or no modification from their original design as formulated for use in salmonids being required. Vaccines against *V. salmonicida* have been available since 1987, and in both cases, use of vaccines has greatly reduced the level of infection. Protection lasts for only a limited period, however, and breakdowns occur 1.5–2 years after vaccination (Lillehaug 1991). Cross pro-tection between the two pathogens, *Vibrio salmonicida* and *Vibrio anguillarum*, so that vaccination against one could prevent clinical infection in the other, does not occur (Lillehaug 1990).

# References

Actis, L.A., Potter, S.A. & Crosa, J.W. (1985) Iron-regulated outer membrane protein OM2 of *Vibrio anguillarum* is encoded by virulence plasmid JM1. *Journal of Bacteriology*, **161**, 736–42.

Aoki, T., Kitao, T., Itabashi, T., Wada, Y. & Sakai, M. (1981) Proteins and polysaccharides in the membrane of *Vibrio anguillarum*. *Developments in Biological Standardization*, **49**, 225–32.

Biosca, E.G., Amaro, C., Esteve, C., Alcaide, E. & Garay, E. (1991) First record of *V. vulnificus* biotype 2 from diseased European eel *Anguilla anguilla* L. *Journal of Fish Diseases*, **14**, 103–111.

Canestrini, G. (1983) La malattia dominate della anguilla. *Atti Istitute Veneto Service*, 7, 809–14.

Chart, H. & Trust, T.J. (1984) Characterization of the surface antigens of the marine fish pathogens *Vibrio anguillarum* and *Vibrio ordalii*. *Canadian Journal of Microbiology*, **30**, 703–10.

Colorni, A., Paperna, I. & Gordin, H. (1981) Bacterial infections in gilthead sea bream (*Sparus aurata*) cultured at Elat. *Aquaculture*, **23**, 257–67.

Crosa, J.H. (1980) A plasmid associated with virulence in the marine fish pathogen *Vibrio anguillarum* specifies an iron sequestering system. *Nature*, **283**, 566−8.

Crosa, J.H., Hodges, Linda, L. & Schiewe, M.H. (1980) Curing of a plasmid is correlated with alteration of virulence in the marine fish pathogen *Vibrio anguillarum*. *Infection and Immunity*, **27**, 891−902.

Egidius, E. & Anderson, K. (1979) Bath immunization − a practical and non-stressing method of vaccinating farmed sea rainbow trout *Salmo gairdneri* Richardson, against vibriosis. *Journal of Fish Diseases*, **2**, 405−10.

Egidius, E., Wiik, R., Anderson, K., Hoff, K.A. & Hjeltnes, B. (1986) *Vibrio salmonicida sp. nov.*, a new fish pathogen. *International Journal of Systematic Bacteriology*, **36**, 518−20.

Espelid, S., Holm, K.O., Hjelmeland, K. & Jørgenson, T. (1988) Monoclonal antibodies against *Vibrio salmonicida*: the causative agent of coldwater vibrioses. (Hitra disease) in Atlantic salmon, *Salmo salar*. *Journal of Fish Diseases*, **11**, 207−14.

Frerichs, G.N. & Roberts, R.J. (1989) The bacteriology of teleosts. In *Fish Pathology* (Ed. by R.J. Roberts), pp. 289−319, Baillière Tindall, London.

Fryer, J.L., Rehovec, J.S. & Garrison, R.L. (1978) Immunization of salmonids for control of vibriosis. *Marine Fisheries Reviews*, **40**, 20−3.

Hacking, M.A. & Budd, J. (1971) *Vibrio* infection in tropical fish in a freshwater aquarium. *Journal of Wildlife Diseases*, **7**, 213−80.

Hayashi, K., Kobayashi, S., Jamata, T. & Ozalai, H. (1964) Studies on the *Vibrio* disease of rainbow trout II. Prophylactic vaccination against the disease. *Journal of the Faculty of Fisheries, Prefectural University, Mie*, **6**, 181−91.

Hjelmeland, K., Streuvag, K., Jørgensen, T. & Espelid, S. (1988) Isolation and characterization of a surface layer antigen from *Vibrio salmonicida*. *Journal of Fish Diseases*, **11**, 197−205.

Hjeltnes, B., Anderson, K. & Egidius, E. (1987) Multiple antibiotic resistance to *Aeromonas salmonicida*. *Bulletin of the European Association of Fish Pathologists*, **7**, 85.

Hofer, B. (1904) *Handbuch der Fisch Krankheiten*. Verlag des Algemeine Fisherei Zeitung, Munich.

Kielm, E.D. & Pacha, R.E. (1969) Characterization and relatedness of marine vibrios pathogenic to fish: deoxyribonucleic acid homology and base composition. *Journal of Bacteriology*, **100**, 1248−55.

Kitao, T., Aoki, T., Kukudome, M., Kawano, K., Wada, Y. & Muzumo, Y. (1983) Serotyping of *Vibrio anguillarum* isolated from diseased freshwater fish in Japan. *Journal of Fish Diseases*, **6**, 175−81.

Kodama, H., Moustafa, M., Ishigura, S., Mikami, T. & Izawa, H. (1984) Extracellular virulence factors of fish *Vibrio*; relationships between toxic material, haemolysins and proteolytic enzyme. *American Journal of Veterinary Research*, **45**, 2203−7.

Lillehaug, A. (1990) A field trial of vaccination against coldwater vibriosis in Atlantic salmon (*Salmo salar* L.). *Aquaculture*, **84**, 1−12.

Lillehaug, A. (1991) Vaccination of Atlantic salmon (*Salmo salar* L.) against coldwater vibriosis − duration of protection and effect on growth rate. *Aquaculture*, **92**, 99−107.

McArdle, J.F. (1973) *Vibrio anguillarum* and its toxin in marine flatfish. MSc Thesis, University of Stirling.

Munn, C.B. (1980) Production and properties of a haemolytic toxin by *Vibrio anguillarum*. In *Fish Diseases* (Ed. by W. Ahne), pp. 69−74. Springer Verlag, Berlin.

Muroga, K., Takahashi, S. & Yamanoe, H. (1979) Non-cholera *Vibrio* isolated from diseased ayu. *Bulletin of the Japanese Society of Scientific Fisheries*, **50**, 591−6.

Olsen, A.B. & Skiewe, V. (1988) *Kaldtransvibriose i Hordaland og Sogn og Fjordane i perioden October 1986 Juni 1987*. *Nördisk Veterinaër Tidjstraft*, **100**, 703−10.

Pacha, R.E. & Kiehn, E.D. (1969) Characterization and relatedness of marine vibrios pathogenic to fish; physiology, serology and epidemiology. *Journal of Bacteriology*, **100**, 1242−7.

Ransom, D.P., Lannon, C.N., Rehovec, J.S. & Fryer, J.L. (1984) Comparison of histopathology caused by *Vibrio anguillarum* and *V. ordalii* in three species of Pacific salmon. *Journal of Fish Diseases*, **7**, 107−15.

Roberts, R.J. (1975) Melanin containing cells of teleost fish and their relation to disease. In *The Pathology of Fishes* (Ed. by W.F. Ribelin & G. Migaki), pp. 399−428. University of Wisconsin Press.

Schiewe, M.H. (1981) Taxonomic status of marine fish vibrios pathogenic for salmonid fish.

*Developments in Biological Standards*, **49**, 149−58.

Schiewe, M.H., Crosa, J.H. & Ordal, E.J. (1977) Deoxyribonucleic acid relationships among marine *Vibrio* pathogens of fish. *Canadian Journal of Microbiology*, **27**, 1011−18.

Schiewe, M.H., Trust, T.J. & Crosa, J.H. (1981) *Vibrio ordalii* sp. nov. A causative agent of vibriosis in fish. *Current Microbiology*, **6**, 343−8.

Schroder, M.J., Espelid, S. & Jørgensen, T.O. (1993) Two serotypes of *Vibrio salmonicida* isolated from diseased cod (*Gadus morhua*); Virulence, immunological studies and vaccination experiments. In press.

Sørensen, U.B.S. & Larsen, J.L. (1986) Serotyping of *Vibrio anguillarum*. *Applied and Environmental Microbiology*, **51**, 593−7.

Tajima, K., Ejura, Y. & Kimura, T. (1990) Serological analysis of thermolabile antigens of *Vibrio anguillarum*. *Journal of Aquatic Animal Health*, **2**, 212−16.

Toranzo, A.E., Barja, J.L., Potter, S.A., Colwell, R.R., Hetrick, F.M. & Crosa, J.H. (1983) Molecular factors associated with virulence of marine vibrios from striped bass in Chesapeake Bay. *Infection and Immunity*, **39**, 1220−7.

West, P.A., Lee, J.V. & Bryant, T.N. (1983) A numerical taxonomical study of species of *Vibrio* isolated from the aquatic environment and birds in Kent, England. *Journal of Applied Bacteriology*, **5**, 203−82.

Wiik, R. & Egidius, E. (1986) Generic relationships of *Vibrio salmonicida* sp. nov. to other fish-pathogenic vibrios. *International Journal of Systematic Bacteriology*, **36**, 521−3.

Wiik, R., Anderson, K., Daae, F.L. & Hoff, F.A. (1989) Virulence studies based on plasmid profiles of the fish pathogen *Vibrio salmonicida*. *Applied and Environmental Microbiology*, **55**, 819−25.

# Chapter 7:
# Furunculosis

The genus *Aeromonas*, within the family Vibrionaceae, consists of Gram-negative rods with rounded ends $0.3-1.0\,\mu m \times 1.0-3.5\,\mu m$. With one exception they are motile with a single polar flagellum. They are non-spore-forming, facultative anaerobes and resistant to the vibriostat 2,4-diamino-6,7-diisopropyl pteridine (0/129). Optimum growth temperature is $22-28°C$ and some do not grow at $35°C$. They occur widely in fresh water and in sewage; some are pathogenic to fish but rarely to man. The molar % G + C of the DNA is $57-63$.

Aeromonas salmonicida is the causative agent of furunculosis of salmonids and related diseases in other species. On commonly used culture media it often produces a diffusable brown pigment which aids identification and unlike other aeromonads it is non-motile. It is an obligate pathogen of fish with limited survival outside the host. Furunculosis is a septicaemic infection, principally of salmonids, which may be acute or chronic with development of furuncles, necrotic swellings in the muscle. Outbreaks are stress-associated and mortality rates may be very high, posing a real threat, in particular, to the salmon farming industry. Control is dependent on good environmental conditions and judicious use of chemotherapeutants pending development of a fully effective vaccine.

## Introduction

The term furunculosis refers to a fatal epizootic disease of salmonids caused by the bacterium currently classified as *Aeromonas salmonicida*. It is now recognised that this bacterium may also cause other disease conditions in salmonids and in other species of fish and these diseases may have other names, such as ulcer disease or carp erythrodermatitis. The presenting gross pathology of these other diseases caused by *A. salmonicida* is often different from furunculosis of salmonids, although it is probable that the pathogeneses have features in common.

The name furunculosis was given by analogy with human furunculosis because of the apparent 'boil-like' character of the clinical lesions found in some cases. This name is not, however, an accurate description as the grotesque necrotic swellings of the musculature, which eventually ulcerate and often characterize the chronic development of the disease in older salmonids, have little in common with the pus-filled swellings of dermal origin in humans. However, the name is too well established world-wide in the fisheries literature to consider correction.

## *Aeromonas salmonicida*

The first authentic report of the bacterium was by Emmerich & Weibel (1894) from a trout hatchery in Germany. They named the bacterium *Bacillus der Forellenseuche* or bacillus of contagious trout disease. In English it was known as *Bacillus salmonicida* until Griffin *et al.* (1953) suggested it should be reclassified in the genus *Aeromonas* currently positioned in the family Vibrionaceae.

## Taxonomy

The taxonomic position of *A. salmonicida* has been reviewed by McCarthy & Roberts (1980), Austin & Austin (1987) and Belland & Trust (1988). Briefly, the position may be summarized thus: DNA homology studies between *A. salmonicida* and the *A. hydrophila* group show a 56–65% degree of binding (McCarthy 1978) indicating a relationship at the generic level which does not support a claim to set up a separate genus, i.e. *Necromonas salmonicida* (Smith 1963). At the species level Schubert's (1974) classification of *A. salmonicida* into three subspecies namely, *salmonicida*, *achromogenes* and *masoucida* based on a variety of properties (see Table 7.1) has been retained in Bergey's Manual of Systematic Bacteriology (Popoff 1984). Skerman *et al.* (1980) also used this classification in their Approved List of Bacterial Names. However, DNA homology studies between many isolates of *A. salmonicida* covering strains that might be classified into all three subspecies have shown that the mean mol % G + C value indicates a very high level of homology, suggesting that

**Table 7.1**  Characteristics of *Aeromonas salmonicida* (after Austin & Austin 1987)

| Character | *A. salmonicida* subsp. *achromogenes* | *A. salmonicida* subsp. *masoucida* | *A. salmonicida* subsp. *salmonicida* |
|---|---|---|---|
| Production of: | | | |
| Brown, diffusible pigment | − | − | + |
| Arginine dihydrolase | + | + | V |
| Catalase | + | + | + |
| β-galactosidase | + | + | + |
| H₂S | − | + | V |
| Indole | − | − | − |
| Lysine decarboxylase | − | + | V |
| Ornithine decarboxylase | − | − | − |
| Oxidase | + | + | + |
| Phenylalanine deaminase | . | . | − |
| Phosphatase | . | . | − |
| Fermentative metabolism | + | + | + |
| Gluconate oxidation | − | + | − |
| Methyl red test | − | + | V |
| Motility | − | − | − |
| Nitrate reduction | + | + | + |
| Voges Proskauer reaction | − | + | − |
| Degradation of: | | | |
| Aesculin | − | + | V |
| Blood (β-haemolysis) | − | + | + |
| Casein | + | − | + |
| Chitin | − | − | − |
| DNA | + | + | + |
| Elastin | . | . | + |
| Gelatin | − | + | + |

*continued*

**Table 7.1**  *Continued.*

| Character | A. salmonicida subsp. achromogenes | A. salmonicida subsp. masoucida | A. salmonicida subsp. salmonicida |
|---|---|---|---|
| Lecithin | . | . | + |
| RNA | + | + | + |
| Starch | . | . | + |
| Tweens | + | + | + |
| Tyrosine | . | . | + |
| Urea | − | − | − |
| Xanthine | − | − | − |
| Growth on/at: | | | |
| 4−5°C | V | V | V |
| 30°C | + | + | + |
| 37°C | − | − | − |
| MacConkey agar | + | + | + |
| Potassium cyanide | − | − | − |
| Thiosulphate citrate bile salt sucrose agar | − | − | − |
| 0−2% (w/v) sodium chloride | + | + | + |
| 3% (w/v) sodium chloride | V | V | V |
| 4% (w/v) sodium chloride | − | − | − |
| Utilization of sodium citrate | − | − | − |
| Production of acid from: | | | |
| Adonitol | − | − | − |
| Amygdalin | − | − | − |
| Arabinose | − | + | + |
| Cellobiose | − | − | − |
| Dulcitol | − | − | − |
| Erythritol | . | . | − |
| Fructose | . | . | + |
| Galactose | + | + | + |
| Glucose | + | + | + |
| Glycerol | . | . | − |
| Glycogen | . | . | + |
| Inulin | . | . | − |
| Lactose | − | − | − |
| Maltose | + | + | + |
| Mannitol | − | + | + |
| Mannose | . | + | + |
| Melibiose | . | . | − |
| Raffinose | − | − | − |
| Rhamnose | − | − | − |
| Salicin | V | V | + |
| Sorbitol | − | − | − |
| Sucrose | + | + | − |
| Trehalose | + | + | + |
| Xylose | − | − | − |
| Guanine plus cytosine ratio (moles %) | | | 57−59 |

V variable
. not reported
− negative
+ positive

subspecies classification is unnecessary (McCarthy 1978, MacInnes *et al.* 1979, Belland & Trust 1988).

McCarthy & Roberts (1980) proposed yet another and different division into three subspecies, based on epizootiological criteria, which is supported by Belland and Trust (1988), namely:

(1)  Group 1 strains. *A. salmonicida* subspecies *salmonicida*. These are strains typically derived from salmonid fish.

(2)  Group 2 strains. *A. salmonicida* subspecies *achromogenes*. These are atypical strains derived from salmonid fish and include the former *achromogenes* and *masoucida*. Two Gram-negative microorganisms associated with specific syndromes in salmonids, ulcer disease (Snieszko *et al.* 1950) and pasteurellosis (Håstein & Bullock 1976) are now recognised as being such atypical strains (Austin & Austin 1987).

(3)  Group 3 strains. *A. salmonicida* subspecies *nova*. These are atypical strains associated with disease in non-salmonid fish.

**Properties**

*A. salmonicida* is a Gram-negative, facultatively anaerobic, non-motile rod, size 1.3−2.0 by 0.8−1.3 μm. Bipolar staining and the presence of coccoid forms aid identification from both tissue smears and culture plates. It grows on nutrient media with 0.85% salt, very often producing a brown diffusable pigment, and is best grown and maintained at 22°C or less. Many more characteristics are presented in Table 7.1, which indicates the criteria used for subspecies identification. Useful phenotypic criteria for the separation of such subspecies are given by McCarthy & Roberts (1980), McCarthy (1978), Popoff (1984) and Böhm *et al.* (1986).

Upon initial isolation from fish, colonies of *A. salmonicida* are extremely friable and may be pushed across the plate with a wire loop. The less common 'smooth' variant produces shiny colonies which are soft when touched with a loop. In broth cultures fresh isolates autoagglutinate and rapidly settle out to produce a sediment, while non-agglutinating smooth variants produce a uniform turbidity. It is probable that all fresh isolates of *A. salmonicida* from clinical cases of disease in fish contain a regular surface protein layer, first described by Udey & Fryer (1978), which they termed the 'additional layer' or 'A layer'. 'A layer-positive' strains are strongly autoagglutinating and virulent, while 'A layer-negative' strains are relatively avirulent and nonagglutinating. Culture at temperatures above 22°C is selective for A− variants, which cannot be induced to revert to A+ (Ishiguro *et al.* 1981). A detailed description of the tetragonally arranged array of the A layer protein responsible for auto-agglutination has been given by Stewart *et al.* (1986).

**Serology**

Studies by McCarthy & Rawle (1975) and Hahnel *et al.* (1983) have confirmed earlier work that serological differences could not be detected among fresh isolates of *A. salmonicida* although older cultures were inclined to lose reactivity. In the light of recent work on the mutability of the A layer it is possible that repeated laboratory culture at too high temperatures with consequent loss of A layer contributed to this finding. Both A layer and lipopolysaccharide, which are major immunogenic components of the outer membrane of *A. salmonicida*, are reported as being structurally and immunologically homogeneous (Chart *et al.* 1984), thus supporting the earlier conclusions on the serological homogeneity of *A. salmonicida* using polyclonal antibodies.

**Phage typing**

Popoff (1971*a,b*) demonstrated that phage typing was useful in epizootiological studies to differentiate isolates. By using eight phages he showed 14 phage types.

**DNA sequencing**

Use of DNA probes to detect restriction fragment length variations did not show significant variation when used to compare seven strains of *A. salmonicida* from widely differing geographical locations (Hennigan *et al.* 1989).

**Plasmid content**

In a study of the plasmid content of 25 isolates of *A. salmonicida* Belland & Trust (1989) showed that typical strains were extremely homogeneous in plasmid content. Atypical strains carried plasmids which were different from plasmids of typical strains and corresponded to isolate source and biotype, suggesting that plasmid content may be a useful epidemiological marker. These results also support the subspecies division proposed by McCarthy & Roberts (1980).

## Furunculosis of salmonids

This is an acute to chronic condition which may affect all species of salmonid. In terms of pathogenesis the disease generally appears to develop as a septicaemia, i.e. an infection of the blood, and it is often fatal. How the bacterium gains entry to the circulation is uncertain, perhaps through the intestine, gills or through skin damage. It rapidly overcomes the leucocytic cell defences of the blood (Klontz *et al.* 1966) and is then free to be transported through the vasculature to localise in any of the organs.

All ages of salmonid fish are vulnerable, although very young fish are less often affected. In chronic cases the slow progression of infection results in a greater degree of localisation in visceral organs, commonly kidney, spleen, blood vessel walls and intestine but also in the liver and gills. It is, however, in the skeletal muscle that the most characteristic lesion is produced, the grotesque swellings known as furuncles, which were referred to previously. The chronic condition manifesting the archetypal furuncles is most often seen in older fish, and these sometimes may recover. Furunculosis may manifest itself in wild riverine populations or in farmed stocks in fresh and sea water. Stressing factors such as crowding, poor water quality, fright, high temperature and trauma are all important in precipitating the disease, especially in farmed populations. The causative agent has been described from most areas where salmonids are found including Europe, North America, Japan, Korea, Australia and South Africa, but apparently not South America.

## Clinical and gross pathology

External signs are dependent on the time course of the disease in individual fish. In a population, a continuum of pathologies may be presented from the most acute to chronic. Acutely dying fish most often show few external signs, whereas in chronic cases one or more of the following may present; darkening, lethargy, inappetence, petechiation at fin bases and sometimes gross swellings (furuncles) which may ulcerate to release necrotic tissue debris and bacteria (Plates 19–23). The gills are very pale. In sea-reared fish, extensive haemorrhage from the gill is common (Miyazaki & Kubota 1975, Bruno *et al.* 1986).

Internally the blood vessels surrounding the lower intestine are inflamed and often those of the pyloric caeca as well. The intestine is devoid of food and may have an exudate of blood, mucus and cellular debris. The spleen is swollen and cherry red, whereas the liver is grey to greenish in hue. Petechiae are common on all serosal surfaces. The swim bladder may be swollen and cloudy. The kidney is convex (swollen) and when cut with a scalpel the contents often appear to be liquefied. The peritoneum and pericardium often have bloody fluid accumulations. Haematocrit measurements often show severely depressed red cell numbers, so explaining the pale appearance of gills and liver. The buffy coat (leucocyte cells) is also reduced or absent in the haematocrit tube.

## Histopathology

The histopathology is fully described by Ferguson & McCarthy (1978) and McCarthy & Roberts (1980). In order to understand the histopathological picture it is important to realise that the bacterium produces very powerful extracellular virulence factors, in particular a leucocidin, which may also act as a neurotoxin, and two proteases (Ellis 1991). When examining histological sections, often the almost total absence of a leucocyte response to colonies of the bacterium and to host tissue damage is remarkable and possibly explained by the presence of the leucocidin which destroys engulfing macrophages and

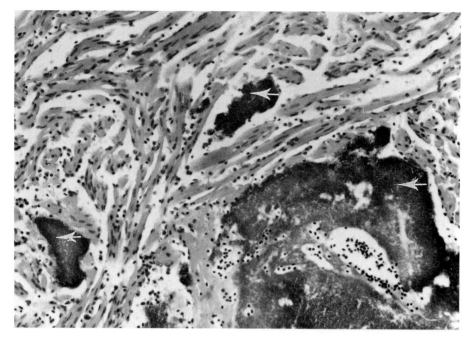

**Fig. 7.1** Large bacterial colonies with minimal host inflammatory response in the cardiac muscle of a brown trout infected with *Aeromonas salmonicida* (H&E × 200) (Courtesy of Dr H.W. Ferguson).

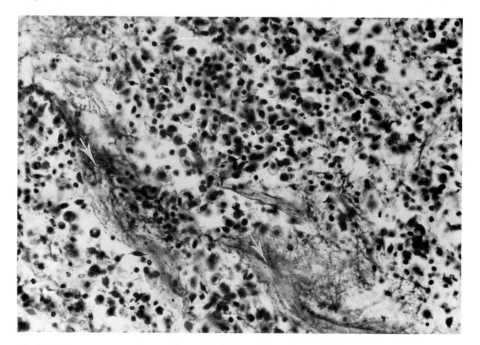

**Fig. 7.2** Section through a mature furuncle. Muscle cells and connective tissue have disappeared and been replaced by necrotic leucocytes, fibrin (arrowed) and bacteria (H&E × 350) (Courtesy Dr T. Hastein).

monocytes and lyses lymphocytes (Fig. 7.1, Plate 22). Mobilization of the leucocytes from the kidney and spleen probably explains their gross depletion from these organs as seen in histological sections. The proteases act most vigorously on connective tissue and their action is seen most clearly in relation to the connective tissues of muscle, but it is common wherever colonies develop, e.g. it induces the petechiation of visceral surfaces and the liquifaction of the kidney by destroying the connective tissues of these sites (Fig. 7.2).

Another feature of pathological interest is the degranulation of the numerous eosinophilic granulocytes (EGC) in the submucosa of the intestine and to a lesser extent in the gill (Vallejo & Ellis 1989).

### Carrier or latent infections

Such infections can occur at any age in salmonid fish whether wild or cultivated. Their importance was recognized very early in studies of furunculosis (Horne 1928). Detection can sometimes be achieved by culture of the bacterium from the tissues (usually kidney or gut) although false negatives are commonplace. The bacterium may also be isolated from the skin or gills of carrier fish, but because these tissues are also populated by other bacterial species detection of low numbers of *A. salmonicida* from these areas is problematical. Detection rates may often be improved by use of 'stress tests'. These use an elevated temperature combined with injection of corticosteroids to stress sample groups of fish (Bullock & Stuckey 1975).

ELISA detection methods may have potential but those developed to date do not appear to offer any greater sensitivity or reliability than conventional bacteriological methods. Nucleic acid probes have even greater prospects but await development of their full potential.

### Significance

Ever since this disease was first described it has caused serious losses in salmonid hatcheries and farms. With the development of antimicrobial therapy in the 1950s, control by the use of therapeutic antimicrobials has been possible in most situations. The commercial development of salmon farming in Scotland has suffered significantly, with increasing numbers of outbreaks (Table 7.2) and estimated losses in sea water running at 15–20% by number (Anon. 1990). The development of resistance to many or all of the licensed antimicrobials has been a major factor contributing to this loss. A similar situation is developing in Norway, the country with the largest Atlantic salmon farming industry.

Furunculosis caused epidemic loss in wild salmonids in the UK in the early part of this century. The major record of that period (Mackie *et al.* 1930, 1933, 1935), although indicating how such outbreaks affect the revenues of the sport fishery for salmonids, does not suggest that losses were ever sufficient to depress population numbers overall.

**Table 7.2**  Outbreaks of furunculosis in Scotland diagnosed by the Marine Laboratory, Aberdeen, from 1979 to 1989

| Year | Number of outbreaks | |
| --- | --- | --- |
| | Fresh water | Sea water |
| 1979 | 4 | 2 |
| 1980 | 3 | 1 |
| 1981 | 2 | 2 |
| 1982 | 6 | 2 |
| 1983 | 3 | 6 |
| 1984 | 0 | 13 |
| 1985 | 3 | 26 |
| 1986 | 2 | 30 |
| 1987 | 1 | 20 |
| 1988 | 13 | 78 |
| 1989 | 15 | 127 |

## Epizootiology

The disease has been known for almost 100 years from its effects in fresh water. With the growth of salmon farming in sea water, particularly in Norway and Scotland, over the last 15 years, its effects have been described in the marine environment too. Despite much investigation the mechanism of transmission is uncertain. Experimentally, disease is achieved by bathing in relatively high concentrations of bacteria, e.g. $10^5$ per ml of a virulent strain. Infection may also be achieved by cohabitation or by traumatizing the skin or gill and subsequently bathing in lower concentrations of bacteria. Disease may be induced in populations with carrier fish by inducing 'stress' (see above).

### Riverine populations

The disease was described by the Furunculosis Committee (Mackie *et al.* 1930, 1933, 1935) as occurring in UK riverine populations of Atlantic salmon (*Salmo salar*). Outbreaks with limited mortality began in June and were associated with rising temperatures. These fish were ascending the river to reach their spawning grounds by November. Epidemic mortality sometimes occurred in August and September if water flows became low, temperatures rose and many fish were contained in river pools. Subsequently Smith (1962) described the occurrence of readily isolable *A. salmonicida* from >40% of dead or dying spent *S. salar* recovered from rivers in December and January, implying that furunculosis caused or contributed to this post-spawning mortality.

### Farmed salmonids in fresh water

There are many reports of the disease in *Salmo*, *Oncorhynchus* and *Salvelinus* species held in tanks, raceways and ponds. A recent account of Swedish experience has been given by Wichardt *et al.* (1989). In Scotland, where a large Atlantic salmon farming industry has developed, *A. salmonicida* infection is significant in fresh water (Table 7.2). Although vertical transmission of *A. salmonicida* via infected ova rarely, if ever, occurs (Bullock & Stuckey 1987) it seems that many Scottish smolt rearing units cannot avoid producing smolts carrying infection with *A. salmonicida*. Current bacteriological and immunological methods to detect carrier fish are unreliable, and in our experience the more time-consuming 'stress test' remains the best, although not infallible, method available. Many smolt producers, however, are disinclined to use any of the tests which are available and there is little current proof which farms are infected. Evidence presented by Munro & Waddell (1984) did suggest that smolt units could be ranked as safest from infection in waters without anadromous salmonids, followed by some freshwater cage sites where dilution factors greatly reduced risks of lateral transfer from wild fish, and that riverine waters with anadromous salmonids were at greatest risk. In some cases sites had become infected through receipt of infected parr or as a consequence of drought when infection-free water supplies had to be augmented by using infected river waters. Escapees from infected farm stocks held in both fresh and sea water are a new source of infection and because of their numbers may be a significant source of the spread of infection.

**Farmed salmonids in sea water**

In many respects the development of clinical disease in individual fish in sea water is similar to fresh water. However, as populations become older the disease often takes a more chronic although nevertheless fatal course. Anaemia is always a feature, but it is especially apparent in sea water because, as the disease progresses, infection regularly localizes in the gills resulting in excessive bleeding and the shedding of large numbers ($> 10^7$ kg fish weight/h) of bacteria (Rose *et al.* 1989). The majority of the released bacteria may die in 2–3 days but some *A. salmonicida* cells will remain viable for up to 10 days in sea water.

Using a hydrographic model to study the fate of *A. salmonicida* released from a hypothetical sea cage farm during a typical furunculosis outbreak, Turrell & Munro (1988) showed that other farms in at least a 10 km radius were at risk of meeting viable bacteria and therefore of suffering infection. It is probable that the bacterium may survive and even grow in faecal and food wastes where these materials collect beneath cages. Resuspension of such material into the upper water layers in relatively shallow sites may pose another disease hazard, and this may persist after the commonly adopted 2–6 week fallow period used as a break when stocking a new year class at a cage site. The disposal of the large numbers of fish carcasses occurring during outbreaks can pose another threat of the spread of *A. salmonicida* unless it is ensured that infection cannot get back from disposal sites into the aquatic environment. Similarly, disposal of solid and liquid wastes from processing plants is increasingly being viewed with concern if some form of disinfection treatment is not employed. The finding of *A. salmonicida* in wild marine fish (e.g. saithe, *Pollachius virens*) which choose to live in and around sea cage sites is yet another example of how the bacterium may be spread (G. Dear, personal communication).

Farming practices and other diseases may contribute to furunculosis outbreaks. It is impossible to rear salmon without causing skin trauma at various stages in the production cycle, e.g. at smolt transfer to sea water, at size grading, at grilse harvest and broodstock selection, during net changes and bath treatments and during involuntary situations when fish are frightened, as in a seal attack, and collide with each other or the net. Salmon lice are another major cause of skin abrasion. All these causes of skin damage are likely to assist the development of furunculosis in individual fish and to induce disease of epizootic proportions when many fish are held together.

## *A. salmonicida*-induced disease in non-salmonids

The bacterium may cause disease in a wide spectrum of freshwater and marine species. Many recent reports are suggestive of lateral transmission from adjacent diseased salmonids held in fish farm systems. However, the older literature shows that in cyprinids, especially carp (*Cyprinus carpio*), infection by *A. salmonicida* subspecies *nova* has been indigenous.

The pathology of cyprinid infections starts as a skin lesion which progresses to multiple skin lesions and then systemic infection. Most often other bacterial species become involved and the cause of death is seldom clear (Antychawicz & Rogulska 1986). Loss of essential ions due to skin lesions or failure of essential organ function is a likely cause. In a study of the pathogenesis of the disease in carp Evenberg *et al.* (1986) found evidence of a marked leuco-penia, suggesting that once infection passes the skin vasculature barrier all *A. salmonicida* infections of fishes may take similar courses, i.e. destruction of the leucocytes of blood and lymphoid organs by the production of leucotoxin(s). Ellis (1991) in reviewing the different virulence factors produced by the sub-species, gives indications as to how these may produce the observed pathologies. The pathology of an atypical *A. salmonicida*-induced disease in Atlantic cod (*Gadus morhua*) described by Morrison *et al.* (1984) and Cornick *et al.* (1984) does show that in some species a very different pathological picture can be presented, i.e. a marked leucocyte response with resultant cyst formation.

Probably much more than salmonids, cyprinids, other ornamental fish and species used as baitfish for angling are transported live around the world. The finding of an atypical *A. salmonicida* in goldfish (*Carassius auratus*) in Australia illustrates how the bacteria most probably arrived there (Hamilton *et al.* 1981). The finding of *A. salmonicida* producing classical furuncles in a baitfish minnow used in salmonid angling waters is another example of a mechanism of the spread of this bacterium by man's activities (Ostland *et al.* 1987). Goldsinny wrasse (*Ctenolabrus rupestris*), now increasingly being used to control sea lice in farmed Atlantic salmon in sea water, are also susceptible to furunculosis, and large numbers of *A. salmonicida* subsp. *salmonicida* have been isolated from wrasse suffering clinical disease in cages of farmed salmon in Scotland (C.G. Mitchell, personal communication).

## Control of disease using antimicrobial agents

To control outbreaks of furunculosis farmers have resorted to treatment with antibiotics. Four types of antibacterial agents are at present licensed for the control of furunculosis in Scotland; oxytetracycline, oxolinic acid and trimethoprim-sulphadiazine (potentiated sulphonamide), which have been in use for a number of years, and amoxycillin, which was first licensed for use in salmon in 1990. A fifth compound, furazolidone, which is not specifically licensed for use in fish, may also be prescribed in limited circumstances.

Antimicrobial agents are usually administered orally, either by incorporation into feed pellets during manufacture or surface-coated onto pellets, usually with a small quantity of fish oil, at the farm. Some antibiotics (e.g. oxytetracycline) can also be administered by intraperitoneal injection. However, because injection of individual animals is labour-intensive and stressful to the fish, use of this method has been limited to occasional treatment of smolts prior to sea water transfer or to valuable broodfish.

### Resistance to antimicrobial agents

In the 1970s and early 1980s, antibiotic resistance posed few problems for the treatment of furunculosis in Scottish salmon farms. Although some isolates of *A. salmonicida* were resistant to oxytetracycline, potentiated sulphonamides or furazolidone (Tsoumas *et al.* 1989, Scottish Office Agriculture and Fisheries Department, SOAFD, unpublished records), resistance to one agent could always be circumvented by treatment with one of the other drugs. During the mid-1980s, however, rising numbers of outbreaks of furunculosis in sea water led to increasing use of antimicrobial agents. In 1985, there was an increase in the number of *A. salmonicida* isolates showing resistance to oxytetracycline, and resistance to oxolinic acid was detected for the first time (Hastings & McKay 1987). In subsequent years, resistance to licensed antibiotics, with the exception of amoxycillin, has become widespread (Table 7.3), and multiple resistance (i.e. resistance of one isolate to two or more antibiotics) is now common (Richards *et al.* 1992). Although resistance of *A. salmonicida* subsp. *salmonicida* to amoxycillin is still rare in Scotland, isolates of *A. salmonicida* subsp. *achromogenes* are usually highly resistant (Barnes *et al.* 1991*b*).

**Table 7.3** Resistance to licensed antimicrobial agents among Scottish *Aeromonas salmonicida* isolates* during 1991

| Antimicrobial agent | Percentage of isolates showing resistance |
|---|---|
| Oxytetracycline | 36 |
| Oxolinic acid | 45 |
| Trimethoprim-sulphadiazine | 29 |
| Amoxycillin | 1 |

* Isolated by Marine Laboratory, Aberdeen

### Mechanisms of resistance

Both plasmid-mediated and mutational drug resistance have been identified in several fish pathogens, including *A. salmonicida*, though the precise biochemical mechanisms involved are as yet poorly understood.

Plasmid-mediated drug resistance has been detected in strains of *A. salmonicida* isolated as early as 1959 (Aoki *et al.* 1971). In a subsequent study, Aoki *et al.* (1983) detected transferable R-plasmids in only two out of 124 resistant strains, but they concluded that many strains harboured non-transferable R-plasmids which conferred drug resistance.

Most R-plasmids found in *A. salmonicida* belong to two incompatibility groups, inc C and inc U. Inc U plasmids conferring multiple drug resistance have been found in a large number of *A. salmonicida* strains from Japan (Aoki *et al.* 1986) and in at least one hatchery in Ireland (Brazil *et al.* 1987). These plasmids, which had molecular weights of 29–34 MDa, were found to confer simultaneous resistance to three, four or five different antibiotics, including tetracycline, trimethoprim and sulphadiazine. The plasmid detected in the Irish hatchery persisted for a period of at least 8 years, probably supported by a reservoir of infection in feral fish in the river. Plasmids similar to those found in *A. salmonicida* have also been detected in other species of bacteria, including *A. hydrophila* (Hedges *et al.* 1985, Aoki *et al.* 1986), and the possibility exists that plasmids conferring drug resistance could be harboured and transferred between these species.

Plasmid-mediated resistance to oxolinic acid, or indeed any of the 4-quinolones, has never been found in any species of bacteria, and the only way that remains for bacteria to become resistant to the 4-quinolones is by chromosomal mutation (Smith 1986). The frequency with which this occurs varies according to the type of 4-quinolone and the concentration of drug to which the bacterium is exposed. With oxolinic acid, sensitive strains of *A. salmonicida* were found to mutate to resistance at frequencies of $1.7 \times 10^{-9}$–$6.5 \times 10^{-8}$ when exposed to the drug at 10 times their MIC (Barnes *et al.* 1991a). It appears that resistance develops in a step-wise fashion, commencing at a low level but increasing on exposure to higher drug concentrations (Tsoumas *et al.* 1989). These workers suggested that resistance may be relatively unstable. However, in a recent study of 20 oxolinic acid resistant isolates from Scottish salmon farms the decline in resistance following repeated passage on drug-free media was so low as to be insignificant (Barnes *et al.* 1990*a*).

Mutants displaying multiple low level antibiotic resistance have been induced following exposure of *A. salmonicida* strains to low concentrations of a number of different antimicrobial agents including the 4-quinolone flumequine (Wood *et al.* 1986). Resistance developed as a result of decreased outer membrane permeability associated with changes in the outer membrane proteins (Griffiths & Lynch 1989). Oxytetracycline-resistant mutants with cross-resistance to oxolinic acid have also been induced (Barnes *et al.* 1990*b*) and similar outer membrane changes have recently been detected in naturally occurring cross-resistant isolates from Scottish salmon farms (Barnes *et al.* 1992).

Resistance to furazolidone is widespread in *A. salmonicida*, but the mechanism(s) by which the bacterium develops resistance to the drug is as yet unclear. Several attempts to demonstrate transferable furazolidone resistance in *A. salmonicida* and other fish pathogens have been unsuccessful (Aoki *et al.* 1983, Brazil *et al.* 1986, Toranzo *et al.* 1983), suggesting that resistance may be conferred by a non-transferable R-plasmid or chromosomal mutation.

**Vaccines**

Attempts to produce an efficacious vaccine have been in progress since the pioneering work of Duff (1942). All of these many vaccines (reviewed by Munro 1984, Hastings 1988) have been at best only modestly successful and it seems from anecdotal comment from industry sources that this conclusion still applies to those vaccines commercially available today. There are, however, successful fish vaccines used in salmonid culture against vibriosis, cold water vibriosis and ERM.

The reasons for the success of these vaccines are poorly understood. They are essentially killed bacterial cultures, each batch of which must be tested for efficacy by immunizing and challenging test fish. There is very limited knowledge of which antigen(s) are important, in what quantity and how to measure whether fish are successfully vaccinated other than by disease challenge. Ellis (1991) reported on the study of the virulence factors possessed by *A. salmonicida*, one of the preliminary areas of study necessary to achieve an understanding of how a more successful vaccine may be made.

**Towards better control**

The severity of the furunculosis problem facing salmon farming in Scotland and Norway cannot be overstated. Losses are increasing, multiple resistance to antibiotics is spreading and persistent and the distribution of farms is so widespread that no area is likely to be free of risk. It is therefore appropriate to review the principal methods of disease control to determine how best to improve the current situation.

## Avoidance

There are two aspects to avoidance, namely avoiding the pathogen altogether and avoiding the multiple resistant antibiotic strains. With some exceptions Scottish smolt units, i.e. the freshwater aspect of salmon farming, have had only minor problems with furunculosis. Although it is probable that infection with *A. salmonicida* is quite common owing to the presence of anadromous salmonids in many water supplies, control of infrequent disease outbreaks by antibiotic therapy in smolt units is realistic because the frequency of antibiotic resistant strains in wild fish is low. The industry has known for a long time that avoidance of infection in fresh water has never been a realistic proposition for some smolt units.

Owing to the high susceptibility of Atlantic salmon in sea water to furunculosis and the ever increasing spread of the pathogen, seawater units are increasingly showing clinical disease. As antibiotic treatments increase, multiple-resistant strains of the bacterium have appeared. Given the enormous numbers of bacteria released during epidemics, the large number of farms around the coastline, the ability of bacteria to survive for several days in sea water and to travel significant distances driven by dispersive forces, as demonstrated in modelling studies, the probable long survival in sediments, in escaped salmon and in some wild species that frequent sea cage sites, it is unlikely that the pathogen will ever be avoided. Escape from sea cages of fish carrying multiple-resistant strains threatens not only sea sites but fresh water sites as well, as escaped carrier fish mature and seek spawning in fresh water. However, hatcheries protected from wild fish in their water supplies would provide a foundation stock of uninfected fish if proof of their infection free status could be obtained. At least they should be free of multiple-resistant strains of *A. salmonicida*. In Scotland stress tested fish from these smolt units are being used increasingly in programmes designed to stock sea areas cleared and fallowed of infected fish. Where smolt units have strains resistant to all the existing licensed antimicrobials, it is considered inadvisable to use their stock. Indeed all carrier smolts whatever their susceptibility to antibiotics should be avoided.

## Eradication

Eradication of multiple-resistant strains of the bacterium should be seriously considered. As these occur very largely in sea cage sites, fallowing not just of individual sites but of large areas covering all adjacent sites and probably adjacent sea lochs/areas of coastline, for periods of perhaps a year, may be necessary to achieve success. It must be emphasized that proof of the effectiveness of fallowing on this scale has not been established but modelling studies on the spread and survival of infection and movements of escaped fish suggest that it is likely to be necessary. Possible survival of *A. salmonicida* for many months in the sediments beneath cages also suggests that exposing the bacteria to aerobic conditions, e.g. by periodic harrowing of the sediment, may also be appropriate in some situations to speed up their eradication.

## Containment

As most of the problem, i.e. multiple-resistant strains, is confined to sea sites from which fish do not leave alive, discussion of containment is restricted to prevention of escapes, broodstock movement to fresh water and parr and smolt movements. Ova can be disinfected and should not be a risk factor. Preventing escapes is essential and in this context all work practices, e.g. net changing, net inspection and appropriateness of net materials, should be reviewed. Broodstock movement should present minimal problems in most situations. As noted under avoidance, movement of parr or smolts carrying multiple-resistant strains should not be allowed to occur.

## Regulation

Use of legislation, such as the powers of the Diseases of Fish Acts 1937 and 1983 in the UK, is currently restricted to preventing movement of salmon with clinical disease. It is difficult to see any extension of this, e.g. regulating the movement of covertly infected fish, because methods of detection of such fish are unreliable.

## Chemotherapy

This has been the major method of control but is now in default owing to the increasing occurrence of multiple-resistant strains. Licensing of new antimicrobials will help; e.g. amoxycillin is now added to the UK list of licensed antimicrobials but with some isolates of *A. salmonicida* already resistant to this compound total reliance on antimicrobials is clearly not a solution. The industry should aim for a situation where several antimicrobials can be effectively used but where the necessity for their use is minimal.

## Vaccines

It is to be expected that vaccines of greater efficacy will shortly be available and that their further development will lead to a degree of control of the disease comparable to the other fish vaccines referred to previously. If this is realized it will result in a much improved measure of control of the disease. However the current situation should be a warning to the industry that the

Atlantic salmon, as currently cultured, that is the methods of husbandry and fish strains presently used, has limitations, and that susceptibility to furunculosis is perhaps the greatest of these.

### Husbandry and the environment of the fish

There is little doubt that *A. salmonicida* awaits periodic stressful and exploits traumatic events in the fish farm system. Covertly infected fish are the probable major on-site reservoirs of infection. As a result of trauma allowing penetration of the pathogen beneath the integument or stressful conditions causing a depression of the humoral and cellular defences of the salmon in ways we do not fully understand, clinical disease is established in individual fish. Some of these causes of trauma and stress are controllable but others never will be, which is why vaccines and antimicrobial drugs will always be a necessary part of the fish farmer's armoury against furunculosis.

Trauma occurs when fish collide with nets and with each other, as a result of storms, transport, grading, vaccine and chemical treatments, and fright reactions as for example, during seal attacks. Lice also damage fish skin when feeding on mucus, skin and blood and may be carriers and spreaders of infection by moving from fish to fish, often selecting the weakest. Containing lice infestation (McHenery *et al.* 1991) is therefore essential in the efforts to control furunculosis outbreaks in sea water.

Stress is often induced simultaneously with incidents causing trauma, and also for other reasons such as establishment of hierarchies or poor water quality due to excessive fish numbers. Cage sites may be unsuitable, e.g. because of excessive or insufficient water flow, poor water quality or production targets too great for the site. Certainly some of these traumatic and stressful events may be minimized but their elimination is unlikely to be feasible.

### Resistance to furunculosis

It is to be anticipated that within each salmonid species strains will exist displaying varying resistance to each subspecies. Olivier *et al.* (1988) reported a genetic basis for such resistance in Atlantic salmon. Selection and breeding of such strains may well offer in the future a practical means of controlling this disease in farmed populations.

## Conclusions

Better control of furunculosis must be found soon; otherwise a significant contraction of the Atlantic salmon farming industry is likely wherever the disease occurs. It is improbable, given the reservoir of infection in wild fish, that *Aeromonas salmonicida* can be eradicated from farms. The advent of multiple-antibiotic-resistant strains of the bacterium in farm stocks is now preventing some farms from effectively controlling the disease. The past success of salmon farming, expanding to the present density of farms, would appear to be the major factor in spreading the infection and more recently leading to the spread of resistant strains.

If disease cannot be contained a lower level of production will be necessary, as the principal management controls left will be reduced stocking (both density of fish per cage and fewer cages per unit area), increased fallow times, greater areas of fallowing and better control of lice infestation. Such extreme measures might be avoided if several more antimicrobials were available for use and/or better vaccines become available.

# References

Anon. (1990) Report of the SOAFD Annual Survey of Fish Farms for 1990. SOAFD Marine Laboratory, Aberdeen. 15pp.

Antychowicz, J. & Rogulska, A. (1986) Preliminary investigations on the bacterial flora of the skin and erythrodermatitis ulcers of carp. *Bulletin of Veterinary Institute of Pulawy*, **28–29**(1–4), 42–5.

Aoki, T., Egusa, S., Kimura, T. & Watanabe, T. (1971) Detection of R factors in naturally occurring *Aeromonas salmonicida* strains. *Applied Microbiology*, **22**, 716–17.

Aoki, T., Kitao, T., Iemura, N., Mitoma, Y. & Nomura, T. (1983) The susceptibility of *Aeromonas salmonicida* strains isolated in cultured and wild salmonids to various chemotherapeutants. *Bulletin of the Japanese Society of Scientific Fisheries*, **49**, 17–22.

Aoki, T., Mitomoa, Y. & Crosa, J.H. (1986) The characterization of a conjugative R-plasmid isolated from *Aeromonas salmonicida*. *Plasmid*, **16**, 213–18.

Austin, B. & Austin, D.A. (1987) *Bacterial Fish Pathogens: Disease in Farmed and Wild Fish*. Ellis, Horwood Ltd, Chichester.

Barnes, A.C., Lewin, C.S., Hastings, T.S. & Amyes, S.G.B. (1990a) In vitro activities of 4-quinolones against the fish pathogen *Aeromonas salmonicida*. *Antimicrobial Agents and Chemotherapy*, **34**, 1819–20.

Barnes, A.C., Lewin, C.S., Hastings, T.S. & Amyes, S.G.B. (1990b) Cross resistance between oxytetracycline and oxolinic acid in *Aeromonas salmonicida* associated with alterations in outer membrane proteins. *FEMS Microbiology Letters*, **72**, 337–40.

Barnes, A.C., Amyes, S.G.B., Hastings, T.S. & Lewin, C.S. (1992) Alterations in outer membrane proteins identified in a clinical isolate of *Aeromonas salmonicida* subsp. *salmonicida*. *Journal of Fish Diseases*, **15**, 279–83.

Barnes, A.C., Lewin, C.S., Hastings, T.S. & Amyes, S.G.B. (1991a) Fluoroquinolones display rapid bactericidal activity and low mutation frequencies against *Aeromonas salmonicida*. *Journal of Fish Diseases*, **14**, 661–7.

Barnes, A.C., Lewin, C.S., Amyes, S.G.B. & Hastings, T.S. (1991b) Susceptibility of Scottish isolates of *Aeromonas salmonicida* to the antibacterial agent amoxycillin. *ICES CM* 1991/F : 28.

Belland, R. & Trust, T.J. (1988) DNA : DNA reassociation analysis of *Aeromonas salmonicida*. *Journal of General Microbiology*, **134**, 307–15.

Belland, R. & Trust, T.J. (1989) *Aeromonas salmonicida* plasmids: Plasmid-directed synthesis of proteins *in vitro* and in *Escherichia coli* minicells. *Journal of General Microbiology*, **135**, 513–24.

Böhm, K.H., Fuhrmann, H., Schlofeldt, H.-J. & Korting, W. (1986) *Aeromonas salmonicida* from salmonids and cyprinids — serological and cultural identification. *Journal of Veterinary Medicine*, **B33**, 777–83.

Brazil, G., Curley, D., Gannon, F. & Smith, P. (1987) Persistence and acquisition of antibiotic resistance plasmids in *Aeromonas salmonicida*. In *Banbury Report*, 24: *Antibiotic Resistance Genes: Ecology, Transfer and Expression* (Ed. by S. Levy & R.P. Novick), pp. 107–14. Cold Spring Harbor, New York.

Bruno, D.W., Munro, A.L.S. & Needham, E.A. (1986) Gill lesions caused by *Aeromonas salmonicida* in sea-reared Atlantic salmon, *Salmo salar* L. ICES CM 1986/F:6.

Buchan, R.E. & Gibbons, N.E. (eds) (1974) *Bergey's Manual of Determinative Bacteriology*, 8th edition. Williams and Wilkins, Baltimore.

Bullock, G.L. & Stuckey, H.M. (1975) *Aeromonas salmonicida*: detection of asymptomatically infected trout. *Progressive Fish-Culturist*, **37**, 237−9.

Bullock, G.L. & Stuckey, H.M. (1987) Studies on vertical transmission of *Aeromonas salmonicida*. *Progressive Fish Culturist*, **49**, 302−3.

Chart, H., Shaw, D.H., Ishiguro, E.E. & Trust, T.J. (1984) Structural and immunochemical homogeneity of *Aeromonas salmonicida* lipopolysaccharide. *Journal of Bacteriology*, **158**, 16−22.

Cornick, J.W., Morrison, C.M., Zwicker, B. & Shum, B. (1984) Atypical *Aeromonas salmonicida* infection in Atlantic cod *Gadus morhua* L. *Journal of Fish Diseases*, **7**, 495−9.

Duff, D.C.B. (1942) The oral immunization of trout against *Bacterium salmonicida*. *Journal of Immunology*, **44**, 87−94.

Ellis, A.E. (1991) An appraisal of the extracellular toxins of *Aeromonas salmonicida* ssp. *salmonicida*. *Journal of Fish Diseases*, **14**, 265−78.

Emmerich, R. & Weibel, E. (1894) Ueber eine durch Bakterien erzengte Seuche unter den Forellen. *Archives für Hygiene und Bakteriologie*, **21**, 1−21.

Evenberg, D., de Graaff, P., Fleuren, W. & van Muiswinkel, W.B. (1986) Blood changes in carp (*Cyprinus carpio*) induced by ulcerative *Aeromonas salmonicida* infections. *Veterinary Immunology and Immunopatholoy*, **12**, 321−30.

Ferguson, H.W. & McCarthy, D.H. (1978) Histopathology of furunculosis in brown trout *Salmo trutta* L. *Journal of Fish Diseases*, **1**, 165−74.

Griffin, P.J., Snieszko, S.F. & Friddle, S.B. (1953) A more comprehensive description of *Bacillus salmonicida*. *Transactions of the American Fisheries Society*, **82**, 241−53.

Griffiths, S.G. & Lynch, W.H. (1989) Characterization of *Aeromonas salmonicida* mutants with low level resistance to multiple antibiotics. *Antimicrobial Agents and Chemotherapy*, **33**, 19−26.

Hahnel, G.B., Gauld, R.W. & Boatman, E.S. (1983) Serological comparison of selected isolates of *Aeromonas salmonicida* ssp. *salmonicida*. *Journal of Fish Diseases*, **6**, 1−11.

Hamilton, R.C., Kalnins, H., Ackland, N.R. & Ashburner, L.D. (1981) An extra layer in the surface layers of an atypical *Aeromonas salmonicida* isolated from Australian goldfish. *Journal of General Microbiology*, **122**, 363−6.

Håstein, T. & Bullock, G.L. (1976) An acute septicaemic disease of brown trout and salmon caused by a *Pasteurella*-like organism. *Journal of Fish Biology*, **8**, 23−6.

Hastings, T.S. (1988) Furunculosis vaccines. In *Fish Vaccination* (Ed. by A.E. Ellis), pp. 93−111. Academic Press.

Hastings, T.S. & McKay, A. (1987) Resistance of *Aeromonas salmonicida* to oxolinic acid. *Aquaculture*, **61**, 165−71.

Hedges, R.W., Smith, P. & Brazil, G. (1985) Resistance plasmids of Aeromonads. *Journal of General Microbiology*, **131**, 2091−5.

Hennigan, M., Vaughan, L.M., Foster, T.J., Smith, P. & Gannon, A.F. (1989) Characterization of *Aeromonas salmonicida* strains using DNA probe technology. *Canadian Journal of Fisheries and Aquatic Science*, **46**, 877−9.

Horne, J.H. (1928) Furunculosis in trout and the importance of carriers in the spread of disease. *Journal of Hygiene*, **28**, 67−78.

Ishiguro, E.E., Kay, W.W., Ainsworth, T., Chamberlain, J., Buckley, J.T. & Trust, T.J. (1981) Loss of virulence during culture of *Aeromonas salmonicida* at high temperature. *Journal of Bacteriology*, **148**, 333−40.

Klontz, G.W., Yasutake, W.T. & Ross, A.J. (1966) Bacterial disease of the salmonidae in the western United States: pathogenesis of furunculosis in rainbow trout. *American Journal of Veterinary Research*, **27**, 1455−60.

McCarthy, D.H. (1978) A study of the taxonomic status of some bacteria currently assigned to the genus *Aeromonas*. Ph.D. Thesis. Council of National Academic Awards, UK.

McCarthy, D.H. & Rawle, C.T. (1975) Rapid serological diagnosis of fish furunculosis caused by smooth and rough strains of *Aeromonas salmonicida*. *Journal of General Microbiology*, **86**, 185−7.

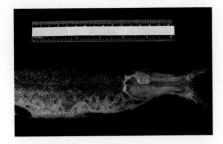

**Plate 1** Classic peduncle lesion on rainbow trout (*Oncorhynchus mykiss*) (Courtesy of late Dr S.F. Snieszko).

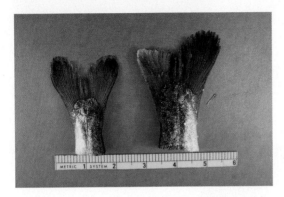

**Plate 2** Early cold water disease lesion on tail of coho salmon (*Oncorhynchus kisutch*) (Courtesy of Dr R.D. Wolke).

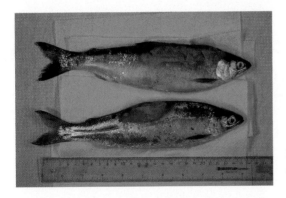

**Plate 3** Severe extensive *Flexibacter psychrophilus* infection in coho salmon (*Oncorhynchus kisutch*).

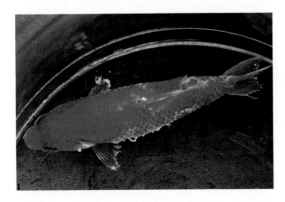

**Plate 4** Columnaris in a goldfish (*Carassius auratus*). The white sloughing exudate is a mixture of mucus, epithelial tissue and *Flexibacter* cells.

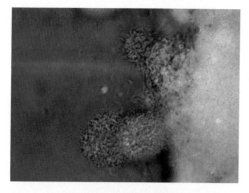

**Plate 5**   Swarm of *Flexibacter columnaris* cells forming the characteristic columns (Courtesy of late Dr S.F. Snieszko).

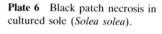

**Plate 6**   Black patch necrosis in cultured sole (*Solea solea*).

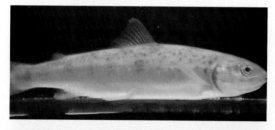

**Plate 7**   Normal dorsal fin on healthy young Atlantic salmon (*Salmo salar*).

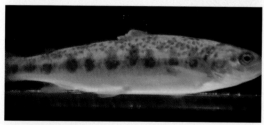

**Plate 8**   Typical thickened and eroded dorsal fin of young Atlantic salmon (*Salmo salar*) associated with the condition 'dorsal fin rot'.

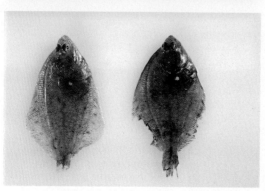

**Plate 9**   Peripheral fin rot in plaice (*Pleuronectes platessa*).

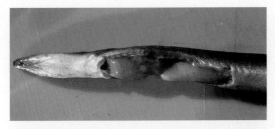

**Plate 10** Japanese eel (*Anguilla japonica*) infected with *Edwardsiella tarda*. There is a focal abscessation of the liver (Courtesy of Dr E.B. Shotts).

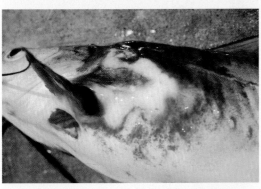

**Plate 11** Large white area of depigmentation with central haemorrhagic ulcer on flank of channel catfish (*Ictalurus punctatus*) infected with *E. tarda* (Courtesy of Dr F.P. Meyer).

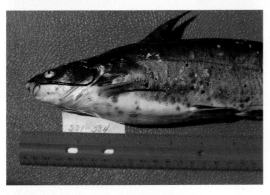

**Plate 12** Petechial haemorrhagic ulcers over the surface of channel catfish (*Ictalurus punctatus*) infected with *E. ictaluri* (Courtesy of Dr T.E. Schwedler).

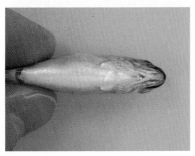

**Plate 13** Ventral reddening and haemorrhage, between opercula, in young rainbow trout (*Oncorhynchus mykiss*) naturally infected with enteric redmouth (ERM) (Courtesy of Dr R. Davies).

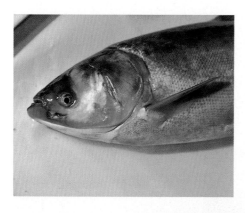

**Plate 14** *Proteus rettgeri* infection in silver carp (*Hypophthalmichthys molitrix*) from ponds fertilized with chicken manure (Courtesy of Dr I. Bejerano).

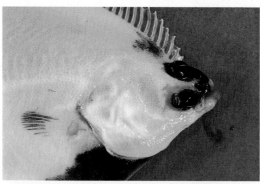

**Plate 15** Oral ulceration in albino plaice (*Pleuronectes platessa*) infected with chronic vibriosis (Courtesy Mr A. Finnie).

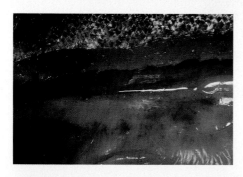

**Plate 16** Deep seated *Vibrio anguillarum* lesion in Atlantic salmon (*Salmo salar*) (Courtesy Dr T. Hastein).

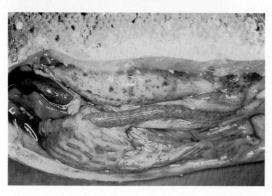

**Plate 17** Generalized petechiation of viscera in Hitra disease or cold-water vibriosis (Courtesy of late Dr E. Egidius).

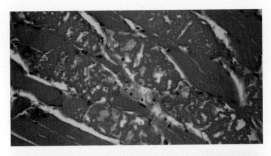

**Plate 18** Typical necrotizing myositis of Hitra disease associated with minimal inflammatory response to the numerous bacteria present (H&E × 600) (Courtesy of late Dr E. Egidius).

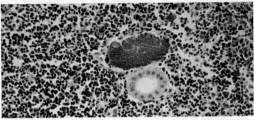

**Plate 19** Colony of *Aeromonas salmonicida* within the anterior kidney of Atlantic salmon (*Salmo salar*) parr (H&E × 100) (Courtesy of Dr T. Hastein).

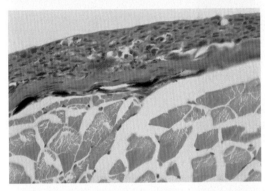

**Plate 20** Colony of *Aeromonas salmonicida* within basal epidermis of Atlantic salmon (*Salmo salar*) parr (H&E × 100) (Courtesy Dr T. Hastein).

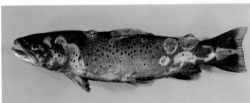

**Plate 21** Furunculosis in brown trout (*Salmo trutta*), with *Saprolegnia* fungus over the surface of furuncles (Courtesy Dr J.E. Thorpe).

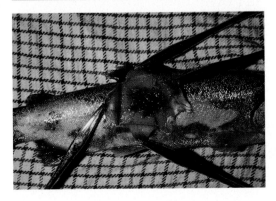

**Plate 22** Furuncle dissected to show the necrotic muscle containing large numbers of *Aeromonas salmonicida* bacteria.

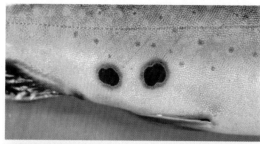

**Plate 23** Ulcer disease in brook trout (*Salvelinus fontinalis*), caused by aberrant *Aeromonas salmonicida*. The characteristic lesion shown here has a ring of melanin around the edge (Courtesy of Dr A. Walker).

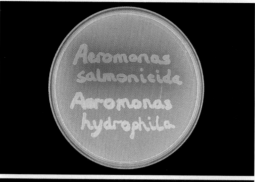

**Plate 24** Cultures of *Aeromonas salmonicida* and *Aeromonas hydrophila*, showing the former secreting brown diffusible pigment into the nutrient agar.

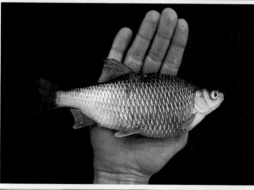

**Plate 25** *Aeromonas hydrophila* septicaemia of a roach (*Rutilus rutilus*) showing generalized hyperaemia and scale-oedema (Courtesy of Dr R. Bootsma).

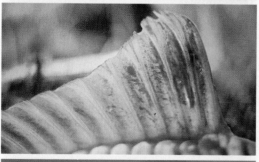

**Plate 26** Chronic aeromonad lesion of dorsal fin of mirror carp (*Cyprinus carpio*) with carp dropsy syndrome (Courtesy Professor N. Fijan).

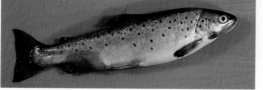

**Plate 27** Female brown trout (*Salmo trutta*) with large haemorrhagic prolapse of the rectum and associated vent lesion due to *Aeromonas hydrophila* infection (Courtesy Mr A. Finnie).

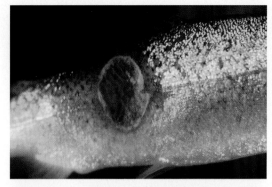

**Plate 28** Shallow ulcer induced by *Pseudomonas fluorescens* in rainbow trout (*Oncorhynchus mykiss*) chronically infected with virus (Courtesy Dr M.T. Horne).

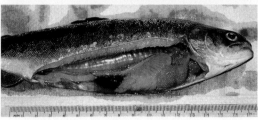

**Plate 29** Granulomata of *Renibacterium salmoninarum* in heart and liver of Atlantic salmon (*Salmo salar*) (Courtesy of Professor R.H. Richards).

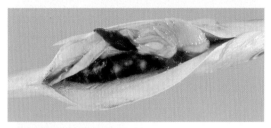

**Plate 30** Granulomata in the kidney and spleen of Atlantic salmon (*Salmo salar*) smolt (Courtesy of Professor R.H. Richards).

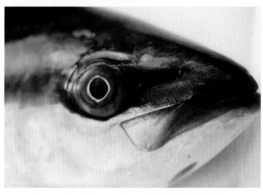

**Plate 31** Yellowtail (*Seriola quinqueradiata*) infected with streptococcosis, showing marked exophthalmia.

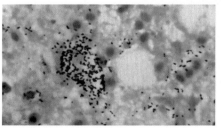

**Plate 32** Direct impression smear from brain of diseased yellowtail (*Seriola quinqueradiata*), showing the arrangement of *Streptococcus* microorganisms (H&E × 540).

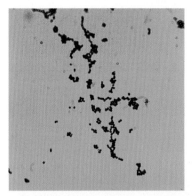

**Plate 33** *Streptococcus* spp. showing Gram-positive staining reaction and characteristic chain formation (Gram × 2000).

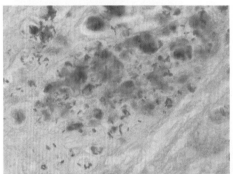

**Plate 34** Tubercle from the liver of a guppy (*Poecilia reticulata*) showing an array of acid fast (red) *Mycobacterium* bacilli in a stroma of caseous necrotic tissue (Z.N. × 2000) (Courtesy of Dr G. Timur).

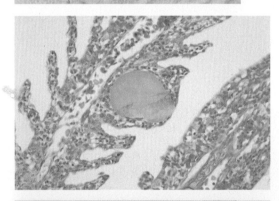

**Plate 35** Epitheliocystis colony between the secondary lamellae of a gilthead bream (*Sparus aurata*) (H&E × 400).

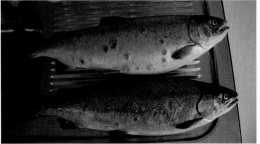

**Plate 36** Skin lesions associated with coho salmon (*Oncorhynchus kisutch*) syndrome attributed to *Piscirickettsia salmonis* (Courtesy of Mr E. Branson).

McCarthy, D.H. & Roberts, R.J. (1980) Furunculosis in fish — the present state of our knowledge. In *Advances in Aquatic Microbiology* (Ed. by M.R. Droop & H.W. Jannasch), pp. 293–341. Academic Press, London.

MacInnes, J.I., Trust, T.J. & Crosa, J.H. (1979) Deoxyribonucleic acid relationships among members of the genus *Aeromonas. Canadian Journal of Microbiology*, **25**, 579–86.

McHenery, J.G., Turrell, W.R. & Munro, A.L.S. (1991) Controlled use of the insecticide dichlorvos in Atlantic salmon farming. In *OIE (Paris) Special Publications Symposium, Problems of Chemotherapy in Aquaculture: From Theory to Reality*. OIE, Paris.

Mackie, T.J., Arkwright, J.A., Pryce-Tannatt, T.E., Mottram, J.C., Johnston, W.D. & Menzies, W.J.M. (1930, 1933, 1935). *Interim, Second and Final Reports of the Furunculosis Committee*. HMSO, Edinburgh.

Miyazaki, T. & Kubota, S.S. (1975) Histopathological studies of furunculosis in Amazo. *Fish Pathology*, **9**, 213–18.

Morrison, C.M., Cornick, J.W., Shum, G. & Zwicker, B. (1984) Histopathology of atypical *Aeromonas salmonicida* infection in Atlantic cod, *Gadus morhua* L. *Journal of Fish Diseases*, **7**, 477–94.

Munro, A.L.S. (1984) A furunculosis vaccine: illusion or achievable objective. In *Symposium on Fish Vaccination* (Ed. by P. de Kinkelin), pp. 97–120. OIE, Paris.

Munro, A.L.S. & Waddell, I.F. (1984) Furunculosis: experience of its control in the sea water culture of Atlantic salmon in Scotland. ICES CM 1984/F:32, 7pp.

Olivier, G., Friars, G.W. & Bailey, J. (1988) Genetic basis for resistance to furunculosis in Atlantic salmon (*Salmo salar* L.). *Bulletin of the Aquaculture Association of Canada*, **88**(2), 88.

Ostland, V.E., Hicks, B.D. & Daly, J.G. (1987) Furunculosis in baitfish and its transmission to salmonids. *Diseases of Aquatic Organisms*, **2**(3), 163–6.

Popoff, M. (1971*a*) Etude sur les *Aeromonas salmonicida*. II Caracterisation des bacteriophages actifs sur les *Aeromonas salmonicida* et lysotopie. *Annales de Recherche Vétérinaire*, **2**, 33–45.

Popoff, M. (1971*b*) Interet diagnostique d'un bacteriophage specifique des *Aeromonas salmonicida. Annales de Recherche Vétérinaire*, **2**, 137–9.

Popoff, M. (1984). Genus III *Aeromonas* Kluyver & van Niel 1936, 398[AL]. In *Bergey's Manual of Systematic Bacteriology*, Vol. 1 (Ed. by N.R. Krieg), pp. 545–8. Williams and Wilkins, Baltimore.

Richards, R.H., Inglis, V., Frerichs, G.N. & Millar, S.D. (1992) Variation in antibiotic resistance patterns of *Aeromonas salmonicida* isolated from Atlantic salmon *Salmo salar* L. in Scotland. In *Chemotherapy in Aquaculture: from Theory to Reality* (Ed. by C. Michel & D.J. Alderman), pp. 276–84. Office International des Epizooties (OIE), Paris.

Rose, A.S., Ellis, A.E. & Munro, A.L.S. (1989) The infectivity by different routes of exposure and shedding rates of *Aeromonas salmonicida* subsp. *salmonicida* in Atlantic salmon, *Salmo salar* L., held in sea water. *Journal of Fish Diseases*, **12**, 573–8.

Schubert, R.H.W. (1974) Genus II. *Aeromonas* Kluyver & van Niel 1936, 398. In *Bergey's Manual of Determinative Bacteriology* 8th edn (Ed. by R.E. Buchanan & N.E. Gibbons), pp. 345–448. Williams & Wilkins, Baltimore.

Skerman, V.B.D., McGowan, V. & Sneath, P.H.A. (1980) Approved lists of bacterial names. *International Journal of Systematic Bacteriology*, **30**, 225–420.

Smith, I. (1962) Furunculosis in kelts. *Freshwater and Salmon Fisheries Research*, No. 27, 12pp. HMSO.

Smith, I.W. (1963) The classification of *Bacterium salmonicida. Journal of General Microbiology*, **33**, 263–74.

Smith, J.T. (1986) The mode of action of 4-quinolones and possible mechanisms of resistance. *Journal of Antimicrobial Chemotherapy*, **18**, Supplement D, 21–9.

Snieszko, S.F., Griffin, P.J. & Friddle, S.B. (1950) A new bacterium (*Haemophilus piscium* n.sp.) from ulcer disease of trout. *Journal of Bacteriology*, **59**, 699–710.

Stewart, M., Beveridge, T.J. & Trust, T.J. (1986) Two patterns in the *Aeromonas salmonicida* A — layer may reflect a structural transformation that alters permeability. *Journal of Bacteriology*, **166**, 120–7.

Toranzo, A.E., Barja, J.L., Colwell, R.R. & Hetrick, F.M. (1983) Characterization of plasmids in bacterial fish pathogens. *Infection and Immunity*, **39**, 184–92.

Tsoumas, A., Alderman, D.J. & Rodgers, C.J. (1989) *Aeromonas salmonicida*: development of resistance to 4-quinolone antimicrobials. *Journal of Fish Diseases*, **12**, 493–507.

Turrell, W.R. & Munro, A.L.S. (1988) A theoretical study of the dispersal of soluble and infectious wastes from farmed Atlantic salmon net cages in a hypothetical sea loch. ICES CM 1988/F:36, 20pp.

Udey, L.R. & Fryer, J.L. (1978) Immunization of fish with bacterins of *Aeromonas salmonicida*. *Marine Fisheries Review*, **40**(3), 12–17.

Vallejo, A.N. & Ellis, A.E. (1989) Ultrastructural study of the response of eosinophil granule cells to *Aeromonas salmonicida* extracellular product and histamine liberations in rainbow trout *Salmo gairdneri* Richardson. *Developmental and Comparative Immunology*, **13**, 133–48.

Wichardt, U.-P., Johnsson, N. & Lyunberg, O. (1989) Occurrence and distribution of *Aeromonas salmonicida* infection on Swedish fish farms, 1951–1987. *Journal of Aquatic Animal Health*, **1**(3), 187–96.

Wood, S.C., McCashion, R.N. & Lynch, W.H. (1986) Multiple low-level antibiotic resistance in *Aeromonas salmonicida*. *Antimicrobial Agents and Chemotherapy*, **29**, 992–6.

# Chapter 8:
# Motile Aeromonad Septicaemia

The motile aeromonads associated with haemorrhagic septicaemia in fresh water fish are
*Aeromonas hydrophila, A. caviae* and *A. sobria*. They are characteristic of the genus, being
Gram-negative facultative anaerobes, non-spore forming, motile with single polar flagella
and resistant to the vibriostat 0/129. Although there is some doubt about whether they act
as primary pathogens, they make a significant contribution to the disease process in those
fish which they do invade. They may cause clinical dropsy, ulceration and widespread tissue
necrosis. Losses may be substantial and control is dependent on eliminating the underlying
factors predisposing to infection.

## Introduction

The aeromonads are characteristically bacteria of fresh water. The motile
species are often ubiquitous members of the aquatic ecosystem, but all can be
components of the microbial flora of aquatic animals and may be pathogens of
poikilotherms, homoiotherms and even man (Fraire 1978, Salton & Schnick
1973), while the non-motile species *A. salmonicida* (formerly *Bacillus salmonicida*) (Griffin *et al.* 1953) is an obligate pathogen of fish (Plate 25).

The motile aeromonads show very considerable heterogeneity and their
taxonomy is confused. Various isolates defined earlier as *Bacillus, Bacterium* or
*Aerobacter* and generally isolated from diseased fish or frogs were brought
together by Kluyver & van Niel (1936) to form the *Aeromonas* genus, and
subsequently characterised as *Aeromonas hydrophila, Aeromonas punctata* and
*Aeromonas liquefaciens* (Snieszko 1957). These descriptions were based principally on pathogenicity and some biochemical tests, and although the legitimacy
of the genus is not now questioned generally, there remains a degree of
confusion over speciation (Ewing & Johnstone 1960, Page 1962, Schubert
1967, 1969, 1974).

Schubert (1974) described five sub-species of motile aeromonads, three of
them subspecies of *Aeromonas hydrophila* and two of *A. punctata*. This stimulated Popoff & Veron (1976) to publish a complex Adansonian analysis of
motile aeromonads which suggested differentiation into three species, *A. hydrophila, A. caviae* and *A. sobria*. Most of the pathogenic strains were encompassed
within the first grouping. This definition of three species has now broadly been
confirmed by analysis of core oligosaccharides (Shaw & Hodder 1978) and
DNA-hybridization (Popoff *et al.* 1981), but it is recognized that within these
nomenspecies there are a number of sub-groups.

For the purposes of the present review the motile aeromonads will be
classified as the three species *A. hydrophila, A. caviae* and *A. sobria*, but
it seems likely that in the fullness of time Austin & Austin's (1987) view

that several distinct species may be masquerading within the specific epithet *Aeromonas hydrophila* may be proved correct.

After the complexity of the taxonomy of the motile aeromonads, that of the non-motile component of the genus is relatively straightforward. It comprises a single species, characterised, within the aeromonads, by lack of motility and a high degree of obligate parasitism on fishes. Two distinct sub-groupings, characterized principally by presence or absence of pigment production, have been suggested as a basis for subdivision into separate species. Biochemical differentiation of strains of oriental origin into a third species *A. masoucida* has also been suggested. DNA homology studies, however, emphasise the close genetic relationship of all three groups (MacInnes *et al.* 1979) and so generally *A. salmonicida* is used as the single specific epithet for all non-motile aeromonads. The subsidiary varietal terms var. *salmonicida*, var. *achromogenes* and var. *masoucida* are used on occasion to delineate below species level but the high level of homology suggested by the mean mol % G + C value suggests that this should be unnecessary (MacInnes *et al.* 1979).

The motile aeromonads and their involvement in diseases of fish will be considered in this chapter.

## Biological characteristics of motile aeromonads

Motile aeromonads are found in all waters except the most saline. Although they may occur in relatively unpolluted water they are much more abundant in waters with a high organic load (Hazen *et al.* 1978, Heuschmann-Brunner 1978, Kaper *et al.* 1981). Thus they are frequently found in waters with high sewage levels (Geldreich 1974).

The motile aeromonads, as the group appellation suggests, are characterized by active motility, achieved by means of a single polar flagellum, and production of gas, as well as acid, from carbohydrates (Fig. 8.1). They are Gram-negative bacilli or cocco-bacilli measuring $0.5\,\mu \times 1.0-1.5\,\mu$. They are aerobic and facultatively anaerobic, fermenting carbohydrates with the formation of acid, and they produce 3-butanediol. They are cytochrome oxidase positive, reduce nitrates, are resistant to the pteridine vibriostat 0/129 and have a G-C ratio of 57–63% (Newman 1982).

Generally the differentiation into species is performed on the basis of carbohydrate and other biochemical reactions, with the three species *A. hydrophila*, *A. caviae* and *A. sobria* being readily distinguished on the basis of the differentiating factors defined by Popoff & Veron (1976) and given in Table 8.1.

## Antigenic structure

In many respects the motile aeromonads are as diverse antigenically as they are biochemically. Despite this diversity of H and O antigens (Ewing *et al.* 1961, Takahashi & Kusuda 1977), Thune, reported by Newman (1982), was able to

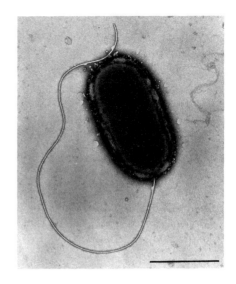

**Fig. 8.1** Electron micrograph of *Aeromonas sobria*, showing the single elongated flagellum (Courtesy of Dr Alicia Toranzo).

show that an antiserum prepared against one particular strain of *A. hydrophila* was effective in removing the haemolytic activity of all other strains examined. He has also observed that heat-labile extracellular proteases of such strains also had common precipitins.

The somatic or O antigens of the motile aeromonads are very heterogeneous (Eddy 1960, Liu 1961). Rao & Foster (1977) found species specific O antigens for the different species although this was not confirmed by Takahashi & Kusuda (1977).

## Extracellular toxin production

Nord *et al.* (1975) showed that strains of *A. hydrophila* produce gelatinase, caseinase, elastase, lipase, lecithinase and deoxyribonuclease in addition to the haemolysins, cytotoxins and enterotoxins which had previously been described

**Table 8.1** Differentiation between the motile *Aeromonas* species by biochemical properties (Adapted from Popoff (1984)

| Characteristics | *A. hydrophila* | *A. caviae* | *A. sobria* |
|---|---|---|---|
| Motility | + | + | + |
| Aesculin hydrolysis | + | + | − |
| Growth in KCN broth | + | + | − |
| L-Histidine & L-arginine utilization | + | + | − |
| L-Arabinose utilization | + | + | − |
| Fermentation of salicin | + | + | − |
| Acetoin production (VP test) | + | − | + |
| Gas from glucose | + | − | + |
| H₂S from cysteine | + | − | + |

(Boulanger *et al.* 1977, Wretlind *et al.* 1971, Donta *et al.* 1978). A dermonecrotic factor, demonstrable in a rabbit skin test, allowed differentiation of *A. hydrophila* from *A. sobria* (Olivier *et al.* 1981). Dermonecrotic strains of *A. hydrophila* caused haemolysis on sheep blood agar plates when incubated at both 10°C and 30°C, whereas *A. sobria* was haemolytic only at 30°C.

The correlation of extracellular toxins and haemolysin production with pathogenicity has been suggested by a number of workers (Hsu *et al.* 1981, Allan & Stevenson 1981, Thune *et al.* 1982) but more recently Thune *et al.* (1986) have found no correlation between β-haemolysin production and pathogenicity, or, for that matter, between protease production and virulence (Chabot & Thune 1991). Shotts *et al.* (1985) found that elastase production exhibited a positive correlation with virulence but found no other correlation. The presence of an S-layer on the surface of cells was strongly correlated with virulence in laboratory challenge (Thune *et al.* 1986), with 95% of isolates from field outbreaks also being associated with the possession of an S-layer. Shotts and his co-workers (Shotts *et al.* 1985, Del Corral *et al.* 1990) in addition to studying proteases and other exotoxins as virulence factors in motile aeromonad infections, have studied the physical capacity of the bacterial cells to adhere to erythrocytes, on the basis that the ability to adhere to host cells is a pre-requisite to infection. They concluded that the ability of particular strains to produce disease was not directly related to adherence capacity but that disease appeared to be related to multiple physiological and biochemical markers. It was difficult to define any single factor or group of factors which could fully account for the degree of virulence.

## Diseases associated with motile aeromonads

Disease associated with this abundant and widespread group of micro-organisms was first recognised in the 19th century when Sanarelli (1891) reported an outbreak of a disease in eels associated with what is presumed to have been either this micro-organism, or *Vibrio anguillarum*. Subsequently Schäperclaus (1930) described a disease of carp (*Cyprinus carpio*), characterized by abdominal swelling, from which he isolated pure cultures of *Bacterium punctatum*. This condition, known as carp dropsy, is now recognised as having a virus as its prime aetiological agent, but *A. hydrophila* (formerly *B. punctatum*) is certainly a component of its pathology. It has also been isolated from diseased frogs (Gibbs 1963), alligators (Shotts *et al.* 1972), snails (Mead 1969), and freshwater prawns (De Figueredo & Plumb 1971).

Its role in human disease is generally in association with other conditions, so that, as in fishes, its pathogenicity often seems to be associated with stressed or compromised hosts. It has been associated with ophthalmitis and ulceration, skin and wound infections, meningitis and septicaemia in man (Dean & Tost 1967, Ketover *et al.* 1973, Joseph *et al.* 1979, Quadri *et al.* 1976).

The principal feature of the pathogenesis of all infections of fishes by the bacterium, whether primary or, much more likely, secondary to some other initiating factor, is generalised dissemination in the form of a bacteraemia, followed by elaboration of toxins, tissue necrosis and the clinical disease known as bacterial haemorrhagic septicaemia. *A. caviae* and *A. sobria* are also on occasion associated with diseases. G.N. Frerichs (unpublished) showed *A. sobria* to be present in the majority of moribund fishes affected with epizootic ulcer disease in Bangladesh, while Toranzo *et al.* (1989) found *A. sobria* to be associated with outbreaks of fatal disease in gizzard shad (*Dorosoma cepedianum*) and showed it to be pathogenic to rainbow trout (*Oncorhynchus mykiss*) in the laboratory.

## Motile aeromonad septicaemia (red pest)

The former and very non-specific name bacterial haemorrhagic septicaemia, which could apply to almost all of the Gram-negative systemic infections of fishes, is no longer used since the term motile aeromonad septicaemia, which was originally applied to the condition in catfish (*Ictaluris punctatus*) culture (Thune *et al.* 1982), is a much more precise and descriptive term. The other epithets used, such as red pest, are a relic of the earlier days of fish bacteriology where little was known of the roles of environmental stressors, host factors such as sexual maturation and other agents of infectious diseases such as viruses and fungi.

Bacterial haemorrhagic septicaemia, whether caused by motile aeromonads, or by other Gram-negatives, is a particular feature of pond fishes such as the cultured cyprinids or catfishes. Seasonal outbreaks of a variety of diseases of cyprinids, now known to be associated with primary viral or parasitic infection, with sudden change of environmental or nutritional status, or with husbandry change, were originally blamed on the motile aeromonad invasion which almost invariably accompanies and exacerbates them (Fijan 1972).

Such secondary invasions with motile aeromonads also characterize a wide range of other diseases, such as epizootic ulcerative syndrome (EUS) of Asian rice-field fishes (Tonguthai 1984), furunculosis of salmonids (Austin & Austin 1987), red-sore disease of large mouth bass (*Microplexus salmoides*) (Hazen *et al.* 1978) and many parasite conditions of tropical farmed fishes which are all characterized by acute haemorrhagic septicaemia and ulceration (Roberts 1989).

There is some dubiety, therefore, as to whether motile aeromonads should even be considered as primary pathogens. There is little doubt however, that once they have invaded a host which has been compromised for whatever reason, they rapidly make the condition worse and can be responsible for ultimate death. The complexity of the situation does make for difficulties of diagnosis and treatment. Unless the underlying primary cause also can be removed, or in the case of a virus or parasitic condition has run its course, treatment specifically for the aeromoniasis will be of little value in the longer term.

*Aeromonas hydrophila*, *Aeromonas caviae* and *Aeromonas sobria* have all been isolated from fish with the clinical signs of bacterial septicaemia, although *A. hydrophila* is by far the most frequently associated. Occasionally other aquatic Gram-negatives such as *Pseudomonas fluorescens* (Roberts & Horne 1978, Schäperclaus 1926) or *Proteus rettgeri* (Bejerano *et al.* 1976) may be isolated in pure culture, or as the dominant component, from such fish.

**Clinical signs**

The pathognomic signs of motile aeromonad septicaemia are, as the name implies, closely linked to the capacity of the relevant species to induce rupture of minor blood vessels (Plate 25). The haemorrhages caused by a soluble haemolysin, which has been cloned and characterized (Aoki & Hirono 1991) may be associated with ulcerative skin lesions, and may be on the surface of organs or deep within tissues. External lesions may vary from an extensive superficial reddening of the surface of a large area of the body, often with necrosis of fins or tail (fin rot), to extensive ulceration over a considerable portion of the flanks or dorsum. If the vent is involved it may also prolapse. The ulcers are usually shallow. They may be punctate (0.5 cm in diameter) and numerous, or take the form of two or three much larger, shallow defects with black edge, white rim and bright red haemorrhagic surface. The surface of the ulcer may go brown as it necrotizes and at cooler temperatures it is common for it to become secondarily infected with the fungus *Saprolegnia diclina* (Thorpe & Roberts 1972).

In cyprinids the condition may be peracute, with few signs, acute, with the typical syndrome described above, or chronic, with large, long-standing ulcers. It is often associated with abdominal oedema or dropsy. This non-specific feature may be associated with primary viral infection which has been exacerbated by the aeromonad, and this is known as the carp dropsy syndrome (Plate 26). Abdominal oedema occurs not infrequently in many cyprinid diseases where virus involvement is not a factor.

Internally there may be an excess of clear or red-tinged ascitic fluid in clinical dropsy, but in most cases the principal feature at post mortem is hyperaemia of viscera with haemorrhage over mesenteries and within visceral and parietal peritoneum. In severe cases the entire viscera may be bright red in colour and fibrinous adhesions may be present. The spleen is visibly enlarged, rounded, and cherry red. The enlarged kidney has often undergone liquefactive necrosis and when it is incised thick necrotic fluid oozes out.

There may be focal myonecrosis, but rarely is this deep within the muscle, as in furunculosis. Usually the necrosis of muscle will be superficial and associated with ulcers, or else around the vent, in the event of rectal prolapse (Plate 27).

Histologically the condition is characterised as a generalised necrotising septicaemia with focal lesions (Fig. 8.2). There are generalized hyperaemic and

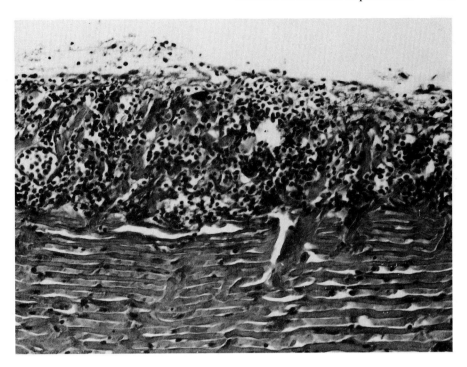

**Fig. 8.2**  Ulcerated aeromonad lesion in brown trout with extensive haemorrhage into the stratum spongiosum of the dermis (H&E × 400) (Courtesy of Dr J.E. Thorpe).

haemorrhagic capillary beds, with a high level of macrophages and other leukocytes within them and migrating from them. The lesions are generally focal areas or zones of acute liquefactive necrosis (Fig. 8.3) and are particularly apparent in the spleen and in the kidney, where haemopoietic tissue may be completely destroyed (Bach *et al.* 1978). Colonies of bacteria are not as frequently observed as in furunculosis but isolated bacterial cells or clusters may be observed within macrophages or in damaged tissue. A particularly characteristic feature is the presence of large amounts of free melanin or lipofuscin, from ruptured haemopoietic melanomacrophage centres. Small, but very distinctive, particles of such pigment are also found with considerable frequency within the macrophages of the circulating blood or within tissue macrophages (Roberts 1989).

In the kidney, tubular epithelial cells are frequently sloughed into the lumen, and often only the glomerulus remains intact, surrounded by a congery of necrotic tubular and haemopoietic tissue. The intestinal vascular bed is usually highly congested, with the submucosa oedematous and rich in macrophages and lymphocytes. The overlying mucosa is generally necrotic and large expanses of mucosal epithelium may have sloughed into the gut lumen (Thorpe & Roberts 1972).

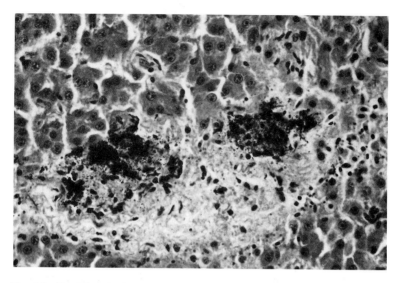

**Fig. 8.3** Focal liquefactive lesion of the liver of brown trout caused by *Aeromonas hydrophila*. Colonies of bacteria are obvious and the absence of a significant cellular inflammatory response (H&E × 600) (Courtesy Dr J.E. Thorpe).

### Fin rot

In farmed pond fishes, it is not uncommon to find, in spring or autumn especially, a condition characterised by brownish necrosis of fins or tail, with chronic haemorrhagic ulceration at the base of the fins or, more frequently, congestions of the subepithelial vessels. *Aeromonas hydrophila* can be isolated from the lesions, and occasionally from internal organs. The condition appears to be totally related to husbandry and water quality practices.

### Scale oedema

Hyperaemia of large areas of the posterior body surface, with protrusion of the scales, can often be seen in pond fishes at times of water shortage or high temperatures. Affected fish may swim normally, or hang in the water, on their sides. The condition is also seen in ornamental goldfish (*Carassius auratus*) and occasionally in cyprinids in stocked fisheries. *Aeromonas sobria* or *A. hydrophila* can be isolated in pure culture from such affected fish. Mortalities are rarely high unless the condition progresses to a full scale epizootic of haemorrhagic septicaemia.

## Epizootiology

The various syndromes with which motile aeromonads are associated vary widely depending on the nature of the initiating stimulus. Thus in cyprinids a very common feature, whether in the case of pond reared carp or ornamental goldfish, is the development of an outbreak in spring, when water temperatures are rising, the fishes' metabolism is increasing, and nutrient level in the water, as well as nutritional status of the fish, is rising. At such times, outbreaks of virus infections such as *Rhabdovirus carpei* (Fijan 1972), sudden changes of temperature, or handling or transfer of fish, can lead to explosive losses with involvement of motile aeromonads.

Similarly, in salmonids outbreaks are characterized by sudden rise in temperature in organic rich water bodies or at sexual maturity. In the epizootic ulcerative syndrome of rice field fishes, the condition generally coincides with lower temperatures and the onset of the dry season.

The inter-relationship between outbreaks of disease and individual strains is an important factor in determining the outcome. Chabot & Thune (1992) have shown that strains with a characteristic 'S-layer' on their surface were likely to be particularly virulent in catfish aeromonad infections, and Torres *et al.* (1990) have shown that strains with a particular heat-stable antigen are likely to be found in association with epizootic ulcer disease affected snakeheads.

## Control

Control of *Aeromonas hydrophila* infection is ideally linked to the control of the underlying factors which have facilitated its invasion of the host. However, when an outbreak occurs, especially among pond fishes, it is generally not possible to determine the underlying stress factors or primary infections, nor is it generally possible to change water flows or stocking densities with any ease. Thus treatment is generally attempted in the form of oral antibiotic therapy.

Chemotherapy for *A. hydrophila* infections depends to a considerable extent on availability and national regulations and corresponds closely to that for *A. salmonicida*. Chloramphenicol and nifurpirinol (Fijan *et al.* 1967), oxytetracycline (Meyer 1964) and sulphamerazine (Seaman 1951) have been used. Generally they are efficacious in the case of fish which are still feeding, but as with any oral treatment, fish which are sufficiently severely affected as to be inappetent, do not receive the treatment. A major problem with antibiotic treatment of *Aeromonas hydrophila*, as indeed with most bacterial infections, is that antibiotic resistance develops readily (Mitchell & Plumb 1980, Aoki & Egusa 1971). It is generally plasmid related, and transferable R-plasmids responsible for multiple drug resistance have been described for most of the antibiotics used to treat aeromonad infections (Ansary *et al.* 1991, Chang & Bolton 1987).

Antibiotics are also used prophylactically in carp culture at times of year when haemorrhagic septicaemia is most likely, i.e. when environmental or husbandry changes are most likely to stress the fish. Thus in central European carp culture many millions of fish are injected with chloramphenicol each year. This is generally implemented immediately before the advent of the spring temperature rise which in conjuction with *Rhabdovirus carpio* infection is so frequently a stimulus to outbreaks of haemorrhagic septicaemia (Schäperclaus 1954, 1959, Fijan 1972).

Vaccination is an alternative method of prophylaxis, and is already a commercial reality in diseases such as vibriosis and enteric redmouth disease. The antigenic diversity of the motile aeromonads suggests that even if resistance to one particular strain was achieved it would be unlikely to protect against the many other potentially pathogenic members of the genus. Thus while there may be some merit in protecting a population against the particular strain(s) in its own environment, a polyvalent vaccine would be necessary if any commercially viable product was to be developed.

The motile aeromonad infections can at times cause devastating losses in both wild and farmed fish populations. Since they are almost invariably associated with the invasion of a pathogenic strain into a stressed population, control, at least in farmed populations, has to be aimed primarily at reducing the level of possible stressors. Since often the stressor is external to the system and may relate to meteorological or agricultural factors beyond the farmers' control, even the most carefully managed systems will be vulnerable at some time, especially in tropical and sub-tropical waters with their high organic loadings.

# References

Allan, B.J. & Stevenson, R.M.W. (1981) Extracellular virulence factors of *Aeromonas hydrophila* in fish infections. *Canadian Journal of Microbiology*, **27**, 1114–22.

Ansary, A., Haneef, R.M., Torres, J.L. & Yadav, M. (1992) Plasmids and antibiotic resistance in *A. hydrophila*. *Journal of Fish Biology*, **15**, 191–6.

Aoki, T. & Egusa, S. (1971) Drug sensitivity of *Aeromonas liquefaciens* isolated from freshwater fishes. *Bulletin of the Japanese Society of Scientific Fisheries*, **37**, 176–85.

Aoki, T. & Hirono, I. (1991) Cloning and characterization of the haemolysin determinants from *Aeromonas hydrophila*. *Journal of Fish Diseases*, **14**, 305–14.

Austin, B. & Austin, D.A. (1987) *Bacterial Fish Pathogens*. Ellis Horwood, Chichester, pp. 11–195.

Bach, R., Chen, P.K. & Chapman, G.B. (1978) Changes in the spleen of the channel catfish *Ictalurus punctatus* Rafinesque induced by infection with *Aeromonas hydrophila*. *Journal of Fish Diseases*, **1**, 205–18.

Bejerano, Y., Sarig, S., Horne, M.T. & Roberts, R.J. (1976) Mass mortalities in silver carp, *Hypophthalmichthys molitrix* (Valenciennes) associated with bacterial infection following handling. *Journal of Fish Diseases*, **2**, 49–56.

Boulanger, Y., Lallier, R. & Cousineau, G. (1977) Isolation of enterotoxigenic *Aeromonas* from fish. *Canadian Journal of Microbiology*, **23**, 1161–4.

Chabot, J.D. & Thune, R.L. (1991) Proteases of the *Aeromonas hydrophila* complex. *Journal of Fish Diseases*, **14**(2), 171–84.

Chang, B.J. & Bolton, S.M. (1987) Plasmids and resistance to antimicrobial agents in *Aeromonas sobria* and *Aeromonas hydrophila* clinical isolates. *Antimicrobial Agents and Chemotherapy*, **31**, 1281–2.

Del Corral, F., Shotts, E.B. & Brown, J. (1990) Adherence haemagglutination and cell surface characteristics of motile aeromonads virulent for fish. *Journal of Fish Diseases*, **13**, 255–68.

Dean, H.M. & Tost, R.M. (1967) Fatal infection with *Aeromonas hydrophila* in a patient with acute myalogenous leukaemia. *Annals of Internal Medicine*, **66**, 1177–9.

Donta, S.T. & Haddow, A.D. (1978) Cytotoxic activity of *Aeromonas hydrophila*. *Infection and Immunity*, **21**, 989−93.

Eddy, B.P. (1960) Cephalotrichous, fermentative Gram-negative bacteria: The genus *Aeromonas*. *Journal of Applied Bacteriology*, **23**, 216−49.

Ewing W.H., Hugh, R. & Johnson, J.G. (1961). *Studies on the* Aeromonas *group*. United States Dept. Health, Education and Welfare. Special Publication, Communicable Disease Centre. Bethesda, Md. USA. 37pp.

Ewing, W.H. & Johnstone, J.G. (1960) Differentiation of *Aeromonas* and C27 cultures from Enterobacteriaceae. *International Bulletin of Bacteriology Nomenclature Taxonomy*, **10**, 223−30.

Fraire, A.E. (1978) *Aeromonas hydrophila* infection. *Journal of the American Medical Association*, **239**, 192.

De Figuereido, J. & Plumb, J.A. (1971) Virulence of different isolates of *Aeromonas hydrophila* in channel catfish. *Aquaculture*, **11**, 349−54.

Fijan, N.F. (1972) Infectious Dropsy of Carp − A disease complex. *Symposium of the Zoological Society of London*, **30**, 39−52.

Fijan, N.N., Kunst, L. & Tomasec, I. (1976) O liceju zarazne boden bolesti sarana nekim antibioticima i furozolidonom. *Veterinary Archives*, **37**, 34−45.

Geldreich, E.E. (1973) Microbiology of Water. *Journal of Water Pollution*, **45**, 1244−59.

Gibbs, E.L. (1963) An effective treatment for red-leg disease in *Rana pipiens*. *Laboratory Animal Care*. **13**, 781−783.

Griffin, P.J., Sniezsko, S.F. & Friddle, S.B. (1953) A more comprehensive description of *Bacterium salmonicida*. *Transactions of the American Fisheries Society*, **82**, 129−38.

Hazen, T.C., Fliermaus, C.P., Hirsch, R.P. & Esch, G.W. (1978) Prevalance and distribution of *Aeromonas hydrophila* in the United States. *Applied Environmental Microbiology*, **36**, 731−8.

Heuschmann-Brunner, G. (1978) Aeromonads of the *hydrophila-punctata* group in freshwater fishes. *Archives für Hydrobiologie*, **83**, 99−125.

Hsu, T.C., Waltman, W.D. & Shotts, E.B. (1981) Correlation of extracellular enzyme activity and biochemical characteristics with regard to virulence of *Aeromonas hydrophila*. *Developments in Biological Standardisation*, **49**, 101−11.

Joseph, S.W., Daily, O.P., Hunter, W.S., Seidler, R.J., Allen, D.A. & Colwell, R.R. (1979) *Aeromonas* primary wound infection of a diver in polluted waters. *Journal of Clinical Microbiology*, **10**, 46−9.

Kaper, J.B., Lockman, H. & Colwell, R.R. (1981) *Aeromonas hydrophila*: Ecology and toxigenicity of isolates from an estuary. *Journal of Applied Bacteriology*, **50**, 359−77.

Ketover, B.P., Young, L.S. & Armstrong, D. (1973) Septicaemia due to *Aeromonas hydrophila*: clinical and immunological aspects. *Journal of Infectious Diseases*, **127**, 284−90.

Kluyver, A.J. & van Niel, C.B. (1936) Prospects for a natural system of classification for bacteria. Zentralblatt für Bakteriologie, *Parasitenkunde Infektionskrankheiten und Hygiene*, **94**, 369−403.

Liu, P.V. (1961) Observations on the specificities of extracellular antigens on the genera *Aeromonas* and *Pseudomonas*. *Journal of General Microbiology*, **24**, 145.

MacInnes, J.H., Trust, T.J. & Crosa, J.H. (1979) Deoxyribonucleic acid relationships among members of the genus *Aeromonas*. *Canadian Journal of Microbiology*, **25**, 579−86.

Mead, A.R. (1969) *Aeromonas hydrophila* in the leukoderma syndrome of *Achatina fulica*. *Malacologia*, **9**, 43.

Meyer, F.P. (1964) Field treatments of *Aeromonas liquefaciens* infections in golden shiners. *Progressive Fish-Culturist*, **26**, 33−35.

Meyer, F.P. (1970) Seasonal fluctuations in the incidence of disease on fish farms. *American Fisheries Society Special Publication*, **5**, 21−9.

Mitchell, A.J. & Plumb, J.E. (1980) Toxicity and efficacy of Furanace on channel catfish infected experimentally with *Aeromonas hydrophila*. *Journal of Fish Diseases*, **3**, 93−100.

Newman, S.G. (1982) *Aeromonas hydrophila* a review. In *Les Antigenes des Micro Organisms des Poissons* (Ed. by D.P. Anderson, M. Dorson & P. Doubouret), pp. 87−117. Symposium International de Tallories Collection, Foundation of Marcel Merieux.

Nord, C.E., Sjoberg, L., Wadstrom, T. & Wretlind, B. (1975) Characterization of three *Aeromonas* and nine *Pseudomonas* species by extracellular enzymes and haemolysins. *Medical Microbiology and Immunology*, **161**, 79−87.

Olivier, G., Lallier, R. & Lariviere, S. (1981) A toxigenic profile of *Aeromonas hydrophila* and *Aeromonas sobria* isolated from fish. *Canadian Journal of Microbiology*, **27**, 330−3.

Page, L.A. (1962) Acetylmethylcarbinol production and the classification of aeromonas associated with ulcerative diseases of ectothermic vertebrates. *Journal of Bacteriology*, **34**, 772−7.

Popoff, M. (1984) Genus III, *Aeromonas* Kluyver & van Niel (1936) I. *Bergey's Manual of Determinative Bacteriology*, Vol. 1 (Ed. by J.G. Holt & N.R. Krieg), pp. 545−8. Williams & Wilkins, Baltimore.

Popoff, M & Veron, M. (1976) A taxonomic study of the *Aeromonas hydrophila*−*Aeromonas punctata* group. *Journal of General Microbiology*, **94**, 11−22.

Popoff, M.Y., Coynault, C., Kiredjian, M. & Lemelin, M. (1981). Polynucleotide sequence relatedness among motile *Aeromonas* species. *Current Microbiology*, **5**, 109−114.

Quadri, S.M.H., Gordon, L.P., Wende, R.D. & Williams, R.P. (1976) Meningitis due to *Aeromonas hydrophila*. *Journal of Clinical Microbiology*, **3**, 102−4.

Rao, V.B. & Foster, B.G. (1977) Antigenic analysis of the genus *Aeromonas*. *Texas Journal of Science*, **29**, 85−91.

Roberts, R.J. (1989) Pathophysiology and Systemic Pathology of Teleosts. In *Fish Pathology* (Ed. by R.J. Roberts), pp. 56−134. Baillière Tindall, London.

Roberts, R.J. & Horne, M.T. (1978) Bacterial meningitis in farmed rainbow trout *Salmo gairdneri* Richardson affected with chronic pancreatic necrosis. *Journal of Fish Diseases*, **1**, 157−64.

Salton, R. & Schnick, S. (1973) *Aeromonas hydrophila* peritonitis. *Cancer Chemotherapy Reports*, **57**, 489−91.

Sanarelli (1891) Über einen neuen Mikroorganismus das Wassers, welcher für Thiere mit veranderlicher und konstater Temperature Pathogen ist. *Zentralblatt für Bakteriologie, Parasitenkunde Infektionskranheiten und Hygiene*, **9**, 193−9.

Schäperclaus, W. (1926) *Bakterium fluorescens* − Infektion und Geschverlstbildungen bei Aalen mit Versuchluckten Angelharken 2. *Fischerei*, **24**, 157.

Schäperclaus, W. (1930) Pseudomonas punctata als Krankheits − erreger bei Fischen. *Zeitung für Fisherei*, **28**, 289−370.

Schäperclaus, W. (1954) *Fishkrankheiten*. Akademisch Verlag, Berlin.

Schäperclaus, W. (1959) Grossversuche mit streptomycin zur Bekamfung der infektionen Bauchwassersucht des Karpfens. *Deutsche Fisherei Zeitung*, **6**, 176−9.

Schubert, R.H.W. (1967). The taxonomy and nomenclature of the genus *Aeromonas* Kluyver and van Niel 1936. I. Suggestions on the taxonomy and nomenclature of the aerogenic *Aeromonas* spp. *International Journal of Systematic Bacteriology*, **17**, 23−7.

Schubert, R.H.W. (1969) Infrasubspecific taxonomy of *Aeromonas hydrophila* (Chester 1901) Stanier 1943. *Zentralblatt fur Bakteriologie Parasitenkunde Infektionskranheiten und Hygiene*, **211**, 406−8.

Schubert, R.H.W. (1974) Genus II. *Aeromonas*. In *Bergey's Manual of Determinative Bacteriology*, 8th edn (Ed. by R.E. Buchanan & N.E. Gibbons), pp. 345−8. William & Wilkins, Baltimore.

Seaman, W.R. (1951) Notes on a bacterial disease of rainbow trout in a Colorado hatchery. *Progressive Fish Culturist*, **13**, 139−41.

Shaw, D.H. & Hodder, A.J. (1978) Lipopolysaccharides of the motile aeromonads; core oligosaccharide analysis as an aid to taxonomic classification. *Canadian Journal of Microbiology*, **24**, 864−8.

Shotts, E.B., Gaines, J.L., Martin, L. & Prestwood, A.K. (1972) *Aeromonas* induced deaths among fish in a eutrophic inland lake. *Journal of the American Medical Association*, **162**, 603−7.

Shotts, E.B., Tsu, T.C. & Waltman, W.D. (1985) Extracellular proteolytic activity of *Aeromonas hydrophila* complex. *Fish Pathology*, **20**, 37−44.

Snieszko, S.F. (1957) Genus IV *Aeromonas* Kluyver & van Niel 1936. In *Bergey's Manual of Determinative Bacteriology*, 7th edn (Ed. by R.S. Breed, E.D.G. Murray & R. Smith), pp. 189−93. Williams & Wilkins, Baltimore.

Takahashi, Y. & Kusuda, R. (1977) Studies on the scale protrusion diseases of carps. *Fish Pathology*, **12**, 15−19.

Thorpe, J.E. & Roberts, R.J. (1972) An aeromonad epidemic in the brown trout (*Salmo trutta* L.). *Journal of Fish Biology*, **4**, 441–51.

Thune, R.L., Graham, T.E., Riddle, L.M. & Amborski, R.L. (1982) Effects of *Aeromonas hydrophila* extracellular products and endotoxins. *Transactions of the American Fisheries Society*, **111**, 749–54.

Thune, R.L., Johnson, M.C., Graham, T.E. & Amborski, R.L. (1986) *Aeromonas hydrophila* β-haemolysin: Purification and examination of its role in virulence of O-group channel catfish *Ictalurus punctatus* Rafinesque. *Journal of Fish Diseases*, **9**, 5–62.

Tonguthai, K. (1984) A preliminary account of ulcerative fish diseases in the Indo-Pacific region. FAO TCP/RAS 4508 Bangkok, 1–39.

Toranzo, A.E., Baya, A.M., Ronalde, J.L. & Herick, F.M. (1989) Association of *Aeromonas sobria* with mortalities in adult gizzard shark *Dorosoma cepedianum* Lesueur. *Journal of Fish Diseases*, **12**, 439–48.

Torres, J.L., Shariff, M. & Tajima, K. (1990) Serological relationships among motile *Aeromonas* spp. associated with healthy and epizootic ulcerative syndrome (EUS) positive fish. Proceedings of the Symposium on Diseases in Asian Aquaculture, Asian Fisheries Society, Bali 25.

Trust, T.J. & Chipman, D.C. (1979) Clinical involvement of *Aeromonas hydrophila*: A Review. *Canadian Medical Association Journal*.

Wretlind, B., Molby, R. & Wadstrom, T. (1971) Separation of two haemolysins from *Aeromonas hydrophila*. Infection and Immunity, **4**, 503–5.

# Part 4:
# Pasteurellaceae

Pasteurellaceae is a family of small coccoid to rod shaped Gram-negative bacteria 0.2−1.0 × 0.4−2.0 µm which may be pleomorphic. Non-motile, non-sporing, aerobic or facultatively anaerobic, they are chemo-organotrophs with both respiratory and fermentative types of metabolism and are cytochrome oxidase-positive. There are three genera in the family, *Pasteurella*, *Haemophilus* and *Actinobacillus* and the mol % G + C of the DNA is 38−47.

# Chapter 9:
# Pasteurellosis

The genus *Pasteurella*, in the Family Pasteurellaceae, consists of Gram-negative cocco-bacilli 0.3–1.0 × 1.0–2.0 μm. They occur singly, sometimes in short chains and frequently exhibit bipolar staining. They are non-motile, non-spore forming, catalase-positive and usually oxidase-positive. Complex media supplemented with yeast extract, blood or serum is used for isolation. They are parasitic in vertebrates, particularly mammals and birds, and the mol % G + C of the DNA is 40–45.

Pasteurellosis, caused by *Pasteurella piscicida* is an important disease of cultured marine fish, particularly in Japan. Granulomatous pseudo-tubercles, composed of masses of bacteria, are formed in the kidney and spleen and there is widespread internal necrosis. Outbreaks may be extensive with heavy losses and are associated with water temperatures going above 25°C. Control depends on good stock management and use of appropriate antibacterial agents. As yet no commercial vaccine is available.

## Introduction

Pasteurellosis, a bacterial disease caused by *Pasteurella*, was first observed in fish in 1963, following a massive kill of white perch (*Roccus americanus*) and striped bass (*R. saxatilis*) on the east coast of Chesapeake Bay in the USA. Thirty cultures of a Gram-negative micro-organism were isolated from the white perch and striped bass and, as a result of clear bipolar-staining and their physiological and biochemical reactions, they were placed in the genus *Pasteurella* (Snieszko *et al.* 1964).

Several years later, 27 of Snieszko's original isolates of *Pasteurella* spp. were submitted for further characterization by Janssen & Surgalla (1968). On the basis of morphological and physiological criteria, this organism was confirmed in the genus *Pasteurella* and identified as the species *P. piscicida*. Subsequently the disease was reported among menhaden (*Brevoortia patronus*) and striped mullet (*Mugil cephalus*) in Galveston Bay, Texas (Lewis *et al.* 1970). A severe outbreak of pasteurellosis of young cultured yellowtail (*Seriola quinqueradiata*) also occurred in the south-western areas of Japan in 1969 (Kubota *et al.* 1970). Subsequently, the micro-organism has been found in many yellowtail farms (Kimura & Kitao 1971, Kusuda & Yamaoka 1972) and has caused serious losses for fish culturists in Japan every year since 1969. Because affected fish show prominent white granules in the kidneys and spleen, Kubota *et al.* (1970) proposed that the condition should be called 'bacterial tuberculoidosis'. At the present time, pasteurellosis among cultured yellowtail is known by this name with the Japanese scientific name of 'Ruiketsusetsu shou'.

## Species specificity and distribution

Although pasteurellosis is one of the most important bacterial diseases among

**Table 9.1**   Species of fish which have been affected by pasteurellosis

| | |
|---|---|
| In Japan | |
| Ayu (*Plecoglossus altivelis*) | Kusuda & Miura (1972) |
| | Matsuoka *et al.* (1990) |
| Black seabream (*Mylio macrocephalus*) | Muroga *et al.* (1977) |
| Young black seabream (*Acanthopagrus schlegeli*) | Oshnishi *et al.* (1982) |
| Red seabream (*Pagrus major*) | Yasunaga *et al.* (1983) |
| Red grouper (*Epinephelus akaara*) | Ueki *et al.* (1990) |
| Snake-head (*Channa maculata*) | Tung *et al.* (1985) |
| Oval fish (*Navodan modestus*) | Yasunaga *et al.* (1984) |
| Yellowtail (*Seriola quinqueradiata*) | Kubota *et al.* (1970) |
| | Kimura & Kitao (1971) |
| | Kusuda & Yamaoka (1972) |
| | |
| In USA | |
| White perch (*Roccus americanus*) | Allen & Pleczar (1967) |
| Striped bass (*Morone saxatilis*) | Snieszko *et al.* (1964) |
| Menhaden (*Brevoortia patronus*) | Lewis *et al.* (1970) |
| | Paperna & Zwerner (1976) |
| | |
| In UK | |
| Rudd (*Scardinius erythrophthalmus*) | Ajmal & Hobbs (1967) |
| Chub (*Coregonus zenithicus*) | |

young cultured marine fish in Japan it is not common elsewhere. Disease outbreaks have been reported in many different species of farmed fish (see Table 9.1).

## Clinical signs and pathology

Gross pathological signs of pasteurellosis vary according to the form of the disease. In acute cases the only external signs may be a darkening of body colour (Muroga *et al.* 1977, Ohnishi *et al.* 1982, Yasunaga *et al.* 1983, Tung *et al.* 1985). Internally, granulomatous-like deposits may develop in the kidney and spleen (Fig. 9.1), the features associated with the descriptive name, bacterial pseudotuberculosis. Histopathological studies of yellowtail have revealed tubercle-like lesions composed of masses of bacteria, epithelial cells and fibroblasts (Kubota *et al.* 1970). In snake-heads, white circumscribed areas 0.5–1.0 mm across appear scattered throughout the spleen and kidneys, with the liver appearing slightly swollen and discoloured (Tung *et al.* 1985). In this study characteristic bipolar stained organisms as well as phagocytes with multiplying engulfed organisms were recovered from impression smears of blood and spleen. The parenchyma of the spleen showed acute necrotic changes together with masses of bacteria lodged embolically within the capillaries and interstitial spaces. There may also be accumulations of purulent material in the abdominal cavity of infected fish (Lewis *et al.* 1970).

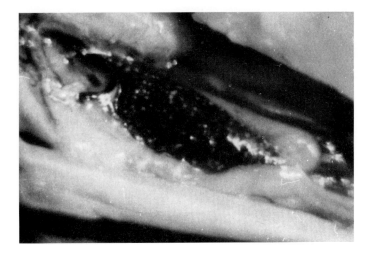

**Fig. 9.1** Yellowtail infected with *Pasteurella piscicida*, showing greyish-white nodules on the spleen, the classical signs of pasteurellosis.

## Aetiological agent

Kimura & Kitao (1971) were the first workers to isolate organisms from young cultured yellowtail suffering from bacterial pseudotuberculosis and they concluded that the organism belonged to *Corynebacterium* or a related genus. They appeared as Gram-positive rods with bipolar staining in young cultures and Gram-negative in older ones, were fastidious in their nutritional requirements and sensitive to penicillin. In contrast, Simidu & Egusa (1972) using the Gram-reaction and some other biochemical characteristics, suggested that the organisms which they had isolated from diseased yellowtails might belong to the genus *Arthrobacter*. Subsequently, Kusuda & Yamaoka (1972) isolated micro-organisms from cultured yellowtail in Japan during an outbreak of pasteurellosis of which the causative organisms were later identified as *Pasteurella piscicida* (Janssen & Surgalla 1968). Comparing the morphological, cultural and physiological characters of *P. piscicida* isolated from diseased white perch in USA and isolates from yellowtail in Japan, Koike *et al.* (1975) showed that they differed in tests for nitrate reduction and arginine dihydrolase, in the Voges-Proskauer and methyl red reactions, in colony appearance and the inability to grow in a medium without sodium chloride or at 37°C. As a result of the differences reported in this study the species name *P. piscicida* was not listed in Bergey's Manual of Systematic Bacteriology (Kreig & Holt 1984).

## Morphology and characteristics

*Pasteurella piscicida* is a Gram-negative short rod (0.6−1.2 × 0.8−2.6 μm) which exhibits characteristic bipolar staining; it is non-motile, non-capsulated and non-spore-forming. However, it shows pleomorphism with cocci and/or long rods being formed on brain-heart infusion agar (BHIA) and blood agar with 1−2.5% sodium chloride (Hashimoto *et al.* 1985). The optimum temperature

**Table 9.2**  Biochemical characteristics of *Pasteurella piscicida*[a]

| | | Acid from | |
|---|---|---|---|
| Oxidase | + | | |
| Catalase | + | Glucose | + |
| H$_2$S production | − | Fructose | + |
| OF | F | Galactose | + |
| MR | d | Mannose | + |
| VP | d | Arabinose | − |
| Indole production | − | Rhamnose | − |
| Nitrate reduction | − | Xylose | − |
| Urease | − | Maltose | d |
| Utilization of | | Trehalose | − |
| Malonate | − | Lactose | − |
| Citrate | − | Sucrose | d |
| Gelatin liquefaction | − | Glycerol | d |
| Hydrolysis of | | Esculin | − |
| Casein | − | Salicin | − |
| Starch | d | | |
| Arginine dihydrolase | d | | |
| Decarboxylation of | | | |
| Ornithine | − | | |
| Lysine | − | | |
| Growth at/on | | | |
| pH 5.5−8.0 | − | | |
| 0.5−3.0% NaCl | − | | |
| 25°C−30°C | − | | |
| Haemolysis | | | |
| (Sheep red blood cells) | − | | |

d: differs from result with U.S. isolates
F: fermentative reaction
[a]: Snieszko *et al.* (1964), Janssen & Surgalla (1968),
Kimura & Kitao (1971), Kusuda & Yamaoka (1972),
Koike *et al.* (1975), Ohnishi *et al.* (1982), Yasunaga *et al.*
(1983).

for growth is 25°C. The bacterium is a facultative anaerobe and is oxidase and catalase positive. Biochemical characteristics are given in Table 9.2.

## Serotypes

Kimura & Kitao (1971) have reported that *P. piscicida* strains isolated in Japan could not be differentiated into serotypes by the slide agglutination test. On the other hand, Kusuda *et al.* (1978) reported that the antigenic structure of *P. piscicida* strains isolated from yellowtails in Japan and the *P. piscicida* strain isolated from white perch in USA could be differentiated by the Ochterlony method and by immuno-electrophoresis.

## Diagnostic test

The presence of white nodules on the kidneys and spleen of diseased yellowtail and the isolation and identification of the causative agent are diagnostic features of pasteurellosis. *P. piscicida* can be isolated by streaking material from the infected kidneys and/or spleen on BHIA supplemented with 1–2% NaCl. Presumptive bacteria are identified as *P. piscicida* if they are Gram-negative, non-motile and rod-shaped with bipolar staining and give a positive oxidase reaction. Serological tests such as slide agglutination using specific antisera (Kimura & Kitao 1971, Kusuda *et al.* 1978, Yasunaga *et al.* 1984, Ueki *et al.* 1990) or direct and indirect fluorescent antibody techniques (Kitao & Kimura 1974, Mori *et al.* 1976) can be used for definitive diagnosis.

## Epizootiology

Every year, when water temperature is raised above 25°C or when salinity is reduced by heavy or long-term rain, bacterial pseudotuberculosis caused by *P. piscicida* appears in fish farms in Japan. If water temperature remains under 25°C, no such outbreaks occur.

At present pasteurellosis is found in the coastal regions of Japan and some areas of the USA and Taiwan. However, as mariculture develops, it is almost certain that the host and geographic range will also increase. It is possible that carrier fish provide a reservoir of infection because *P. piscicida* does not survive for more than 4–5 days in estuarine waters (Toranzo *et al.* 1982). Transmission is probably horizontal from fish to fish. Oral infection seems to be a most important entry route (Wakabayashi *et al.* 1977) although there are also possibilities of both perbranchial and percutaneous infections. Pasteurellosis can occur in acute and chronic forms and acute epizootics may result in massive losses over relatively short periods of time.

## Control

Avoidance of overcrowding and good management may prevent outbreaks of this disease. Ampicillin (Kusuda & Inoue 1976, 1977), amoxicillin (Kitao *et al.* 1989), novobiocin (Shimizu & Egusa 1972), thiamphenicol, florfenicol (Fukui *et al.* 1987, Yasunaga & Yasumoto 1988, Yasunaga & Tsukahara 1988), oxolinic acid, flumequin and sodium nifurstyrenate have all been used to control bacterial pseudotuberculosis in yellowtails in Japan. However, drug-resistant strains of *P. piscicida* carrying transferable R-plasmids were reported in yellowtail farms in 1980 (Aoki & Kitao 1985). The following year, multiple drug-resistant strains with ampicillin resistant R-plasmids were also isolated from yellowtail farms in various districts of Japan (Takashima *et al.* 1985). Recently, treatment of this infection has become even more difficult. For this reason a rapid detection method for ampicillin resistant strains of *P. piscicida* has been developed (Kitao & Aoki 1983, Yasunaga *et al.* 1985, Matsuoka *et al.* 1986). There have been several reports in Japan of vaccines effective against bacterial pseudotuberculosis (Wakabayashi *et al.* 1977, Fukuda & Kusuda 1981*a,b*, 1985, Hamaguchi & Kusuda 1988, Kusuda & Hamaguchi 1988, Kusuda *et al.* 1988) although a commercially available vaccine has not yet been developed.

## References

Ajmal, M. & Hobbs, B.C. (1967) Species of *Corynebacterium* and *Pasteurella* isolated from diseased salmon, trout and rudd. *Nature*, **215**, 142–3.

Allen, N. & Pelczar, M.J., Jr (1967) Bacteriological studies on the white perch, *Roccus americanus*. *Chesapeake Science*, **8**, 135–54.

Aoki, T. & Kitao, T. (1985) Detection of transferable R plasmids in strains of the fish-pathogenic bacterium *Pasteurella piscicida*. *Journal of Fish Diseases*, **8**, 345–50.

Fukuda, Y. & Kusuda, R. (1981*a*) Efficacy of vaccination for pseudotuberculosis in cultured yellowtail by various routes of administration. *Bulletin of the Japanese Society of Scientific Fisheries*, **47**, 147–50.

Fukuda, Y. & Kusuda, R. (1981*b*) Acquired antibody against pseudotuberculosis in yellowtail. *Fish Pathology*, **15**, 263–9.

Fukuda, Y. & Kusuda, R. (1985) Vaccination of yellowtail against pseudotuberculosis. *Fish Pathology*, **20**, 421–5.

Fukui, H., Fujihara, Y. & Kano, T. (1987) *In vitro* and *in vivo* antibacteriological activities of florfenicol, a new fluorinated analog of thiamphenicol, against fish pathogens. *Fish Pathology*, **22**, 201–7.

Hamaguchi, M. & Kusuda, R. (1988) The effect of various cultivation periods on the efficacy of formalin killed cell vaccine of *Pasteurella piscicida* in yellowtail. *Bulletin of the Japanese Society of Scientific Fisheries*, **54**, 1847.

Hashimoto, S., Muraoka, A., Mihara, S. & Kusuda, R. (1985) Effects of cultivation temperature, NaCl concentration and pH on the growth of *Pasteurella piscicida*. *Bulletin of the Japanese Society of Scientific Fisheries*, **51**, 63–8.

Janssen, W.A. & Surgalla, M.J. (1968) Morphology, physiology, and serology of a *Pasteurella* species pathogenic for white perch (*Roccus americanus*). *Journal of Bacteriology*, **96**, 1606–10.

Kimura, M. & Kitao, T. (1971) On the etiological agent of 'Bacterial tuberculosis' of *Seriola*. *Fish Pathology*, **6**, 8–14.

Kitao, T. & Aoki, T. (1983) Evaluation of rapid slide β-lactamase test, a modified iodometric method, for detecting ampicillin resistance strains of *Pasteurella piscicida*. *Fish Pathology*, **18**, 103–6.

Kitao, T. & Kimura, M. (1974) Rapid diagnosis of pseudotuberculosis in yellowtail by means of the fluorescent antibody technique. *Bulletin of the Japanese Society of Scientific Fisheries*, **40**, 889–93.

Kitao, T., Nakauchi, R., Saito, R. & Tanaka, I. (1989) *In vivo* studies of amoxicillin on antibacterial activity for some fish pathogens. *Fish Pathology*, **24**, 83–7.

Koike, Y., Kuwahara, A. & Fujiwara, H. (1975) Characterization of '*Pasteurella piscicida*' isolated from white perch and cultivated yellowtail. *Japanese Journal of Microbiology*, **19**, 241–7.

Kreig, H.R. & Holt, J.C. (1984) *Bergey's Manual of Systematic Bacteriology. Family III Pasteurellaceae*, pp. 550–70.

Kubota, S., Kimura, M. & Egusa, S. (1970) Studies on 'bacterial tuberculoidosis' in cultured yellowtail — I. Symptomatology and histopathology. *Fish Pathology*, **4**, 111–18.

Kusuchi, R. & Hamaguchi, M. (1988) The efficacy of attenuated live bacterin of *Pasteurella piscicida* against Pseudotuberculosis in yellowtail. *Bulletin of the European Society of Fish Pathologists*, **8**, 50–2.

Kusuda, R. & Inoue, K. (1976) Studies on the application of ampicillin for pseudotuberculosis of cultured yellowtails — I. *In vitro* studies on sensitivity, development of drug-resistance and reversion of acquired drug-resistance characteristics of *Pasteurella piscicida*. *Bulletin of the Japanese Society of Scientific Fisheries*, **42**, 969–73.

Kusuda, R. & Inoue, K. (1977) Studies on the application of ampicillin for pseudotuberculosis in cultured yellowtail. III. Therapeutic effect of ampicillin on yellowtails artificially infected with

*Pasteurella piscicida. Fish Pathology*, **12**, 7−10.

Kusuda, R. & Miura, W. (1972) Characteristics of a *Pasteurella* sp. pathogenic for pondcultured ayu. *Fish Pathology*, **7**, 51−6.

Kusuda, R. & Yamaoka, M. (1972) Etiological studies on bacterial pseudotuberculosis in cultured yellowtail with *Pasteurella piscicida* as causative agent. I. On the morphology and biochemical properties. *Bulletin of the Japanese Society of Scientific Fisheries*, **38**, 1325−32.

Kusuda, R., Kawai, K. & Masui, T. (1978) Etiological studies on bacterial pseudotuberculosis in cultured yellowtails with *Pasteurella piscicida* as the causative agent. II. On the serological properties. *Fish Pathology*, **13**, 79−83.

Kusuda, R., Ninomiya, M., Hamaguchi, M. & Muraoka, A. (1988) The efficacy of ribosomal vaccine prepared from *Pasteurella piscicida* against pseudotuberculosis in cultured yellowtail. *Fish Pathology*, **23**, 191−6.

Lewis, D.H., Crumbles, L.C., McConnell, S. & Flowers, A.I. (1970) Pasteurella-like bacteria from an epizootic in menhaden and mullet from Galveston bay. *Journal of Wildlife Diseases*, **6**, 160−3.

Matsuoka, M., Wada, Y. & Takai, S. (1986) A rapid β-lactamase test using dead fish kidney for detecting ampicillin resistance strains of *Pasteurella piscicida. Fish Pathology*, **21**, 57−8.

Matsuoka, M., Wada, Y., Kawamoto, I. & Doi, S. (1990) *Pasteurella piscicida* infection in juvenile ayu (*Plecoglossus altivelis*). *Fish Pathology*, **25**, 253−4.

Mori, S., Kitao, T. & Kimura, M. (1976) A field survey by means of the direct fluorescent antibody technique for diagnosis of pseudotuberculosis in yellowtail. *Fish Pathology*, **11**, 11−16.

Muroga, K., Sugiyama, T. & Ueki, N. (1977) Pasteurellosis in cultured black seabream (*Mylio macrocephalus*). *Journal of the Faculty of Fisheries and Animal Husbandry of Hiroshima University*, **16**, 17−21.

Ohnishi, K., Watanabe, K. & Jo, Y. (1982) *Pasteurella* infection in young black seabream. *Fish Pathology*, **16**, 207−10.

Paperna, I. & Zwerner, D.E. (1976) Parasites and diseases of striped bass *Morone saxatilis* (Walbaum) from the lower Chesapeake Bay. *Journal of Fish Biology*, **9**, 267−81.

Simidu, U. & Egusa, S. (1972) A re-examination of the fish-pathogenic bacterium that had been reported as a Pasteurella species. *Bulletin of the Japanese Society of Scientific Fisheries*, **38**, 803−12.

Snieszko, S.F., Bullock, G.L., Hollis, E. & Boone, J.G. (1964) *Pasteurella* sp. from an epizootic of white perch (*Roccus americanus*) in Chesapeake Bay tidewater areas. *Journal of Bacteriology*, **88**, 1814.

Takashima, N., Aoki, T. & Kitao, T. (1985) Epidemiological surveillance of drug-resistant strains of *Pasteurella piscicida. Fish Pathology*, **20**, 209−17.

Toranzo, A.E., Barja, J.L. & Hetrick, F.M. (1982) Survival of *Vibrio anguillarum* and *Pasteurella piscicida* in estuarine and fresh waters. *Bulletin of the European Association of Fish Pathologists*, **3**, 43−5.

Tung, M.C., Tsai, S.S., Ho, L.F., Huang, S.T. & Chen, S.C. (1985) An acute septicemic infection of *Pasteurella* organism in pond-cultured Formosa snake-head fish (*Channa maculata* Lacepede) in Taiwan. *Fish Pathology*, **20**, 143−8.

Ueki, N., Kayano, Y. & Muroga, K. (1990) *Pasteurella piscicida* infection in juvenile red grouper (*Epinephelus akaara*). *Fish Pathology*, **25**, 43−4.

Wakabayashi, H., Toyoda, H. & Egusa, S. (1977) Artificial infection of yellowtail with a gastric administration of cultured *Pasteurella piscicida* cells. *Fish Pathology*, **11**, 207−12.

Yasunaga, N. & Tsukahara, J. (1988) Dose titration study of florfenicol as therapeutic agent in naturally occurring pseudotuberculosis. *Fish Pathology*, **23**, 7−12.

Yasunaga, N. & Yasumoto, S. (1988) Therapeutic effect of florfenicol on experimentally induced pseudotuberculosis in yellowtail. *Fish Pathology*, **23**, 1−5.

Yasunaga, N., Hatai, K. & Tsukahara, J. (1983) *Pasteurella piscicida* from an epizootic of cultured red sea bream. *Fish Pathology*, **18**, 107−10.

Yasunaga, N., Yasumoto, S., Hirakawa, E. & Tsukahara, J. (1984) On a massive mortality of oval filefish (*Navodan modestus*) caused by *Pasteurella piscicida. Fish Pathology*, **19**, 51−5.

Yasunaga, N., Hirakawa, E. & Tsukahara, J. (1985) A rapid β-lactamase test by acidometric method for detecting ampicillin resistance strains of *Pasteurella piscicida. Fish Pathology*, **20**, 501−2.

# Part 5:
# Pseudomonadaceae

Pseudomonadaceae are strictly aerobic, Gram-negative, straight or curved rods, $0.5-1.0 \times 1.5-5.0\,\mu m$. Metabolism is respiratory, never fermentative. Motile by polar flagella, they grow well at low temperatures with a range from below $4-43°C$. The DNA base ratio is $58-71\%$ G + C. Recently the family has been extensively reclassified and reduced to the present three genera, *Pseudomonas*, *Xanthomonas* and *Frateuria* (with a tentative fourth, *Zoogloea*).

# Chapter 10:
# *Pseudomonas* and *Alteromonas* Infections

*Pseudomonas*, the type genus of the Pseudomonadaceae is composed of Gram-negative straight or slightly curved rods, non-spore forming, $0.5-1.0 \times 1.5-5.0\,\mu m$, usually motile with one or more polar flagella. They have simple growth requirements and are strictly aerobic with respiratory metabolism, although nitrate may be used as an alternative electron acceptor in some cases. Generally oxidase-positive, but oxidase-negative strains occasionally occur, they may produce yellow-green, green or blue water soluble diffusible pigments. The temperature range for growth is $4-43°C$ with good growth at low temperatures. The mol % G + C in the DNA is $55-64$, and they are widely distributed in the environment, in soil and water, and may be opportunistic pathogens of man, animals and plants. Frequently they are isolated from the surface and the intestine of fish and may cause disease. Three species are pathogenic for fish, namely *Pseudomonas fluorescens*, *P. chlororaphis*, and *P. anguilliseptica*, causing haemorrhagic bacteraemias associated with elevated temperatures and improper management.

Some *Alteromonas* species, common in the marine environment, also have been implicated in fish disease. Although similar in many characteristics to *Pseudomonas* species, the mol % G + C in the DNA is lower, $38-50$, and they are not known to produce any fluorescent pigments.

## Introduction

The name *Pseudomonas* appears in the earliest descriptions of disease conditions in fish as a causative agent, but with increased knowledge of bacterial taxonomy and improved methods of identification many have now been assigned to other genera. Circumscription of the Family Pseudomonadaceae had undergone many changes. In the classification proposed by Kluyver & van Niel (1936) 25 genera were included, grouped into three tribes with the Pseudomonadaceae comprising *Pseudomonas* and three other genera. On the basis of detailed metabolic studies and on results from tests such as IMViC, a number of them, including some important fish pathogens, were excluded from *Pseudomonas* and now are placed in the genus *Aeromonas*.

It was not until the seventh edition of Bergey's Manual (Snieszko 1957) that *Aeromonas* first appeared as a genus. It is now more readily distinguished from *Pseudomonas* by being fermentative in the glucose O-F test (Hugh & Leifson 1953) and the family Enterobacteriaceae by being oxidase-positive (Kovacs 1956). Substantial re-classification has since been carried out, based on extensive biochemical tests, single carbon source utilization, DNA base ratios and more recent nucleic acid hybridization data (Palleroni *et al.* 1973, Swings *et al.* 1980), and the Family has been limited further. It now consists of closely related genera of aerobic pseudomonads, *Pseudomonas*, *Xanthomonas* and *Frateuria*, with the tentative inclusion of a fourth genus *Zoogloea* (Palleroni 1984). Among these the genus *Pseudomonas* can be differentiated by the lack of requirement for organic growth factors and inability to grow at pH 3.3. Many species produce diffusible pigments which may fluoresce green in ultra-violet light or are non-fluorescent blue-green, red brown or orange. The G + C content of the DNA is 58–70 mol %.

The number of *Pseudomonas* species increased from 12 in the fifth edition of Bergey's Manual of Determinative Bacteriology (Bergey *et al.* 1939) to approximately 150, many of which were host specific plant pathogens. At present it is restricted to around 100 species from all sources (Palleroni 1984). Detailed information on species associated with fish and their habitat is far from complete since many workers dealing with pseudomonads have been content to identify bacteria to the genus level only. This has been complicated further by several species involved in fish disease being subjected to the taxonomic shifts discussed. The organism isolated by Schäperclaus (1930) from haemorrhagic septicaemia in freshwater fish for example, was identified as *P. punctata* and later classified as *Aeromonas punctata* by Snieszko in the seventh edition of Bergey's Manual (1957), retained as such by Schubert (1974) in the eighth edition, but now is included in the species *A. hydrophila*, e.g. in the current edition (Krieg & Holt, 1984). Similarly *Pseudomonas ichthyodermis* (Wells & ZoBell 1934, ZoBell & Upham 1944) was first reclassified as *Vibrio ichthyodermis* (Shewan *et al.* 1960) and then as *V. anguillarum* (Hendrie *et al.* 1971). This complex background is continuing to affect the current literature. The causative organism of an outbreak of disease in rabbit fish (*Sigamus rivulatus*) has been identified as *Pseudomonas putrefaciens* (Saeed *et al.* 1990) when, in the light of earlier taxonomic studies by Lee *et al.* (1977) and MacDonnell & Colwell (1985), it should have been named *Shewanella putrefaciens*.

## *Pseudomonas* species in fish disease

*Pseudomonas* species are frequently associated with fish (Cahill 1990) and are found on eggs (Bell *et al.* 1971, Sugita *et al.* 1988), the skin and gills (Colwell 1962, Horsley 1973) and the intestine (Trust & Sparrow 1974, Austin & Al-Zahrani 1988). Generally the bacterial flora of fish, including *Pseudomonas*, *Cytophaga*, *Flavobacterium*, *Micrococcus*, and *Acinetobacter* species and others reflects the microbial population of the aquatic habitat and is influenced by factors such as bacterial load in the water and salinity. As *Pseudomonas* species are so widespread and numerous they may become involved in disease processes and act as secondary invaders of fish compromised by pathogens or other factors. Some have been reported as primary pathogens, principally *P. anguilliseptica* and *P. fluorescens*, and there has been one report of *P. chlororaphis*, an organism very similar to *P. fluorescens*, causing heavy mortalities among farmed amago trout (*Oncorhynchus rhodorus*) in Japan (Hatai *et al.* 1975).

## Pseudomonas anguilliseptica

*Pseudomonas anguilliseptica* was first described as the causative agent of a destructive haemorrhagic bacteraemia of cultured eels (*Anguilla japonica*) in Japan by Wakabayashi & Egusa (1972) and Muroga *et al*. (1972). The appearance of a remarkable petechial haemorrhage in the skin gave rise to the name Sekiten-byo which means literally red-spot disease. Small haemorrhages are produced in the skin around the mouth and opercula and along the ventral surfaces. The body surface may ooze blood and slime in severe cases but there is no reddening of the fins or the anus. Gross symptoms are usually absent from the viscera although occasionally there are small petechiae in the peritoneum as well as liver congestion. Severe bacteriaemia occurs in moribund eels.

The causative agent *Pseudomonas anguilliseptica* can be isolated from the liver, spleen, kidney, heart and blood of infected eels, with small colonies forming on nutrient agar after 72 h incubation at 25°C. Growth can be enhanced by the addition of 10% horse blood to the medium but lysis does not occur. The bacteria isolated are Gram-negative, non-acid-fast, non-sporing bacilli 0.4 µm by 2 µm although long filamentous cells occur in young cultures. Motility, due to a single polar flagellum, can be demonstrated in cultures grown at 15°C but not in those grown at 25°C. Organisms are catalase- and oxidase-positive and do not ferment glucose. No soluble pigment is produced.

The Japanese eel (*Anguilla japonica*) is more susceptible to infection by *P. anguilliseptica* than the European eel (*A. anguilla*) (Muroga *et al*. 1975), but the disease does occur outside Japan. A severe outbreak was reported in Scotland (Stewart *et al*. 1983) in which 67,000 elvers died. Carp (*Cyprinus carpio*), crucian carp (*Carassius carassius*), ayu (*Plecoglossus altevelis*), goldfish (*Carassius auratus*), loach and bluegill (*Lepomis macrochirus*) have been found susceptible to experimental infection (Muroga *et al*. 1975).

Sekiten-byo is controlled in Japan by raising the water temperature to 26−27°C for about 2 weeks before allowing it to return to ambience (Muroga *et al*. 1973). This procedure was effective also in Scotland (Stewart *et al*. 1983). A formalin-killed vaccine has been developed by Nakai & Muroga (1979) which was effective in producing agglutinating antibodies and protective immunity after a single intramuscular injection. The immunity persisted for over 5 months at 20°C so that eels vaccinated in the late autumn were protected in the early spring, the most likely time for the disease to occur in Japan. Field trials in pond cultured eels confirmed the efficacy of this vaccine (Nakai *et al*. 1982).

## Pseudomonas fluorescens

Pseudomonad septicaemia is a haemorrhagic condition of fish usually associated with stress or improper management. Many species, but particularly cultured or aquarium fish, have been affected, and although numerous members of the genus *Pseudomonas* have been implicated, isolates most closely resemble *P. fluorescens*, which now is considered the aetiological agent (Bullock & McLaughlin 1970).

*P. fluorescens* can be isolated from the kidney or lesions of affected fish. It grows well on the nutrient agar at 22−25°C and produces a diffusible yellow-green pigment which fluoresces under ultra-violet light. Cetrimide added to the medium inhibits other Gram-negative bacteria and prevents overgrowth of *P. fluorescens*. The isolates are Gram-negative rod shaped bacteria 0.5 μm by 1.5−4 μm, motile by one or occasionally three polar flagella. Most are cytochrome oxidase positive and oxidize but do not ferment glucose.

Probably all species of fish are vulnerable to pseudomonad septicaemia under adverse environmental conditions or when compromised by other factors. Superficial ulcers on rainbow trout (*Oncorhynchus mykiss*) chronically infected with infectious pancreatic necrosis virus were shown to be caused by *P. fluorescens* (Roberts & Horne 1978) (Plate 28). The condition is best prevented by good stock management, ensuring high water quality and reducing stocking densities. Disinfection to eliminate an underlying cause has been used successfully in conjunction with antibiotic therapy. White catfish (*Ictalurus catus*) were treated with formalin to control a protozoan disease caused by *Ichthyophthirius* before being treated with kanamycin as an intraperitoneal injection at 25 mg/kg or oxytetracycline at 55 mg/kg body weight/day in the diet (Meyer & Collar 1964).

### *Alteromonas* and related organisms

Although most *Pseudomonas* species in aquatic habitats are found in fresh water, marine species do exist and these must be differentiated from members of the genus *Alteromonas*, which are similar in many characteristics but rare in terrestrial habitats. They are common, however, in the marine environment, and have a growth requirement for over 100 mM Na$^+$. They are differentiated by having a lower DNA base ratio, being 38−50 mol % G + C compared with 55−64 mol % G + C in marine *Pseudomonas* species.

*Alteromonas putrefaciens*, associated with fish spoilage, has a DNA base composition somewhat high for the genus and has been reclassified as *Shewanella*. *Alteromonas piscicida* was originally classified as *Flavobacterium piscicida* and later *Pseudomonas piscicida* (Buck *et al.* 1963), but with the DNA base composition of 43−46 mol % G + C is now placed in this genus. It was originally isolated from an area of dead fish associated with discoloration of the sea, a Red Tide, and is pathogenic for marine fish and crabs (Bein 1954, Meyers *et al.* 1959). *Alteromonas haloplanktis* has been found pathogenic for oysters (Colwell & Sparks 1967).

# References

Austin, B. & Al-Zahrani, A.M.J. (1988) The effect of antimicrobial compounds on the gastro-intestinal microflora of rainbow trout *Salmo gairdneri* Richardson. *Journal of Fish Biology*, **33**, 7–14.

Bein, S.J. (1954) A study of certain chromogenic bacteria isolated from 'Red Tide' water with a description of a new species. *Bulletin of Marine Science of the Gulf Carribean*, **4**, 110–19.

Bell, G.R., Hoskins, G.E. & Hodgkiss, W. (1971) Aspects of characterization, identification and ecology of the bacterial flora associated with the surface of the stream-incubating Pacific salmon (*Oncorhynchus*) eggs. *Journal of the Fisheries Research Board of Canada*, **28**, 1511–25.

Bergey, D.H., Breed, R.S., Murray, E.G.D. & Parker, A.H. (1939) *Bergey's Manual of Determinative Bacteriology*, 5th edition. Ballière, Tindall and Cox, London.

Buck, J.D., Meyers, S.P. & Leifson, E. (1963) *Pseudomonas Flavobacterium piscicida* Bein comb. nov. *Journal of Bacteriology*, **86**, 1125–6.

Bullock, G.L. & McLaughlin, J.J.A. (1970) Advances in knowledge concerning bacteria pathogenic to fishes (1954–1968). In *A Symposium on Diseases of Fishes and Shellfishes* (Ed by S.F. Snieszko), pp. 231–42. American Fisheries Society Special Publications (5), Washington, DC.

Cahill, M.M. (1990) Bacterial flora of fishes: a review. *Microbial Ecology*, **19**, 21–41.

Colwell, R.R. (1962). The bacterial flora of Puget Sound fish. *Journal of Applied Bacteriology*, **28**, 147–58.

Colwell, R.R. & Sparks, A.K. (1967) Properties of *Pseudomonas enalia*, a marine bacterium pathogenic for the invertebrate *Crassotrea gigas* (Thunberg). *Applied Microbiology*, **15**, 980–6.

Hatai, K., Egussa, S., Nakajima, M. & Chikahata, H. (1975) *Pseudomonas chlororaphis* as a fish pathogen. *Bulletin of the Japanese Society of Scientific Fisheries*, **41**, 1203–7.

Hendrie, M.S., Hodgkiss, W. & Shewan, J.M. (1971) Proposal that the species *Vibrio anguillarum*, *Vibrio piscium* and *Vibrio ichthyodermis* be combined as a single species *Vibrio angiullarum*. *International Journal of Systematic Bacteriology*, **21**(1), 64–8.

Horsley, R.W. (1973) The bacterial flora of Atlantic salmon (*Salmo salar* L.) in relation to its environment. *Journal of Applied Bacteriology*, **36**, 377–86.

Hugh, R. & Leifson, E. (1953) The taxonomic significance of fermentative versus oxidative metabolism of carbohydrates by various Gram-negative bacteria. *Journal of Bacteriology*, **66**, 24–6.

Kluyver, A.J. & van Niel, C.B. (1936) Prospects for a natural system of classification of bacteria. *Zentralblatt für Bacteriologie Parasitenkunde, infektions — krankheiten und hygiene abteilung* II., **94**, 369–403.

Kovacs, N. (1956) Identification of *Pseudomonas pyrocyanea* by the oxidase reaction. *Nature*, **178**, 703.

Kreig, N.R. & Holt, J.G. (1984) Bergey's Manual of Systematic Bacteriology Vol. 1. Williams and Wilkins, Baltimore.

Lee, J.V., Gibson, D.M. & Shewan, J.M. (1977) A numerical taxonomic study of some Pseudomonas-like bacteria. *Journal of General Microbiology*, **98**, 439–51.

MacDonnell, M.T. & Colwell, R.R. (1985) Phylogeny of the Vibrionaceae and recommendation for two new genera *Listonella* and *Shewanella*. *Systematic and Applied Microbiology*, **6**, 171–82.

Meyer, F.P. & Collar, J.D. (1964) Description and treatment of *Pseudomonas* infection in white catfish. *Applied Microbiology*, **12**, 201–3.

Meyers, S.P., Baslow, M.H., Bein, S.J. & Marks, C.E. (1959) Studies on *Flavobacterium piscicida* Bein. I Growth, toxicity and ecological considerations. *Journal of Bacteriology*, **78**, 225–30.

Muroga, K., Jo, Y. & Gam, M. (1973) Studies on red spot disease of pond-cultured eels I. The occurrences of the disease in eel culture ponds in Tokushima prefecture in 1972. *Fish Pathology*, **8**, 1–9.

Muroga, K., Jo, Y. & Sawada, T. (1975) Studies on red spot disease of pond cultured eels II. Pathogenicity of the causative bacterium *Pseudomonas anguillaseptica*. *Fish Pathology*, **9**, 107–14.

Nakai, T. & Muroga, K. (1979) Studies on red spot disease of pond cultured eels. V Immune response of the Japanese eel to the causative bacterium *Pseudomonas anguillaseptica. Bulletin of the Japanese Society of Scientific Fisheries*, **45**, 817−21.

Nakai, T., Muroga, K., Ohnishi, K., Jo, Y. & Tanimoto, H. (1982) Studies on red spot disease of cultured eels. IX A field vaccination trial. *Aquaculture*, **30**, 131−5.

Palleroni, N.J. (1984) Family 1 Pseudomonadaceae Winslow, Broadhurst, Buchanan Krumwiede, Rodgers and Smith 1917, 555. In *Bergey's Manual of Systematic Bacteriology*, Vol. 1. (Ed. by N.R. Kreig & J.G. Holt), pp. 141−99. Williams and Wilkins, Baltimore.

Palleroni, N.J., Kunisawa, R., Contopoulou, R. & Doudoroff (1973) Nucleic acid homologies in the genus *Pseudomonas. International Journal of Systematic Bacteriology*, **23**, 333−9.

Roberts, R.J. & Horne, M.T. (1978) Bacterial meningitis in farmed rainbow trout *Salmon gairdneri* Richardson affected with chronic pancreas necrosis. *Journal of Fish Diseases*, **1**, 157−64.

Saeed, M.O., Alamoudi, M.M. & Al-Harbi, A.H. (1990) Histopathology of *Pseudomonas putrefaciens* associated with disease in cultured rabbit fish *Siganus rivulatus* (Forskal). *Journal of Fish Diseases*, **13**(5), 417−22.

Schäperclaus, W. (1930) *Pseudomonas punctata* abs Kranksheitserreger bei Fischen. *Zeitschrift für Fisherei und deren Hilfwissenschaften*, **28**, 289−370.

Schubert, R.H.W. (1974) Genus II *Aeromonas* Kluyver and van Niel 1936, 398. In *Bergey's Manual of Determinative Bacteriology*, 8th edn (Ed. by R.E. Buchanan & N.E. Gibbons), pp. 345−8. Williams and Wilkins, Baltimore.

Shewan, J.M., Hobbs, G. & Hodgkiss, W. (1960) A determinative scheme for the identification of certain genera of Gram-negative bacteria, with special reference to the Pseudomonadaceae. *Journal of Applied Bacteriology*, **23**(3), 379−90.

Snieszko, S.F. (1957) Genus IV *Aeromonas* Kluyver and van Niel 1936. In *Bergey's Manual of Determinative Bacteriology*, 7th ed (Ed. by R.S. Breed, E.D.G. Murray & N.R. Smith), pp. 189−93. Williams and Wilkins, Baltimore.

Stewart, D.J., Woldemarian, K., Dear, G. & Mochaba, F.M. (1983) An outbreak of 'Sekiten-byo' among cultured European eels, *Anguilla anguilla* L., in Scotland. *Journal of Fish Diseases*, **6**, 75−6.

Sugita, H., Tsunohara, M., Ohkoshi, T. & Degachi, Y. (1988) The establishment of an intestinal microflora in developing goldfish (*Carassius auratus*) of culture ponds. *Microbial Ecology*, **15**, 333−44.

Swings, J., Gillis, K., Kersters, K., De Vos, P., Gosselé, F. & De Ley, J. (1980) *Frateuria* a new genus for *Acetobacter aurantius. International Journal of Systematic Bacteriology*, **30**, 547−56.

Trust, T.J. & Sparrow, R.A.H. (1974) The bacterial flora in the alimentary tract of freshwater salmonid fishes. *Canadian Journal of Microbiology*, **20**, 1219−28.

Wakabayashi, H. & Egusa, S. (1972) Characteristics of a *Pseudomonas* and pond-cultured eels (*Anguilla japonica*). *Bulletin of the Japanese Society of Scientific Fisheries*, **38**, 577−87.

ZoBell, C.E. & Upham, H.C. (1944) A list of marine bacteria including descriptions of sixty new species. *Bulletin of Scripps Institute of Oceanography, University of California, Technical Series*, **5**, 239−92.

# Part 6:
# Gram-Positive Fish Pathogens

The Gram-positive fish pathogens fall into three separate groups, *Renibacterium salmoninarum*, *Streptococcus* species and *Clostridium botulinum* type E

*Renibacterium* is grouped with the aerobic regular non-sporing Gram-positive rods. It is distinguished from the other aerobic genera *Kurthea* and *Caryophanon* by its host specificity and by a high mol % of G + C in the DNA, 55. This and the composition of the cell wall differentiates it from some pathogenic corynebacteria to which it is also similar. *Renibacterium salmoninarum* is the only member of the genus and an obligate pathogen of salmonid fish.

*Streptococcus* in the Family Deinococceaceae is grouped with the facultative anaerobic Gram-positive cocci, within which it has been distinguished by mode of cell division, to give chains or pairs and by the major products of glucose fermentation. The mol % G + C of the DNA is 34−46. This system of classification is no longer considered entirely satisfactory and the genus *Streptococcus* is under review. Classification of the fish pathogens is still being developed but includes alpha-haemolytic species similar to enterococci, the beta-haemolytic *Streptococcus iniae* and non-haemolytic species.

*Clostridium* is a genus of anaerobic endospore-forming, Gram-positive rods with a wide diversity of metabolic activity. The mol % G + C of the DNA is 22−55 but species tend to fall into two groups, 22−34 and 40−55, indicating that the genus may later be split into two. *Clostridium botulinum* type E is a relatively rare fish pathogen.

# Chapter 11:
# Bacterial Kidney Disease — BKD

*Renibacterium salmoninarum* grows as short rods (0.5 × 1.0 μm) forming pairs and short chains; it is aerobic, strongly Gram-positive, periodic acid Schiff positive, non-acid-fast, non-sporing and non-motile. Growth is slow, taking 3−5 weeks for colonies to appear with an optimum temperature of 15−18°C and growth inhibited at 25°C. Blood or serum in the medium enhances growth and l-cysteine is required for growth. *R. salmoninarum* is catalase positive and oxidase-negative. Mol % G + C of the DNA 55.5 (Banner *et al.* 1991).

    *R. salmoninarum* is an obligate pathogen causing bacterial kidney disease in salmonid fish, a major problem in seawater farming of salmon in the Pacific Northwest of America. It is transmitted both horizontally and vertically. The bacteria are able to penetrate and survive in host phagocytic cells and eggs, making it difficult both to treat and to eradicate. A group of morphologically similar bacteria is responsible for pseudokidney disease in fish; they are of low virulence and relatively unimportant as fish pathogens. These are *Carnobacterium piscicola*, *Lactococcus piscium* and *Vagococcus salmoninarum*. They were originally classified as lactobacilli, which as part of the normal flora of fish may be opportunist pathogens. It is important to differentiate these other Gram-positive rods from *R. salmoninarum* and this can be done easily by their growth characteristics and serology.

## Introduction

Bacterial kidney disease (BKD), caused by *Renibacterium salmoninarum* (Sanders & Fryer 1980), is a serious infection of cultured (Earp *et al.* 1953) and apparently also of feral salmonids (Mitchum *et al.* 1979, Banner *et al.* 1986). The disease, initially recorded in freshwater situations, is now recognized as a costly problem in the seawater farming of salmonids, particularly in the Pacific Northwest of North America, and the disease has recently been the subject of four excellent reviews (Fryer & Sanders 1981, Klontz 1983, Munro & Bruno 1988, Elliott *et al.* 1989).

## The disease

BKD was first described in the early 1930s in wild Atlantic salmon (*Salmo salar*) in Scotland (Smith 1964). Shortly thereafter, it was observed in the United States in three species of cultured trout (*Oncorhynchus mykiss*, *Salmo trutta* and *Salvelinus fontinalis*) in Massachusetts (Belding & Merrill 1935) and California (work of J.H. Wales, cited by Earp *et al.* 1953). In Canada, BKD was first observed in 1937 in mature cutthroat trout (*Oncorhynchus clarki*) in a hatchery at Cultus Lake, British Columbia (work of D.C.B. Duff, cited by Evelyn 1986).

    To date, natural outbreaks of BKD have been reported only in salmonids. The disease is a systemic infection that is normally slowly progressive and frequently fatal. It seldom shows up in fish until they are 6−12 months old. For this reason it is a costly problem in the seawater farming of salmonids, where the practice is to market fish at large size.

Fish severely affected with BKD may show no obvious external signs, or may show one or more of the following: pale gills indicative of anaemia, exophthalmia, abdominal distension (due to the accumulation of ascitic fluid), skin blisters filled with clear or turbid fluid, shallow ulcers (the results of broken skin blisters), haemorrhages (particularly around the vent), and, more rarely, cavitations in the musculature, filled with blood-tinged caseous or necrotic material (Fig. 11.1). Internally, there may be turbid fluid in the abdominal and pericardial cavities, varying amounts of haemorrhage on the walls of the abdominal cavity and in the viscera, a membranous layer on one or more of the visceral organs, and most characteristically, creamy-white granulomatous lesions (Fig. 11.2) in the kidney and, less frequently, in the spleen and liver (Plate 29). Interestingly, these last-named lesions can be well encapsulated and may even be resolved in species such as Atlantic salmon (*Salmo salar*) (Plate 30), which appear to be fairly resistant to BKD (Munro & Bruno 1988). In the more susceptible Pacific salmon, however, the granulomas are rarely well encapsulated (T.P.T. Evelyn, unpubl. data).

Histopathologically the lesion is a chronic granulomatosis, principally of haemopoietic tissue, but extending to liver, cardiac and skeletal muscle and indeed to virtually any organ *in extremis*. The granuloma is often large, with a central caseous zone bounded by epithelioid cells and infiltrating lymphoid cells. Presence of a capsule is variable and lack of encapsulation is often associated with more aggressive infections (Figs 11.3, 11.4).

## The pathogen

The bacterium responsible for BKD is *Renibacterium salmoninarum* (Sanders & Fryer 1980). It is a small ($0.5 \times 1.0 \mu m$), Gram positive, non-acid-fat, PAS-positive, non-sporing, non-motile, fastidious rod that grows best at 15–18°C and not at all at 25°C. It is likely to be mistaken for only one other group of fish-pathogenic bacilli, and then only if the diagnosis is based entirely on an examination of Gram-stained tissue smears. Under such circumstances it could be confused with members of a group of small, asporogenous, Gram-positive bacilli that are responsible for a condition named pseudokidney disease (Ross & Toth 1974). The pseudokidney disease bacilli do not appear to be highly virulent (Ross & Toth 1974, Michel *et al*. 1986) and have been reported as causing problems in fish only that have undergone stress, such as that due to handling or spawning (Hiu *et al*. 1984). In North America pseudokidney disease usually affects adult salmonids, but in Europe infections have also been reported in trout fry and fingerlings and in carp (*Cyprinus carpio*) (Michel *et al*. 1986). The infections are systemic and frequently chronic, with pathological signs including one or more of the following: abdominal distension due to ascites formation, splenomegaly, muscle granulomata, internal haemorrhages, sub-

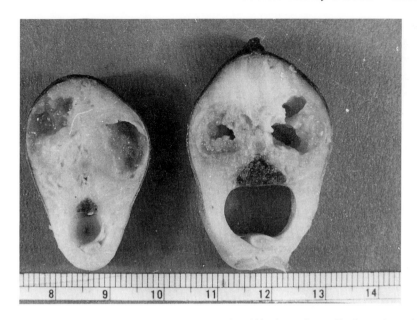

**Fig. 11.1**  Cavitation of the muscle of cultured Pacific salmon due to *Renibacterium salmoninarum* (Courtesy Dr R.E. Wolke).

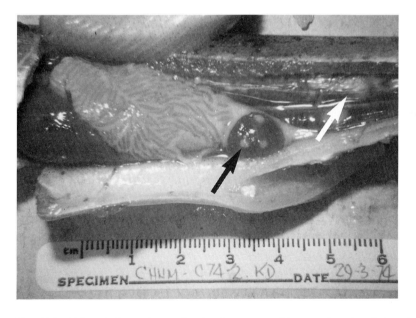

**Fig. 11.2**  Cultured chum salmon, showing the creamy white granulomatous lesions typical of bacterial kidney disease in the spleen (black arrow) and kidney (white arrow). Note also the swollen kidney (Courtesy of J.E. Ketcheson).

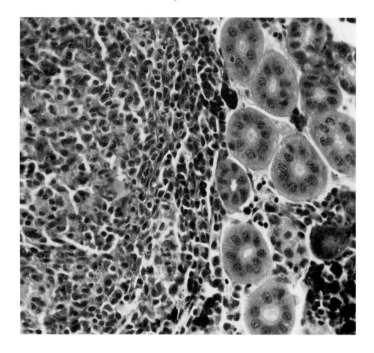

**Fig. 11.3** (above) Early BKD lesion in the kidney of Atlantic salmon, showing displacement of renal tubules by epithelial tissue (H&E × 100) (Courtesy of Dr R.H. Richards).

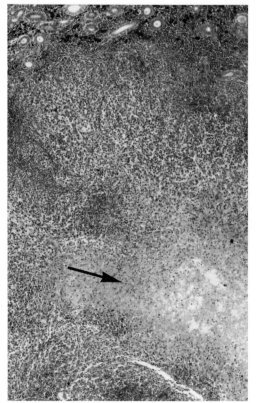

**Fig. 11.4** (left) Extensive BKD lesion in kidney of Atlantic salmon. Much of the renal tissue is replaced by the large chronic inflammatory granuloma with a caseating centre (arrow) (H&E × 100) (Courtesy of Dr R.H. Richards).

cutaneous sanguineous vesiculation and renal granulomata (Hiu *et al.* 1984, Michel *et al.* 1986). The causative bacilli were initially identified as *Lactobacillus piscicola* (Hiu *et al.* 1984), but a re-examination of the isolates obtained from various cases of pseudokidney disease indicates that *L. piscicola* should be renamed *Carnobacterium piscicola* (Collins *et al.* 1990) and that at least two other species of Gram-positive bacilli are also sometimes involved, *Lactococcus piscium* (Williams *et al.* 1990) and *Vagococcus salmoninarum* (Wallbanks *et al.* 1990). These bacteria are, however, easily distinguished from *Renibacterium salmoninarum* because, unlike it, they grow readily on standard laboratory media such as tryptic soy agar or brain heart infusion agar, grow well at 30°C, are biochemically active with a number of substrates including carbohydrates, and fail to react with anti-*R. salmoninarum* sera.

The slow-growing and fastidious properties of *Renibacterium salmoninarum*, as well as the chronic nature of the disease that it usually causes, have contributed to the slowness with which information on it has developed. In addition, other properties of the pathogen, particularly its ability to enter and survive in phagocytic cells and eggs of its hosts, have greatly complicated the task of developing methods for controlling renibacterial infections.

Isolates from widely separated sources are uniform in their phenotypic characteristics (Austin *et al.* 1983, Goodfellow *et al.* 1985, Bruno & Munro 1986*a*) but the response obtained for a given test can vary depending on the testing system used. Thus, although the pathogen is positive for the gelatinase and DNAse reactions by standard methods (Bruno & Munro 1986*a*), it is negative for these features by the API-ZYM (API Laboratory Products) system (Goodfellow *et al.* 1985). Using the latter system, it can be distinguished from all other fish pathogens tested as well as from other Gram-positive bacteria with which it might conceivably be mistaken. In addition, *Renibacterium salmoninarum* is unique among Gram-positive fish pathogens in its requirement for L-cysteine (Austin & Austin 1987).

Serologically, isolates also appear to be homogeneous when tested against polyclonal antisera (Bullock *et al.* 1974, Getchell *et al.* 1985), but serological differences among strains are detectable using monoclonal antibodies (Arakawa *et al.* 1987, Wiens & Kaattari 1987). It has been established that different monoclonal antibodies recognize epitopes that are isolate-specific on a 57 kd surface protein (Wiens & Kaattari 1987). This protein, the major surface antigen, occurred on all isolates examined by Getchell *et al.* (1985) and Wiens and Kaattari (1987). It is heat stable and its presence in the tissues of renibac-terial-infected fish is thought to form the basis of a number of serological tests for detecting such infections: the immunodiffusion test (Chen *et al.* 1974), the coagglutination test (Kimura & Yoshimizu 1981), the counter-immunoelec-trophoresis test (Cipriano *et al.* 1985) and various forms of the enzyme-linked immunosorbent assay (ELISA) (Sakai *et al.* 1987, Pascho & Mulcahy 1987, Turaga *et al.* 1987*a*). The antigen is released to the culture medium during growth, is associated with virulence (Bruno 1988, 1990) and the auto-aggregating properties of the microorganism (Daly & Stevenson 1987, Bruno 1988, 1990), and can be dissociated from the cell surface with distilled water (Daly & Stevenson 1987) or saline (Bruno 1990). This protein also occurs, along with other renibacterial proteins, in the serum with BKD fish (Turaga *et al*. 1987*a*, Wiens & Kaattari 1987), the concentration of the proteins being positively correlated with the degree of anaemia exhibited by the fish (Turaga *et al*. 1987*b*). These proteins, referred to as the soluble proteins also inhibit antibody production by fish lymphocytes *in vitro* (Turaga *et al*. 1987*b*).

Chemical analysis shows *Renibacterium salmoninarum* to be unique and to justify its placement in its present taxon. The cell wall contains a unique polysaccharide, which is covalently linked to the peptidoglycan and accounts for 60–70% of the dry weight of the cell wall. It contains galactose as the major sugar and smaller amounts of rhamnose, N-acetylglucosamine and N-acetylfucosamine. The last-named compound is rare in Gram-positive bacteria and is therefore of diagnostic value for the bacterium (Fiedler & Draxl 1986). In addition, the peptidoglycan contains a peptide bridge composed of glutamic acid, lysine, alanine and glycine (molar ratio $1:1:4:1$), the sequence of these amino acids in the bridge being unique among the Gram-positive bacteria (Kusser & Fiedler 1983). The mol. % G + C of the DNA is 55.5% (Banner *et al*. 1991).

Lipid analysis also showed renibacterial cells to be different from those of other Gram-positive bacteria (Embley *et al*. 1983). The fatty acids were virtually all methyl-branched rather than straight-chained, and several unsaturated menaquinones and a distinctive pattern of polar lipids composed of diphosphatidylglycerol, two major and six or seven minor glycolipids, and two unidentified minor phospholipids were present. In addition, it lacked components found in a number of other Gram-positive bacteria, mycolic acid, diaminobutyric acid, and phosphatidylinositol and its related dimannosides.

## Epizootiology of BKD

### Geographic range

BKD has been reported from most areas of the world where salmonids occur, notable exceptions being Australia, New Zealand and the Soviet Union. The disease has been reported in the United Kingdom, a number of European countries (France, Germany, Italy, Norway, Spain, Sweden, Yugoslavia and Iceland), Japan, North America and, most recently, South America (Chile) (Amos 1985, Bylund 1987). The infection is widely distributed in North America. In Canada, for example, it has been found in all but two regions (Newfoundland and the Yukon Territory), the lack of reports from these regions probably reflecting inadequate sampling rather than the absence of the infection.

### Sources of infection

It has generally been held that *Renibacterium salmoninarum* is an obligate pathogen of salmonid fishes and that the reservoir of infection is the infected salmonid (Fryer & Sanders 1981). It seems that water or aquatic sediments are unlikely as reservoirs of *Renibacterium salmoninarum* because of the poor survival of the pathogen outside of the host. Tests in the author's laboratory, for example, show that the pathogen exhibits only limited survival in sterile soft and hard fresh water and in sea water (Table 11.1), and that in situations such as salmon farms there are organisms such as mussels (*Mytilus edulis*) that remove the pathogen from the water column and digest it (T.P.T. Evelyn, unpublished data). In addition, Austin & Rayment (1985) have shown the survival of viable cells in non-sterile fresh water and freshwater sediments to be only approximately 4 and 21 days, respectively, and they failed to detect the pathogen in fresh water and sediments of trout farms in which BKD was known to be enzootic.

It also appears unlikely that non-salmonid fishes serve as a source of reni-bacterial infections because documented reports of the pathogen in non-salmonid fishes, commercially important or otherwise, do not exist. In contrast, certain other salmonid pathogens are frequently recovered in non-salmonid fishes. For example, the virus responsible for infectious pancreatic necrosis and the bacterium causing furunculosis in salmonids have both been isolated from a large number of non-salmonids (Hill 1982, Paterson 1983). Notwithstanding the foregoing, infections can be established in non-salmonid fishes under special conditions. Such infections have been accomplished experimentally in five of the six species of non-salmonid fishes tested to date (Table 11.2). In addition, Pacific herring (*Clupea harengus pallasi*) living in net pens with BKD-affected coho salmon have been reported as infected (Eunice Lam, personal communication). It is possible, therefore, that Pacific herring and other non-salmonids, which occur incidentally on salmon farms, could become accidental carriers of the pathogen by virtue of prolonged exposure to it on the farms. Such infections must, however, be rare because a survey of Pacific herring and other non-salmonid fishes living in and adjacent to netpens with BKD-affected salmon failed to reveal the presence of any such infections (Paclibare *et al.* 1988a) and

**Table 11.1** Survival of *Renibacterium salmoninarum* (Rs) in various filter-sterilized suspending media at 15°C

| Suspending medium | % Survival at indicated times (days)[a] | | | | |
|---|---|---|---|---|---|
| | 2 | 5 | 7 | 12 | 16 |
| Saline (0.9% NaCl) | 0.01 | 0 | 0 | 0 | 0 |
| Hard fresh water[b] | 97.0 | 70.0 | 59.0 | 17.0 | 0.01 |
| Soft fresh water[c] | 87.0 | 3.0 | 0.02 | 0 | 0 |
| Sea water[d] | 63.0 | 19.0 | 10.0 | 3.0 | 0 |

[a] Initial viable cell population: $1.71 \times 10^5$ Rs cells/ml
[b] A hatchery water supply: Hardness 224 ppm as $CaCO_3$
[c] A hatchery water supply: hardness 22 ppm as $CaCO_3$
[d] Salinity 32‰.

**Table 11.2**   Susceptibility of various non-salmonid fishes to *Renibacterium salmoninarum* (Rs)

| Non-salmonid | Susceptibility[a] | Author(s) |
|---|---|---|
| Pacific herring | | Traxler & Bell (1988) |
| (*Clupea harengus pallasi*) | + | |
| Sablefish | | |
| (*Anoplopoma fimbria*) | + | Bell et al. (1990) |
| Pacific lamprey | | |
| (*Lampetra tridentata*) | – | Bell & Traxler (1986) |
| Shiner perch | | |
| (*Cymatogaster aggregata*) | + | T.P.T. Evelyn, unpublished data |
| Common shiner | | |
| (*Notropis cornutus*) | + | Hicks et al. (1986) |
| Flathead minnow | | |
| (*Pimephales promelas*) | + | Hicks et al. (1986) |

[a] Based on the response to an intraperitoneally injected challenge with Rs (first four species) and to infection by lavage (last two species)

because tests with one of these non-salmonids, the shiner perch (*Cymatogaster aggregata*), indicated that it was refractory to infection when held in tanks for periods up to 5 months with renibacterial infected fish (T.P.T. Evelyn, unpublished data).

**Mode of transmission**

It is now clear that the pathogen is transmitted both horizontally and vertically, perhaps explaining why the pathogen persists in salmon populations as well as it does. Horizontal transmission in fresh water has been shown to occur in the wild in several species of trout (Mitchum & Sherman 1981) as well as in the laboratory in sockeye salmon (*Oncorhynchus nerka*) (Bell *et al.* 1984). In the sockeye study, fish which were known to be *Renibacterium*-free and which had been fed various experimental diets intended to reduce their susceptibility to *Renibacterium salmoninarum* were tested for their resistance by holding them in freshwater tanks with fish deliberately infected with *Renibacterium*. In every case the uninfected sockeye became infected and died of BKD. Horizontal transmission also occurs in sea water, and (Murray *et al.* (1992)) using 12 g chinook salmon (*Oncorhynchus tshawytscha*) held in sea water, showed in a diet experiment analogous to that of Bell *et al.* (1984) that transmission of the pathogen readily occurred when deliberately infected fish were held in the same tank as uninfected fish (the time to 50% mortality in the latter fish was approximately 145 days at an average temperature of 9.9°C).

Horizontal transmission in sea water was also taken advantage of on two occasions by T.P.T. Evelyn (unpublished data) to assess the efficacy of various experimental anti-BKD vaccines in sockeye salmon. On these occasions, variously vaccinated sockeye salmon fingerlings that had been tested by Gram stain and culture and been found to be free of the bacterium were placed in netpens alongside other salmon that were known to be affected with the BKD. Within 12 months of exposure, 66—78% of the test sockeye that had survived the initial outbreaks of vibriosis had died of BKD. That horizontal transmission of the bacterium can occur in salmonids held in close proximity to each other in fresh or sea water should not be too surprising when one considers the survival times found for the microorganism in these media (see Table 11.1).

Using rainbow trout and chinook salmon, Bullock *et al.* (1978) showed that the bacterium could be transmitted from parent to progeny via the egg. Because the transmission occurred even with surface-disinfected eggs, it seemed likely that the pathogen was located within the egg, where it would have been out of reach of the disinfectant. The intra-ovum location of the pathogen has now been firmly established (Evelyn *et al.* 1984*a*,*b*, 1986*a*), the pathogen occurring in the yolk where it is out of reach of surface disinfectants (Evelyn *et al.* 1986*a*). *Renibacterium*-infected coelomic fluid has been shown to be an important source of infection for the egg (Evelyn *et al.* 1986*b*, Lee & Evelyn 1989), the infections occurring via the micropyle and being favoured by high numbers of bacterial cells in the coelomic fluid. There are indications, however, that intra-ovum infections may also occur prior to ovulation and directly from the ovarian tissue. Observations supporting the latter conclusion were the presence of egg and progeny infections in situations where the coelomic fluid was unlikely to account for them, i.e. the coelomic fluid appeared free of renibacterial cells or contained such low numbers of the cells as to make egg infections unlikely (Lee & Gordon 1987, Lee & Evelyn 1989). In addition, it has been established experimentally that eggs can become infected while still in the ovarian tissue and before exposure to coelomic fluid (Bruno & Munro 1986*b*). In short, *Renibacterium salmoninarum* appears to be particularly well adapted for ensuring that it is vertically transmitted. It is small enough to pass through the micropyle, it appears to induce uptake by cells not normally considered to be strongly phagocytic (e.g. thrombocytes (Lester & Budd 1979), endothelial cells of the collecting ducts in the kidney (Bruno 1986), and, important for vertical transmission, oocytes), and it does not produce toxins that are acutely lethal. The last property means that many infected fish survive to spawn or to serve as sources of eggs for propagative purposes while carrying the high numbers of bacterial cells that favour egg infections.

## Control of BKD

### Chemotherapy

Control of BKD by chemotherapy leaves much to be desired because treatment provides only temporary relief. The poor control of BKD by chemotherapy has been attributed to the intracellular nature of the pathogen (Fryer & Sanders 1981). It appears to survive and multiply within the phagocytic cells of the host (Young & Chapman 1978, Bruno 1986), and in this location, judging by the inability of chemotherapy to effect cures, it appears to be out of reach of antimicrobial agents (in this respect, phagocytic cells of fish appear to differ from those in humans which are said to concentrate erythromycin (Brittain 1987)). In fish, phagocytosed bacterial cells thus survive to initiate new problems once chemotherapy is stopped.

Studies on chemotherapy for BKD, recently reviewed by Elliott *et al.* (1989), began in the early 1950s and focused largely on the sulphur drugs. When, by the late 1950s it became evident that these drugs provided only temporary control of BKD, attention turned to the antibiotics. Erythromycin was identified as the antibiotic of choice for combating BKD, and a 21-day oral regimen was recommended for treating young hatchery fish (Wolf & Dunbar 1959). In addition, injected erythromycin has increasingly been used in adult salmonids to prevent prespawning mortalities due to BKD (Peterson 1982, Groman & Klontz 1983, Sakai *et al.* 1986). Use of erythromycin for broodstock injection carried with it the advantage that there were no untoward effects in the progeny of the treated fish (Sakai *et al.* 1986). However, broodstock injection with the potentially teratogenic antibiotic mixtures of penicillin, streptomycin and terramycin evaluated by DeCew (1972) probably provides more broad-spectrum protection than treatment with erythromycin alone.

As with the sulphur drugs, treatment with erythromycin often must be repeated to effect control of BKD even though the level of the drug attained in orally treated fish (Moffit & Schreck 1988) can be many times the *in vitro* minimum lethal concentration determined for the drug ($<0.3\,\mu g/ml$) by Evelyn *et al.* (1986*c*). Austin (1985) therefore carried out an extensive search for new antimicrobial drugs that might be orally administered to salmonids for controlling BKD. His study showed that sodium penicillin and, not surprisingly, the macrolide antibiotics, specifically erythromycin phosphate, erythromycin thiocyanate, clindamycin and spiramycin, were the antibiotics of choice for therapeutic purposes. Antibiotics of potential value for prophylaxis were erythromycin phosphate, erythromycin thiocyanate, rifampicin, clindamycin and kitasamycin.

Austin's results also confirmed that treatment of *Renibacterium*-infected fish with antibiotics cannot be relied upon to entirely eliminate infections but they suggested that treatment for 10 days was almost as effective as treatment for 21. This finding should be investigated further because of the reduced costs that would result and because there are indications that prolonged treatment with erythromycin can seriously impair kidney function in salmonids (Hicks & Geraci 1984). Another finding of Austin requiring further study was that the efficacy of chemotherapy may be reduced and even abolished by feeding antibiotics with lipoidal carriers such as phosphatidylcholine liposomes, or with fatty acid-containing surfactants such as the Tweens. This was demonstrated using clindamycin. For the time being, therefore, it would probably be advisable to incorporate antibiotics, particularly macrolide antibiotics, into fish diets directly or by using products like gelatin rather than lipoidal products such as fish or vegetable oil.

**Vaccination**

Vaccination would be the ideal approach for preventing or controlling BKD because the disease is widespread and control by means of chemotherapy is unsatisfactory. Unfortunately, the prognosis for an effective anti-BKD vaccine does not appear good. Evelyn (1971) showed that sockeye salmon produced agglutinins in response to injection of heat-killed cells plus Freund's complete adjuvant. The response was, however, slow to develop, and two injections or large doses of antigen were required before all animals responded. Subsequent studies by Evelyn *et al.* (1984*c*) with sockeye and coho salmon showed that the agglutinin response did not translate into protection against the pathogen. In the latter studies, various cell-associated and extracellular products were tested following administration by injection (with and without adjuvant), immersion, spraying and feeding. Lack of protection was also noted by Baudin Laurencin *et al.* (1977) in coho salmon (*Oncorhynchus kisutch*) following injection of killed (presumably) bacterial cells in Freund's complete adjuvant, even though an elevated agglutinin response occurred. In an effort to produce an effective anti-BKD vaccine, Kaattari *et al.* (1987, 1988) utilized the highly immunogenic fish pathogen *Vibrio anguillarum* and a strongly mitogenic substance (probably lipopolysaccharide) derived from it (Yui & Kaattari 1987) as adjuvants in various renibacterial vaccines. Efficacy tests in coho salmon were conducted on a number of the injected vaccine preparations, including killed renibacterial cells, killed vibrio cells to which soluble renibacterial antigen was covalently linked, and killed renibacterial cells to which the soluble vibrio fraction was covalently linked. Again, however, the results were disappointing and the protection observed was feeble and inconsistent.

The most promising anti-BKD vaccine studies were those using Atlantic salmon (Paterson *et al.* 1981) and rainbow trout (McCarthy *et al.* 1984) rather than Pacific salmon. With the former species, high titres of agglutinins resulted in under-yearling and post-yearling parr following a single injection of killed renibacterial cells in FCA. With the post-yearling parr, the response lasted to the smolt stage and appeared to confer protection from natural challenge, the protection being measured in terms of the reduction of BKD lesions evident in the vaccinated fish. In Atlantic salmon vaccinated by injection without adjuvant or by immersion, the immune response was feeble or non-existent. With rainbow trout, the most promising vaccine was a pH-lysed renibacterial cell preparation. This preparation conferred protection against an injected *Renibacterium salmonicida* challenge when administered by injection (without adjuvant) but not by immersion. The foregoing results with Atlantic salmon and rainbow trout must, however, be tempered by the findings of others with these species. Bruno & Munro (1984), for example, were unable to demonstrate any increased survival in injection-challenged Atlantic salmon that had been previously exposed to renibacterial infection or that had been vaccinated by injection with killed bacterial cells in Freund's complete adjuvant when these groups were compared with a naive lot of Atlantic salmon. This held true even though the vaccinates produced elevated anti-renibacterial agglutinins. Similarly, Sakai *et al.* (1989) obtained only feeble protection in rainbow trout vaccinated by injection with killed bacterial cells, with or without-Freund's complete adjuvant. In these fish, agglutinins were only slightly elevated but phagocytic activity of the macrophages was markedly enhanced.

Future work on BKD vaccines might emphasize using purified bacterial products to avoid the possibility that the vaccines contain immunosuppressive substances such as those reported by Turaga *et al.* (1987*b*). In addition the role of a number of immunomodulators should be investigated because it may be that renibacterial immunogens are only feebly immunogenic.

### Avoidance

At the moment, control of BKD is best achieved by avoidance. Avoidance measures must take into account that the disease is spread vertically as well as horizontally.

It should be possible to prevent vertical transmission by using seedstock (eggs and smolts) derived from broodstock that have been screened and found to be free of the bacterium. The male fish is not believed to pose a significant risk of vertical transmission, because it has not been possible to infect eggs with heavily contaminated milt or to increase the egg infection rate by fertilizing eggs while they are immersed in heavy suspensions of renibacterial cells (Evelyn *et al.* 1986*b*). For this reason, broodstock inspection should concentrate on females. The screening procedure used should be rapid, adapted to the mass processing of samples, and, above all, sensitive. For this reason an ELISA, such as described by Pascho & Mulcahy (1987), or perhaps the filtration-fluorescent antibody technique of Elliott & Barila (1987) should be used. ELISA, adapted for use on membrane substrates (see Sakai *et al.* 1987), has not proved suitably sensitive (Paclibare *et al.* 1988*b*) and so cannot be recommended for renibacterial screening at present. Until recently, the immuno-fluorescent antibody technique was the procedure used for broodstock screening in British Columbia, but it proved ineffective in preventing vertical transmission, perhaps because it was too insensitive to detect infected fish. In coelomic fluid samples containing $10^4$ renibacterial cells per ml, for example, it was apt to miss the infection approximately 50% of the time (Lee & Evelyn 1991). The sample of choice for broodstock screening is coelomic fluid because it is known to be a source of infection for eggs and because its *Renibacterium* load appears to reflect the infection status of ovarian tissue, the other likely source of infection for eggs (Lee & Gordon 1987, Lee & Evelyn 1989).

To help ensure that vertical transmission does not occur, female broodstock should be injected with erythromycin (20 mg/kg fish) prior to spawning. Other drugs that have been evaluated experimentally and have shown promise for this purpose are penicillin G, oxytetracycline, cephradine and rifampicin (Brown *et al*. 1990). Broodstock injection decreases the chances that egg infections will occur because it reduces the number of viable bacterial cells present in the fish. In addition, it also arms the eggs with therapeutic levels of non-leachable erythromycin (Evelyn *et al*. 1986*c*, Armstrong *et al*. 1989), thus helping to ensure that any viable bacterial cells within the eggs are killed. The drug is detectable in alevins hatching from eggs of treated fish, and tests on the efficacy of the procedure indicate that it is likely to be of significant benefit. In one experiment utilizing eggs from erythromycin-injected broodstock that had been micro-injected with *Renibacterium salmoninarum* (10 bacterial cells per egg), the infection rate was reduced by 62% by the hatch stage. When cephradine and rifampicin were used, the analogous reductions were 81 and 78%, respectively (Brown *et al*. 1990). In a second experiment, eggs and alevins from experimentally infected mature coho salmon were completely freed of the pathogen by injecting the fish with erythromycin prior to spawning. In comparison, eggs and alevins from the control (uninjected) brood coho had infection rates averaging 15 and 22%, respectively (Lee & Evelyn 1991).

The broodstock injection is given medially between the epaxial muscles, just anterior to the dorsal fin, and its timing is important if therapeutic levels of erythromycin are to accumulate in the eggs (Evelyn *et al*. 1986*c*). Initially it was shown that injections given between 30 and 56 days before spawning (but not earlier) resulted in the necessary antibiotic accumulation. However, injections given as close as 9 days prior to spawning also result in the required intra-ovum levels of the antibiotic (Armstrong *et al*. 1989). As an added precaution, following spawning, eggs from treated broodfish should be surface-disinfected with an iodophore to eliminate any surface-borne renibacterial cells. In addition, smolts produced from the above eggs should be grown in ground water or in surface water that has been treated to kill fish pathogens (see Elliott *et al*. 1989) or that is devoid of salmonids. Consideration should also be given to treating fry with orally administered erythromycin shortly after first feeding. At this stage, the cost of treatment should be minimal, and the infection level should be low. *Renibacterium* infections at this stage might thus be reasonably amenable to treatment.

In attempting to avoid horizontal infections, two important actions should be taken in addition to the routine sanitary precautions normally carried out on salmon farms. First, the farm should be located well away from major salmon rivers or from other salmonid farms. Second, it is highly advisable that only one age group of fish be held on any given farm at any given time. This procedure prevents one age group of fish (usually the older fish) from infecting another age group (usually the younger fish), and it provides an opportunity for disinfection of the farm during its fallow period. If, however, circumstances force the holding of more than one age group on the farm, then the different age groups should be held as far apart as possible and they should be arranged so that they are abreast of the dominant line of current flow.

**Detection methods**

Central to the control of BKD by avoidance is the need for a convenient and sensitive method for detecting renibacterial infections. This is particularly important where one is attempting to identify pathogen-free fish for propagative purposes and where these fish must be drawn from populations in which the pathogen is known to be present. Mention has been made earlier of a number of serological methods for detecting the microorganism. Of these, only those listed in the previous section are convenient and sensitive enough for routine surveys. Ideally, however, if the dot blot ELISA procedures evaluated by Sakai *et al.* (1987) can be shown to be as sensitive in the hands of others, these procedures would probably be adopted for renibacterial screening work because the equipment needed for their execution is minimal.

Culture techniques for routine screening are probably contra-indicated because of the lengthy incubation periods required to grow the microorganism and because of contamination problems with faster growing bacteria that may be present in the samples. Notwithstanding this, an ability to culture the pathogen has been essential in gaining an understanding of how it manages to persist as well as it does in salmonids. In addition, culture can be expected to play an important role in the evaluation of techniques developed for controlling BKD and in studies on the epizootiology of the disease. Two advances in the ability to culture the pathogen deserve special mention. These are an improved ability to grow it selectively (Austin *et al.* 1983) and the development of a new technique, based on the use of a nurse culture or its metabolite(s), for accelerating growth of the microorganism and for increasing the sensitivity with which it can be detected (Evelyn *et al.* 1989, 1990). By combining the positive features of these two techniques, a more powerful tool for studying *Renibacterium salmoninarum* will be available.

## Conclusions

With the present technology, it should be possible to have a productive salmon farming industry even in regions where BKD is widely distributed. To accomplish this, however, strict adherence to measures for avoiding the infection is required.

Future research on BKD should aim, in part, to determine whether present approaches to avoiding the infection are entirely adequate. This research should include studies to (1) determine whether there are reservoirs of the bacterium other than salmonid fishes, (2) evaluate, and if necessary improve on, the broodstock injection procedure, (3) develop methods for treating eggs directly to free them of the pathogen, (4) evaluate the dot blot form of the ELISA to see whether it is as sensitive as it is has been reported to be, and (5) to determine whether immunity to *Renibacterium salmoninarum* can be enhanced using vaccines containing immunomodulators.

Research on nutrition should also be undertaken because the ability of fish to cope with BKD may also be enhanced by improved diets. Tests with synthetic diets clearly indicate that this may be so (Lall *et al.* 1985, Bowser *et al.* 1988), but further work is needed to determine whether similar results can be reproducibly obtained with commercial feeds.

In the long term, breeding programmes are likely to provide the most important answer to the BKD problem because resistance to BKD is clearly genetically based (Suzumoto *et al.* 1977, Winter *et al.* 1980). This will be especially important for farmers wishing to grow BKD-susceptible species such as Pacific salmon. Domesticated strains of such species with resistance to BKD similar to that of rainbow trout should be one of the goals of the breeding programs. In the Pacific Northwest of North America, the process of producing BKD resistant strains of Pacific salmon has begun only recently, but already strains with increased resistance to BKD have been identified and the heritability of the trait established (Withler & Evelyn 1990).

# References

Amos, K.H. (Ed.) (1985) *Procedures for the Detection and Identification of Certain Fish Pathogens*, 3rd edition. Fish Health Section, American Fisheries Society, Corvallis, Oregon.

Arakawa, C.K., Sanders, J.E. & Fryer, J.L. (1987) Production of monoclonal antibodies against *Renibacterium salmoninarum*. *Journal of Fish Diseases*, **10**, 249–53.

Armstrong, R.D., Evelyn, T.P.T., Martin, S.W., Dorward, W. & Ferguson, H.W. (1989) Erythromycin levels within eggs and alevins derived from spawning broodstock chinook salmon (*Oncorhynchus tshawytscha*) injected with the drug. *Diseases of Aquatic Organisms*, **6**, 33–6.

Austin, B. (1985) Evaluation of antimicrobial compounds for the control of bacterial kidney disease in rainbow trout, *Salmo gairdneri* Richardson. *Journal of Fish Diseases*, **8**, 209–20.

Austin, B. & Austin, D. (1987) *Bacterial Fish Pathogens: Disease in Farmed and Wild Fish*. Ellis Horwood Ltd, Chichester.

Austin, B. & Rayment, J.N. (1985) Epizootiology of *Renibacterium salmoninarum*, the causal agent of bacterial kidney disease in salmonid fish. *Journal of Fish Diseases*, **8**, 505–9.

Austin, B., Embley, T.M. & Goodfellow, M. (1983) Selective isolation of *Renibacterium salmoninarum*. *FEMS Microbiology Letters*, **17**, 111–14.

Banner, C.R., Rohovec, J.S. & Fryer, J.L. (1991) A new value for mol percent guanine + cystosine of DNA for the salmonid fish pathogen *Renibacterium salmoninarum*, *FEMS Microbiology Letters*, **79**, 57–60.

Banner, C.R., Long, J.J., Fryer, J.L. & Rohovec, J.S. (1986) Occurrence of salmonid fish infected with *Renibacterium salmoninarum* in the Pacific Ocean. *Journal of Fish Diseases*, **9**, 273–5.

Baudin Laurencin, F., Vigneulle, M. & Mevel, M. (1977) Premières observations sur la corynebacteriose des salmonides en Bretagne. *Bulletin de l'Office International des Epizooties*, **87**, 505–7.

Belding, D.L. & Merrill, B. (1935) A preliminary report upon a hatchery disease of the Salmonidae. *Transactions of the American Fisheries Society*, **65**, 76–84.

Bell, G.R. & Traxler, G.S. (1986) Resistance of the Pacific lamprey, *Lampetra tridentata* (Gairdner), to challenge by *Renibacterium salmoninarum*, the causative agent of kidney disease in salmonids. *Journal of Fish Diseases*, **9**, 277–9.

Bell, G.R., Higgs, D.A. & Traxler, G.S. (1984) The effect of dietary ascorbate, zinc, and manganese on the development of experimentally induced bacterial kidney disease in sockeye salmon (*Oncorhynchus nerka*). *Aquaculture*, **36**, 293–311.

Bell, G.R., Hoffman, R.W. & Brown, L.L. (1990) Pathology of experimental infections of the sablefish (*Anoplopoma fimbria*) with *Renibacterium salmoninarum*, the agent of bacterial kidney disease in salmonids. *Journal of Fish Diseases*, **13**, 355–67.

Bowser, P.R., Landy, R.B. & Wooster, G.A. (1988) Efficacy of elevated dietary fluoride for the control of *Renibacterium salmoninarum* infection in rainbow trout *Salmo gairdneri*. *Journal of the World Aquaculture Society*, **19**, 1–7.

Brittain, D.C. (1987) Uptake of antibiotics I. Erythromycin. *Medica Clinica North America*, **71**, 1147–54.

Brown, L.L., Albright, L.J. & Evelyn, T.P.T. (1990) Control of vertical transmission of *Renibacterium salmoninarum* by injection of antibiotics into maturing female coho salmon *Oncorhynchus kisutch*. *Diseases of Aquatic Organisms*, **9**, 127–31.

Bruno, D.W. (1986) Histopathology of bacterial kidney disease in laboratory infected rainbow trout, *Salmo gairdneri* Richardson, and Atlantic salmon, *Salmo salar* L., with reference to naturally infected fish. *Journal of Fish Diseases*, **9**, 523–37.

Bruno, D.W. (1988) The relationship between autoagglutination, cell surface hydrophobicity and virulence of the pathogen *Renibacterium salmoninarum*. *FEMS Microbiology Letters*, **51**, 135–40.

Bruno, D.W. (1990) Presence of a saline-extractable protein associated with virulent strains of the fish pathogen, *Renibacterium salmoninarum*. *Bulletin of the European Association of Fish Pathologists*, **10**(2), 8–10.

Bruno, D.W. & Munro, A.L.S. (1984) Epidemiological studies of bacterial kidney disease in Scotland. In *International Seminar on Fish Pathology for the 20th Anniversary of the Japanese Society of Fish Pathology*, pp. 57–8. Tokyo, Japan.

Bruno, D.W. & Munro, A.L.S. (1986*a*) Uniformity in the biochemical properties of *Renibacterium salmoninarum* isolates obtained from several sources. *FEMS Microbiology Letters*, **33**, 247–50.

Bruno, D.W. & Munro, A.L.S. (1986*b*) Observations on *Renibacterium salmoninarum* and the salmonid egg. *Diseases of Aquatic Organisms*, **1**, 83–7.

Bullock, G.L., Stuckey, H.M. & Chen, P.K. (1974). Corynebacterial kidney disease of salmonids: growth and serological studies on the causative bacterium. *Applied Microbiology*, **28**, 811–14.

Bullock, G.L., Stuckey, H.M. & Mulcahy, D. (1978) Corynebacterial kidney disease: egg transmission following iodophore disinfection. *Fish Health News*, **7**, 51–2.

Bylund, G. (1987) Aspects on fish disease problems in Scandinavian countries. In *Parasites and Diseases in Natural Waters and Aquaculture in Nordic Countries* (Ed. by A. Stenmark and G. Malmberg), pp. 102–11. Naturiska Riksmuseets, Stockholm.

Chen, P.K., Bullock, G.L., Stuckey, H.M. & Bullock, A.C. (1974) Serological diagnosis of corynebacterial kidney disease of salmonids. *Journal of the Fisheries Research Board of Canada*, **31**, 1939–40.

Cipriano, R., Starliper, C.E. & Schachte, J.H. (1985) Comparative sensitivities of diagnostic procedures used to detect bacterial kidney disease in salmonid fishes. *Journal of Wildlife Diseases*, **21**, 144–8.

Collins, M.D., Farrow, J.A.E., Philips, B.A., Ferusu, S. & Jones, D. (1990) Classification of *Lactobacillus divergens*, *Lactobacillus piscicola*, and some catalase-negative, asporogenous, rod-shaped bacteria from poultry in a new genus, *Carnobacterium*. *International Journal of Systematic Bacteriology*, **37**, 310–16.

Daly, J.G. & Stevenson, R.M.W. (1987) Hydrophobic and haemagglutinating properties of *Renibacterium salmoninarum*. *Journal of General Microbiology*, **133**, 3575–80.

DeCew, M.G. (1972). Antibiotic toxicity, efficacy, and teratogenicity in adult spring chinook salmon (*Oncorhynchus tshawytscha*). *Journal of the Fishery Research Board of Canada*, **29**, 1513–17.

Earp, B.J., Ellis, C.H. & Ordal, E.J. (1953) Kidney disease in young salmon. State of Washington Department of Fisheries, Special Report Series, Number 1.

Elliott, D.G. & Barila, T.Y. (1987) Membrane filtration-fluorescent antibody staining procedure for detecting and quantifying *Renibacterium salmoninarum* in coelomic fluid of chinook salmon (*Oncorhynchus tshawytscha*). *Canadian Journal of Fisheries and Aquatic Sciences*, **44**, 206–10.

Elliott, D.G., Pascho, R.J. & Bullock, G.L. (1989) Developments in the control of bacterial kidney disease of salmonid fishes. *Diseases of Aquatic Organisms*, **6**, 201–15.

Embley, T.M., Goodfellow, M., Minnikin, D.E. & Austin, B. (1983) Fatty acids, isoprenoid quinone and polar lipid composition in the classification of *Renibacterium salmoninarum*. *Journal of Applied Bacteriology*, **55**, 31–7.

Evelyn, T.P.T. (1971) The agglutinin response in sockeye salmon vaccinated intraperitoneally with a heat-killed preparation of the bacterium responsible for salmonid kidney disease. *Journal of Wildlife Diseases*, **7**, 328–35.

Evelyn, T.P.T. (1986) A historical note on bacterial kidney disease (BKD) in Canada. Fish Health Section, *American Fisheries Society Newsletter*, **14**(4), 6.

Evelyn, T.P.T., Ketcheson, J.E. & Prosperi-Porta, L. (1984*a*) Further evidence for the presence of *Renibacterium salmoninarum* in salmonid eggs and for the failure of povidone-iodine to reduce the intra-ovum infection rate in water-hardened eggs. *Journal of Fish Diseases*, **7**, 173–82.

Evelyn, T.P.T., Prosperi-Porta, L. & Ketcheson, J.E. (1984*b*) The salmonid egg as a vector of the kidney disease bacterium, *Renibacterium salmoninarum*. In *Fish Diseases*, 4th COPRAQ Session (Ed. ACUIGRUP, Editora ATP), Madrid, pp. 111–17.

Evelyn, T.P.T., Ketcheson, J.E. & Prosperi-Porta, L. (1984*c*) On the feasibility of vaccination as a means of controlling bacterial kidney disease in Pacific salmon. Abstracts, International Conference on Biology of Pacific Salmon, 5–12 September 1984, Victoria/Agassiz, British Columbia.

Evelyn, T.P.T., Prosperi-Porta, L. & Ketcheson, J.E. (1986*a*) Persistence of the kidney disease bacterium, *Renibacterium salmoninarum*, in coho salmon, *Oncorhynchus kisutch* (Walbaum), eggs treated during water-hardening with povidone-iodine. *Journal of Fish Diseases*, **9**, 461–4.

Evelyn, T.P.T., Prosperi-Porta, L. & Ketcheson, J.E. (1986*b*) Experimental intra-ovum infection of salmonid eggs with *Renibacterium salmoninarum* and vertical transmission of the pathogen with such eggs despite treatment with erythromycin. *Diseases of Aquatic Organisms*, **1**, 197–202.

Evelyn, T.P.T., Ketcheson, J.E. & Prosperi-Porta, L. (1986*c*) Use of erythromycin as a means of preventing vertical transmission of *Renibacterium salmoninarum*. *Diseases of Aquatic Organisms*, **2**, 7–11.

Evelyn, T.P.T., Bell, G.R., Prosperi-Porta, L. & Ketcheson, J.E. (1989) A simple technique for accelerating the growth of the kidney disease bacterium *Renibacterium salmoninarum* on a commonly used culture medium (KDM2). *Diseases of Aquatic Organisms*, **7**, 231–34.

Evelyn, T.P.T., Prosperi-Porta, L. & Ketcheson, J.E. (1990) Two new techniques for obtaining consistent results when growing *Renibacterium salmoninarum* on KDM2 culture medium. *Diseases of Aquatic Organisms*, **9**, 209–12.

Fiedler, F. & Draxl, R. (1986) Biochemical and immunological properties of *Renibacterium salmoninarum*. *Journal of Bacteriology*, **168**, 799–804.

Fryer, J.L. & Sanders, J.E. (1981) Bacterial kidney disease of salmonid fish. *Annual Review of Microbiology*, **35**, 273–98.

Getchell, R.G., Rohovec, J.S. & Fryer, J.L. (1985) Comparison of *Renibacterium salmoninarum* isolates by antigenic analysis. *Fish Pathology*, **20**, 149–59.

Goodfellow, M., Embley, T.M. & Austin, B. (1985) Numerical taxonomy and emended description of *Renibacterium salmoninarum*. *Journal of General Microbiology*, **131**, 2739–52.

Groman, D.B. & Klontz, G.W. (1983) Chemotherapy and prophylaxis of bacterial kidney disease with erythromycin. *Journal of the World Mariculture Society*, **14**, 226–35.

Hicks, B.D. & Geraci, J.R. (1984) A histological assessment of damage in rainbow trout, *Salmo gairdneri* Richardson, fed rations containing erythromycin. *Journal of Fish Diseases*, **7**, 457–465.

Hicks, B.D., Daly, J.G. & Ostland, V.E. (1986) Experimental infection of minnows with the bacterial kidney disease bacterium *Renibacterium salmoninarum*. Abstract, Third Annual Meeting, Aquaculture Association of Canada, July 1986, Guelph, Ontario.

Hill, B.J. (1982) Infectious pancreatic necrosis virus and its virulence. In *Microbial Diseases of Fish, Special Publications of the Society for General Microbiology*, 9 (Ed. by R.J. Roberts), pp. 91–114. Academic Press, London, New York.

Hiu, S.F., Holt, R.A., Sriranganathan, N., Seidler, R.J. & Fryer, J.L. (1984) *Lactobacillus piscicola*, a new species from salmonid fish. *International Journal of Systematic Bacteriology*, **34**, 393–400.

Kaattari, S.L., Holland, N., Turaga, P. & Wiens, G. (1987) Development of a vaccine for bacterial kidney disease. Bonneville Power Administration, Project 84–46, Annual Report 1986, Portland, Oregon.

Kaattari, S.L., Chen, D., Turaga, P. & Wiens, G. (1988) Development of a vaccine for bacterial kidney disease. Bonneville Power Administration, Project 84–46, Annual Report 1987, Portland, Oregon.

Kimura, T. & Yoshimizu, M. (1981) A coagglutination test with antibody sensitized staphylococci for rapid and simple diagnosis of bacterial kidney disease (BKD). *Developments in Biological Standards*, **49**, 135–48.

Klontz, G.W. (1983) Bacterial kidney disease in salmonids: an overview. In *Antigens of Fish Pathogens* (Ed. by D.P. Anderson, M. Dorson & P.H. Dubourget), pp. 177–99. Collection Fondation Marcel Merioux.

Kusser, W. & Fiedler, F. (1983) Murein type and polysaccharide composition of cell walls from *Renibacterium salmoninarum*. *FEMS Microbiology Letters*, **20**, 391–394.

Lall, S.P., Paterson, W.D., Hines, J.A. & Adams, N.J. (1985) Control of bacterial kidney disease in Atlantic salmon, *Salmo salar* L., by dietary modification. *Journal of Fish Diseases*, **8**, 113–24.

Lee, E.G.-H. & Evelyn, T.P.T. (1989) Effect of *Renibacterium salmoninarum* levels in ovarian fluid of spawning chinook salmon on the prevalence of the pathogen in their eggs and progeny. *Diseases of Aquatic Organisms*, **7**, 179–84.

Lee, E.G.-H. & Evelyn, T.P.T. (1991) Broodstock erythromycin injection prevents Renibacterium vertical transmission. *Fish Health Section American Fisheries Society Newsletter*, **19**(4), 1.

Lee, E.G.-H. & Gordon, M.R. (1987) Immunofluorescence screening of *Renibacterium salmoninarum* in the tissues and eggs of farmed chinook salmon spawners. *Aquaculture*, **65**, 7–14.

Lester, R.J.G. & Budd, J. (1979) Some changes in the blood cells of diseased coho salmon. *Canadian Journal of Zoology*, **57**, 1458–64.

McCarthy, D.H., Croy, T.R. & Amend, D.F. (1984) Immunization of rainbow trout, *Salmo gairdneri* Richardson, against bacterial kidney disease: preliminary efficacy evaluation. *Journal of Fish Diseases*, **7**, 65–71.

Michel, C., Faivre, B. & Kerouault, B. (1986) Biochemical identification of *Lactobacillus piscicola* strains from France and Belgium. *Diseases of Aquatic Organisms*, **2**, 27–30.

Mitchum, D.L. & Sherman, L.E. (1981) Transmission of bacterial kidney disease from wild to stocked hatchery trout. *Canadian Journal of Fisheries and Aquatic Sciences*, **38**, 547–51.

Mitchum, D.L., Sherman, L.E. & Baxter, G.T. (1979) Bacterial kidney disease in feral populations of brook trout (*Salvelinus fontinalis*), brown trout (*Salmo trutta*), and rainbow trout (*Salmo gairdneri*). *Journal of the Fisheries Research Board of Canada*, **36**, 1370–6.

Moffitt, C.M. & Schreck, J.A. (1988) Accumulation and depletion of orally administered erythromycin thiocyanate in tissues of chinook salmon. *Transactions of the American Fisheries Society*, **117**, 394–400.

Munro, A.L.S. & Bruno, D.W. (1988) Vaccination against bacterial kidney disease. In *Fish Vaccination* (Ed. by A.E. Ellis), pp. 124–34. Academic Press, London.

Murray, C.B., Evelyn, T.P.T., Beacham, T.D., Banner, L.W., Ketcheson, J.E. & Prosperi-Porta, L. (1992) Experimental induction of bacterial kidney disease in chinook salmon by immersion and cohabitation challenges. *Diseases of Aquatic Organisms*, **12**, 91–6.

Paclibare, J.O., Albright, L.J. & Evelyn, T.P.T. (1988a) Investigations on the occurrence of the kidney disease bacterium *Renibacterium salmoninarum* in non-salmonids on selected farms in British Columbia. *Bulletin of the Aquaculture Association of Canada*, **88**(4), 113–15.

Paclibare, J.O., Evelyn, T.P.T. & Albright, L.J. (1988b) A comparative evaluation of various methods for detecting the kidney disease bacterium *Renibacterium salmoninarum* in salmonids. *Bulletin of the Aquaculture Association of Canada*, **88**(4), 110–12.

Paterson, W.D. (1983) Furunculosis and other associated diseases caused by *Aeromonas salmonicida*. In *Antigens of Fish Pathogens* (Ed. by D.P. Anderson, M. Dorson & P.H. Dubourget), pp. 119–36. Collection Fondation Marcel Merioux.

Paterson, W.D., Desautels, D. & Weber, J.M. (1981) The immune response of Atlantic salmon, *Salmo salar* L., to the causative agent of bacterial kidney disease, *Renibacterium salmoninarum*. *Journal of Fish Diseases*, **4**, 99–111.

Pascho, R.J. & Mulcahy, D. (1987) Enzyme-linked immunosorbent assay for a soluble antigen of *Renibacterium salmoninarum*, the causative agent of salmonid bacterial kidney disease. *Canadian Journal of Fisheries and Aquatic Sciences*, **44**, 183–91.

Peterson, J.E. (1982) Analysis of bacterial kidney disease (BKD) and BKD control measures with erythromycin phosphate among cutthroat trout (*Salmo clarki* Bouveri). *Salmonid*, **5**(6), 12−15.

Ross, A.J. & Toth, R.J. (1974) *Lactobacillus* — a new fish pathogen? *Progressive Fish Culturist*, **36**, 191.

Sakai, D.K., Nagata, M., Iwami, T., Kiode, N., Tamiya, Y., Ito, Y. & Atoda, M. (1986) Attempt to control BKD by dietary modification and erythromycin chemotherapy in hatchery-reared masu salmon *Oncorhynchus masou* Brevoort. *Nippon Suisan Gakkaishi*, **52**, 1141−7.

Sakai, M., Koyama, G., Atsuta, S. & Kobayashi, M. (1987) Detection of *Renibacterium salmoninarum* by a modified peroxidase-antiperoxidase (PAP) procedure. *Fish Pathology*, **22**, 1−5.

Sakai, M., Atsuta, S. & Kobayashi, M. (1989) Attempted vaccination of rainbow trout *Oncorhynchus mykiss* against bacterial kidney disease. *Nippon Suisan Gakkaishi*, **55**, 2105−9.

Sanders, J.E. & Fryer, J.L. (1980) *Renibacterium salmoninarum* gen. nov., sp. nov., the causative agent of bacterial kidney disease in salmonid fishes. *International Journal of Systematic Bacteriology*, **30**, 496−502.

Smith, I.W. (1964) The occurrence and pathology of Dee disease. *Freshwater and Salmon Fishery Research*, **34**, 1−12.

Suzumoto, B.K., Schreck, C.B. & McIntyre, J.B. (1977) Relative resistances of three transferrin genotypes of coho salmon (*Oncorhynchus kisutch*) and their hematological responses to bacterial kidney disease. *Journal of the Fisheries Research Board of Canada*, **34**, 1−8.

Traxler, G.S. & Bell, G.R. (1988) Pathogens associated with impounded Pacific herring *Clupea harengus pallasi*, with emphasis on viral erythrocytic necrosis (VEN) and atypical *Aeromonas salmonicida*. *Diseases of Aquatic Organisms*, **5**, 93−100.

Turaga, P.S.D., Wiens, G.D. & Kaattari, S.L. (1987a) Analysis of *Renibacterium salmoninarum* antigen production *in situ*. *Fish Pathology*, **221**, 209−14.

Turaga, P., Wiens, G. & Kaattari, S. (1987b) Bacterial kidney disease: the potential role of soluble protein antigen(s). *Journal of Fish Biology*, **31**(Supplement A), 191−4.

Wallbanks, S., Martinez-Murcia, A.J., Fryer, J.L., Philips, B.A. & Collins, M.D. (1990) 16S rRNA sequence determination for members of the genus *Carnobacterium* and related lactic acid bacteria and description of *Vagococcus salmoninarum* sp. nov. *International Journal of Systematic Bacteriology*, **40**, 224−30.

Wiens, G.D. & Kaattari, S.L. (1987) Monoclonal antibody analysis of common surface protein(s) of *Renibacterium salmoninarum*. *Fish Pathology*, **24**, 1−7.

Williams, A.M., Fryer, J.L. & Collins, M.D. (1990) *Lactococcus piscium* sp. nov. a new *Lactococcus* species from salmonid fish. *FEMS Microbiology Letters*, **68**, 109−14.

Winter, G.W., Schreck, C.B. & McIntyre, J.D. (1980) Resistance of different stocks and transferrin genotypes of coho salmon, *Oncorhynchus kisutch*, and steelhead trout, *Salmo gairdneri*, to bacterial kidney disease and vibriosis. *Fisheries Bulletin US*, **77**, 795−802.

Withler, R.E. & Evelyn, T.P.T. (1990) Genetic variation in resistance to bacterial kidney disease within and between two strains of coho salmon from British Columbia. *Transactions of the American Fisheries Society* (in press).

Wolf, K. & Dunbar, C.E. (1959) Test of 34 therapeutic agents for control of kidney disease in trout. *Transactions of the American Fisheries Society*, **88**, 117−34.

Young, C.L. & Chapman, G.B. (1978) Ultrastructural aspects of the causative agent and renal histopathology of bacterial kidney disease in brook trout (*Salvelinus fontinalis*). *Journal of the Fisheries Research Board of Canada*, **35**, 1234−48.

Yui, M.A. & Kaattari, S.L. (1987) *Vibrio anguillarum* antigen stimulates mitogenesis and polyclonal activation of salmonid lymphocytes. *Developmental and Comparative Immunology*, **11**, 530−49.

# Chapter 12:
# Streptococcal Infections

*Streptococcus* is a large, complex genus of Gram-positive spherical or oval bacteria less than 2 μm in diameter, which occur in pairs or chains when grown in liquid media. They do not form endospores, most are non-motile and some form capsules. Most are facultative anaerobes and chemo-organotrophic with fermentative metabolism and complex growth requirements, e.g. medium supplemented with blood enhances isolation and demonstrates haemolytic activity. Mol % G + C of DNA is 34–46.

Streptococci may occur as commensals or parasites in man and animals, a few are saprophytes in the natural environment and some have been identified from diseased fish in fresh and salt water in Japan and the United States. Serology, particularly the Lancefield group system based on cell wall antigens, is important in classification of streptococci, although of limited use with fish pathogens. Disease affects a wide variety of fish and presents as a streptococcal septicaemia. It is most severe when the water temperature rises above 20°C and other environmental stressors are present. Transmission is horizontal between fish or by contaminated food. Control is mainly by chemotherapy and eradication is very difficult. In Japan in particular it is a source of serious economic loss.

## Introduction

Streptococcal septicaemia was reported first among cultured rainbow trout (*Oncorhynchus mykiss*) in the Shizuoka Prefecture in Japan in April 1957 (Hoshina *et al.* 1958). Somewhat later, Robinson & Meyer (1966) reported two epizootics, both involving infections of golden shiner (*Notemigonus crysoleucas*) with *Streptococcus* sp. Subsequently, Plumb *et al.* (1974) isolated *Streptococcus* sp. from over 50% of the diseased fish during an epizootic in estuarine bays along the Florida and Alabama Gulf Coast of Mexico in the United States in 1972. Since then, the disease has occurred both sporadically and epizootically among cultured freshwater and saltwater fish in many parts of the world. In Japan in particular, streptococcosis has been associated with serious economic losses in cultured yellowtail (*Seriola quinqueradiata*) since 1974 (Kusuda *et al.* 1976, Kitao *et al.* 1979).

## Species specificity and distribution

Outbreaks have been reported in cultured freshwater fish in the United States (Robinson & Meyer 1966, Pier *et al.* 1978), South Africa (Boomker *et al.* 1979) and Japan (Hoshina *et al.* 1958, Kitao *et al.* 1981) and in cultured marine fish in Japan (Kusuda *et al.* 1976, Iida *et al.* 1986) and Singapore (Foo *et al.* 1985). Severe epizootics have also occurred in several species of marine fish in the Gulf of Mexico (Plumb *et al.* 1974) and in the Chesapeake Bay (Baya *et al.* 1990) in the United States.

Some host specificity exists in so far as trout suffer from heavy mortalities

**Table 12.1**  Species which have been affected by streptococcosis

|  |  |
|---|---|
| Natural infections |  |
| Rainbow trout | *Oncorhynchus mykiss* |
| Sea trout | *Cynoscion regalis* |
| Silver trout | *Cynoscion nothus* |
| Golden shiner | *Notemigonus crysoleucas* |
| Yellowtail | *Seriola quinqueradiata* |
| Menhaden | *Brevoortia patronus* |
| Sea catfish | *Arius felis* |
| Striped mullet | *Mugil cephalus* |
| Pinfish | *Lagodon rhomboides* |
| Atlantic croaker | *Macropogon undulatus* |
| Spot | *Leiostomus xanthus* |
| Stingray | *Dasyatis sp.* |
| Freshwater dolphin | *Inia geoffrensis* |
| Eel | *Anguilla japonica* |
| Ayu | *Plecoglossus altivelis* |
| Amago salmon | *Oncorhynchus rhodurus* |
| Jacopever | *Paralichthys olivaceus* |
| Striped bass | *Morone saxatilis* |
| Blue fish | *Pomatomous saltatix* |
| Siganids | *Siganus cahaliculatus* |
| Seabream | *Pagrus major* |
| Tilapia | *Oreochromis sp.* |
| Experimental infections |  |
| Green sunfish | *Lepomis cyanellus* |
| Blue gill | *Lepomis macrochirus* |
| American toad | *Bufo americanus* |
| Blue minnow | *Fundulus grandis* |
| Jack mackerel | *Trachurus japonicus* |

while some tilapia species (*Sarotherodon mossambicus* and *Tilapia sparrmanii*), carp (*Cyprinus carpio*) and largemouth bass (*Micropterus salmoides*) are not affected (Boomker *et al.* 1979).

Species affected naturally and by experimental intervention are shown in Table 12.1.

## Clinical signs and pathology

Clinical signs vary among species of affected fish. However, erratic swimming, darkening of body colour, unilateral or bilateral exophthalmia, corneal opacity, haemorrhages on the opercula and the bases of the fins, and ulceration of body surface are the most common symptoms.

The haemorrhagic lesions, which gradually extend and ulcerate to release necrotic material, are generally raised and have a darkened zone around them. They are more superficial than the lesions of furunculosis or vibriosis. Areas particularly affected are the dorsum, just anterior to the caudal peduncle, the operculum, around the mouth, and, unusually, the underside of the operculum.

Lesions are frequently seen in the anal area, involving the anal fin and also the vent itself (Fig. 12.1).

In many species the eyes are affected with high frequency. The initial lesion may be restricted to exophthalmia resulting from retrobulbar congestion and oedema, but this usually extends to inflammatory infiltration and frank necrosis involving the optic nerve and choroid and extending into the orbit and eye proper (Plates 31, 32). In the eye there is hyperaemia, then haemorrhage of retinal vessels into the vitreous humour, followed by lenticular necrosis and even evulsion of the necrotic material through ulceration of the cornea.

There may be hyperaemia of branchial vessels, infiltration with macrophages and necrosis leading to massive haemorrhage and death. The intestinal tract also may be hyperaemic, with significant sloughing of the mucosa.

The principal visceral organs affected are the spleen and liver and to a more limited degree the heart and kidney. The liver is generally pale, with numerous areas of focal necrosis, while the spleen is enlarged, with rounded edges, and cherry red in colour. It has most of its haemopoietic architecture destroyed and the ellipsoids are thus very prominent, being swollen and usually associated with numbers of bacteria. The heart often manifests pericarditis (Fig. 12.2) and the peritoneal cavity is often distended with blood tinged serous exudate which only rarely has a fibrinous component leading to adhesions (Robinson & Meyer 1966, Plumb *et al.* 1974, Kusuda *et al.* 1976, 1978, Kitao *et al.* 1981, Jo 1982, Miyazaki 1982, Baya *et al.* 1990).

## Aetiological agent

There are few descriptions of the biochemical characteristics of isolates. The *Streptococcus* species described by Robinson & Meyer (1966), Plumb *et al.* (1974) and Rasheed & Plumb (1984) all proved to belong to the same category, namely non-haemolytic or gamma haemolytic, and Lancefield's B group. In contrast the *Streptococcus* species reported by Boomker *et al.* (1979) was identified as a Lancefield's D group enterococcus. Beta-haemolytic *Streptococcus iniae* (Pier & Madin 1976) is described as a separate species in Bergey's Manual (Hardie, 1986) because it did not react with any of the Lancefield's group antisera and furthermore the guanine and cytosine (G + C%) ratio of its DNA was 32.9%. From the results in Table 12.2, the beta-haemolytic streptococci isolated from yellowtail by Minami *et al.* (1979), from ayu salmon by Ohnishi & Jo (1981), from flounder by Nakatsugawa (1983), from yellowtail by Kaige *et al.* (1984) and from jacopever by Sakai *et al.* (1986), all have similar biochemical characteristics. In particular, the beta-haemolytic streptococcus isolated by Kitao *et al.* (1981) has been reported to show strong cross-agglutination with the antiserum of *Streptococcus iniae* (unpublished data). Kawahara & Kusuda (1987), using a direct fluorescent antibody technique, showed that the beta-haemolytic *Streptococcus* species isolated from diseased ayu is antigenically the same as *Streptococcus iniae*. Based on those results, it has been

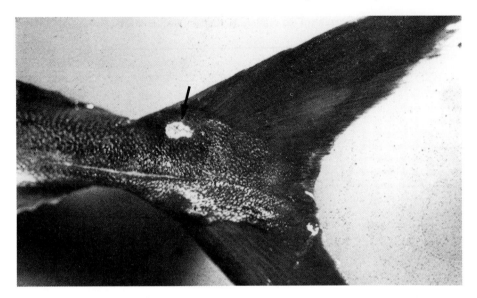

**Fig. 12.1**   Yellowtail infected with streptococcosis, showing necrotic ulcer formation on the caudal peduncle (arrowed).

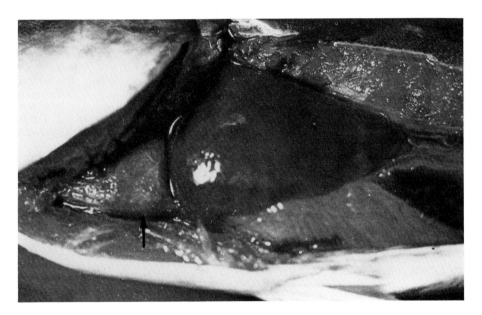

**Fig. 12.2**   Yellowtail infected with *Streptococcus* sp. showing marked pericarditis (arrowed).

proposed that the strains described as beta-haemolytic *Streptococcus* species by Japanese researchers should be classified as a subspecies of *Streptococcus iniae*.

In contrast classification of alpha-haemolytic strains of *Streptococcus* isolated from fish is more problematic. Kusuda *et al.* (1976) and Kitao (1982) reported that the morphological and biochemical characteristics of alpha-haemolytic

**Table 12.2**  Comparative results of the cultural, biochemical and serological characteristics of pathogenic fish *Streptococcus*

| Test | *Streptococcus sp.* Hoshina et al. 1958 | *Streptococcus sp.* Kusuda et al. 1976 | *Streptococcus sp.* Kitao 1982 | *Streptococcus sp.* Kusuda et al. 1978 | *S. faecalis* ATCC19433 | *S. faecium* ATCC19434 | *S. iniae* Pier & Madin (1976) |
|---|---|---|---|---|---|---|---|
| Haemolytic type | α/γ | α | α | α | α | α | β |
| Growth at 10°C | − | + | + | + | + | + | + |
| at 45°C | + | + | + | + | + | + | − |
| NaCl 6.5% | + | + | + | + | + | + | − |
| pH 9.6 | + | + | + | + | + | + | ND |
| 0.1% MB milk | + | + | + | + | + | + | − |
| 40% Bile | ND | + | + | + | + | + | − |
| Hydrolysis of | | | | | | | |
| Gelatin | − | − | − | − | ± | − | − |
| Starch | − | − | − | − | − | − | + |
| Hippurate | − | − | − | − | + | − | − |
| Esculin | + | + | + | + | + | + | + |
| Arginine | ND | + | + | ND | + | + | ND |
| Decarboxylation of | | | | | | | |
| Arginine | ND | ND | ND | ND | + | + | ND |
| 0.01% TTC | ND | + | ND | + | + | − | ND |
| 0.04% PT | ND | − | ND | − | + | − | ND |
| Arabinose | + | − | − | − | − | − | − |
| Glycerol | + | − | − | − | + | − | − |
| Inulin | − | ND | ND | ND | ND | ND | − |
| Lactose | + | − | − | ± | + | + | − |
| Salicin | + | + | + | + | + | + | + |
| Sorbitol | + | + | − | + | + | d | − |
| Sucrose | + | − | − | ± | d | + | + |
| Trehalose | + | + | + | + | + | + | + |
| Lancefield type | | | | | D | D | |
| G + C% | ND | ND | ND | ND | ND | ND | 32.9 |
| Antiserum*[1] (yellowtail strain) | ND | ND | + | ND | − | − | − |
| Antiserum*[2] (Beta-haemolytic *Streptococcus sp.*) | ND | ND | − | ND | − | − | + |
| *S. iniae* antiserum | ND | ND | − | ND | − | − | + |

**Table 12.2** *Continued*

| Test | Isolates of *Streptococcus sp.* | | | | | | |
|---|---|---|---|---|---|---|---|
| | *Streptococcus sp.* Minami et al. 1979 | *Streptococcus sp.* Kitao et al. 1981 | *Streptococcus sp.* Ohnishi & Jo (1981) | *Streptococcus sp.* Nakatsugawa (1983) | *Streptococcus sp.* Sakai et al. 1986 | American strains* | *Streptococcus sp.* Baya et al. 1990 |
| Haemolytic type | β | β | β | β | β | γ | γ |
| Growth at 10°C | − | − | − | − | − | − | ND |
| at 45°C | − | − | − | − | − | − | − |
| NaCl 6.5% | − | − | − | − | − | − | − |
| pH 9.6 | − | − | − | − | − | − | ND |
| 0.1% MB milk | − | − | − | − | − | − | ND |
| 40% Bile | − | − | − | − | − | d | ND |
| Hydrolysis of | | | | | | | |
| Gelatin | − | − | − | − | − | − | ND |
| Starch | + | + | + | + | + | − | − |
| Hippurate | − | − | − | − | − | + | ND |
| Esculin | + | + | + | + | + | − | ND |
| Arginine | + | + | + | + | + | d | + |
| Decarboxylation of | | | | | | | |
| Arginine | − | − | ND | + | ND | d | − |
| 0.01% TTC | ND | ND | ND | ND | ND | ND | ND |
| 0.04% PT | ND | ND | ND | ND | ND | ND | ND |
| Arabinose | − | − | − | − | − | − | − |
| Glycerol | + | − | − | − | − | − | ND |
| Inulin | − | − | − | − | − | ND | ND |
| Lactose | + | − | − | − | − | − | ND |
| Salicin | + | + | + | + | + | d | − |
| Sorbitol | − | − | − | − | − | − | − |
| Sucrose | + | + | + | + | + | d | + |
| Trehalose | + | + | + | + | + | + | − |
| Lancefield type | | | | | | B | B |
| G + C% | ND | ND | ND | ND | ND | ND | ND |
| Antiserum*[1] (yellowtail strain) | ND | − | ND | ND | ND | ND | − |
| Antiserum*[2] (Beta-haemolytic Streptococcus sp.) | ND | + | ND | ND | ND | ND | − |
| *S. iniae* antiserum | ND | + | ND | ND | ND | ND | − |

* American strains were isolated from various fish in USA and the tests were performed by Kusuda & Komatsu (1978). American strains involved Arkansas strain (Robinson & Meyer 1966) and strains isolated by Plumb *et al.* (1974)

Nd = not done

d = different

*Streptococcus* species isolated from cultural yellowtail in Japan were very similar to those of *Streptococcus faecalis* and *Streptococcus faecium* (*Enterococcus* group) but did not react with Lancefield's group D antiserum (Kitao 1982). Therefore these strains still have no species designation. Recently, following DNA/DNA hybridization studies, it has been suggested that the fish derived alpha-haemolytic *Streptococcus* species are in fact genetically distinct from *S. faecalis* and *S. faecium* (T. Kitao *et al.*, unpublished data).

Kusuda *et al.* (1992) have identified isolates from streptococcal infection of yellowtails and eels in Japan as *Enterococcus seriolicida* sp. nov., as a result of detailed biochemical and DNA/DNA hybridization studies, and proposed that the disease caused by this aetiological agent be called 'enterococcal infection'. This work relates a collection of isolates made in Japan in 1973 and 1974 and it remains to be seen whether it is of general application.

## Morphology

*Streptococcus* cells are usually spherical or ovoid (diameter $0.7 \times 1.4\,\mu m$) in shape and arranged singly or in pairs in vivo. In liquid culture they usually occur in chains (Plate 33). Cells are Gram-positive, non-acid fast, non-motile, non-capsule-forming and non-sporulating

## Cultivation

The pathogen is easily grown on trypticase soy agar supplemented with 0.5% glucose (Ohnishi & Jo 1981, Kitao 1982), brain heart infusion agar (Plumb *et al.* 1974, Nakatsugawa 1983), Todd-Hewitt broth agar (THBA) (Kitao 1982) and horse blood agar (Nakatsugawa 1983). Colonies develop after 24−48 h of incubation at 20−30°C. The colonies on agar plates are small (0.5−1.0 mm diameter), yellowish, translucent, rounded and slightly raised (Fig. 12.3). Beta-haemolytic *Streptococcus* species isolated from freshwater and saltwater fish in Japan produce very small viscous colonies on THBA in primary culture.

## Cultural and biochemical characteristics

The pathogenic streptococci of fish show considerable variation in biochemical properties between isolates. Unfortunately their taxonomic position is still unresolved. The mol% guanine plus cytosine of the DNA has been described only for *Streptococcus iniae* and is 32.9 (Pier & Madin 1976). Some of the other cultural, biochemical and serological characteristics of this genus are illustrated in Table 12.2.

## Serology

Lancefield's classification of beta-haemolytic streptococci can be made by ring

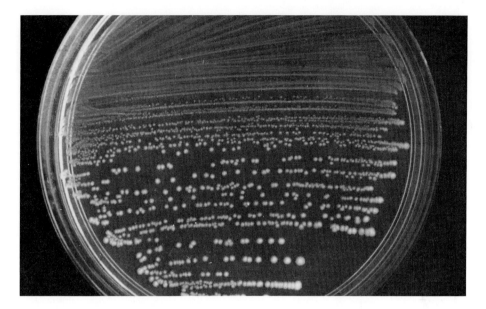

**Fig. 12.3**  Appearance of alpha-haemolytic *Streptococcus* sp. on Todd-Hewitt agar media.

precipitin, gel diffusion precipitation (Rotta *et al*. 1971) and countercurrent electrophoresis (Dajani 1973), in each case by using an extract of the group-specific carbohydrate antigen. There are four methods of extraction, the hot acid method of Lancefield (1933), the hot formamide method of Fuller (1938), the autoclave method of Rantz & Randall (1955) and the enzyme method of Maxted (1948). Co-agglutination (Christensen *et al*. 1973) and immuno-fluorescent techniques (Cars *et al*. 1975) can also be used.

Isolated streptococcal strains may be serotyped using commercially available Lancefield's group antisera. Usually the bacteria derived from fish fall into either group B (Robinson & Meyer 1966, Plumb *et al*. 1974, Rasheed & Plumb 1984, Baya *et al*. 1990) or group D (Boomker *et al*. 1979). As mentioned above, however, none of the *Streptococcus iniae* and alpha-haemolytic *Streptococcus* species isolated from cultured yellowtail in Japan react with any of the known Lancefield's group antisera; they react only with antisera raised to each specifically.

## Antigenic variations

Kitao (1982) stated that there were two antigenic types: the KG$^+$ type agglutin-ates with antiserum of the *Streptococcus* KG7409 strain, and the KG$^-$ type strain possesses a specific envelope-like substance which inhibits agglutination with antisera of *Streptococcus* species KG7409. Variants exist which may lose this envelope-like substance, usually after culture on agar plates containing TTC (2,3,5-Triphenyltetrazolium chloride) (Fig. 12.4), and as a consequence

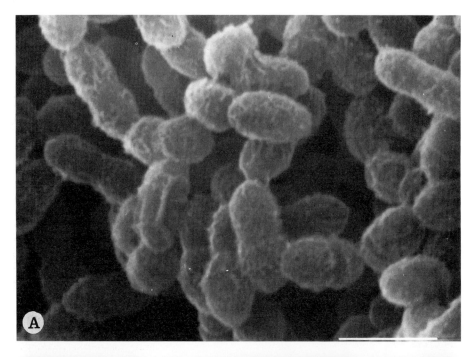

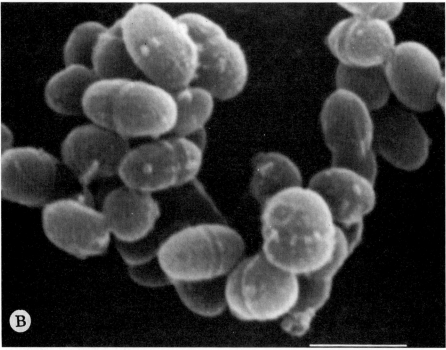

**Fig. 12.4** Scanning electron micrograph of *Streptococcus* sp. strains. (A) — Rough cells of KG⁻ strain (original strain), showing the presence of surface substances around the cells.
(B) — Smooth cells of KG⁺ strain (variant strain) denuded of the extracellular substances which surround the cells of KG⁻ type strain. Bar equals 1 μm.

they may act as KG$^+$. Antisera prepared against KG$^-$ type strains agglutinate both KG$^-$ and KG$^+$ strains.

## Diagnosis

The presence of typical clinical signs and demonstration of Gram-positive cocci from the brains (Plate 32), kidneys and/or other internal organs constitutes a presumptive diagnosis. Sugiyama *et al.* (1981) reported that the causative bacteria are best detected in brains of diseased fish.

Isolation is usually carried out following culture in Todd Hewitt broth or on brain heart infusion or heart infusion agar containing 0.5% glucose for 24−36 h at 25−30°C. Confirmatory diagnosis is by determining cultural characteristics and serological identification of the isolates. Fluorescent antibody techniques are the most rapid and effective methods for diagnosis of streptococcal infection (Kawahara *et al.* 1986).

## Epizootiology

### Sources and reservoir of infection

In Japan, it has been shown that *Streptococcus* species, causally associated with streptococcosis, remain in sea water and mud around fish farms throughout the year, but during the summer months somewhat higher numbers of organisms are detected in sea water than in mud. In contrast, during autumn and winter, Kitao *et al.* (1979) found that the organisms were more easily isolated in mud. Microorganisms released from diseased fish seem to be the most important source of infection in the aquatic environment. Minami (1979) recovered *Streptococcus* species from several species of wild fish, including the sardine (*Sardinops melanosticta*), anchovy (*Engraulis japonica*) and round-herring (*Etrumeus micropus*). The bacteria were shown to survive for 6 months in frozen sand-lance (*Ammodytes personatus*), which is the primary wet fish used in the diets for farmed yellowtail (Minami 1979, Yasunaga 1982). These facts indicate that contaminated diets may be the principal source of streptococcal infections in farmed fish. Fish which survive epizootics may also serve as reservoirs of infection.

### Mode of transmission

Transmission of streptococcosis in fish is horizontal with infection occurring from direct contact with infected fish or contaminated fish food. Robinson & Meyer (1966) showed that the disease could be readily transmitted experimentally by introducing infected golden shiners to healthy aquarium fish. Infection could also be induced by placing healthy fish in a suspension of 10$^6$ cells per ml for 10 min. Experimental infections following intraperitoneal or intramuscular injections of bacteria have also been reported by many workers (Hoshina *et al.* 1958, Robinson & Meyer 1966, Cook & Lofton 1975, Ohnishi & Jo 1981, Sugiyama *et al.* 1981, Iida *et al.* 1986, Sakai *et al.* 1986). In contrast, Rasheed & Plumb (1984) failed to induce any mortalities amongst gulf killifish dipped in bacterial suspensions for different time periods or among fish immersed in a hyperosmotic solution prior to being dipped in a bacterial suspension. However, the fish became infected when they were injured prior to dipping in the bacterial suspension. Taniguchi (1982) reported that oral infection was successful when fish were given a thawed fish food mixed with the organisms.

Although streptococcosis of cultured yellowtail occurs throughout the year in Japan, the most severe epizootics occur between August and November (Fig. 12.5). Generally, in freshwater fish such as the rainbow trout, ayu and tilapia, epizootics of streptococcosis caused by beta-haemolytic *Streptococcus* species occur when water temperatures exceed 20°C.

**Pathogenicity**

The mechanisms of pathogenicity are not yet fully understood. However, Kusuda & Kimura (1978) reported that the pathogenicity of alpha-haemolytic *Streptococcus* species towards yellowtail is enhanced by in vivo passage through yellowtail. Kitao (1983) found that the KG$^-$ type of *Streptococcus* species was more virulent than the KG$^+$ type strains in causing streptococcosis in cultured yellowtails.

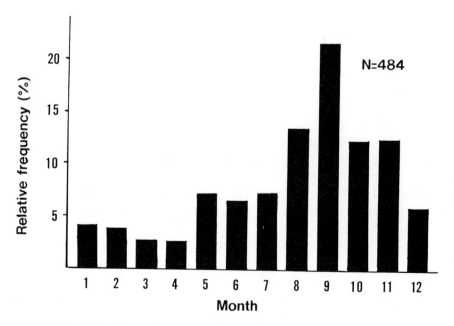

**Fig. 12.5**  Monthly incidence of streptococcosis among cultured yellowtail in Japan during 1989.

The pathogenicity of streptococci in yellowtail has been attributed to an exotoxin (Watson 1960), the development of which is related to disease and death (Kimura & Kusuda 1979, 1982, Kusuda & Hamaguchi 1988, 1989).

Robinson & Meyer (1966) found that injections of group B (gamma-haemolytic) *Streptococcus* species were lethal to golden shiners, bluegills, green sunfish and American toads. In contrast big-mouth buffalo (*Ictiobus cyprinellus*), goldfish (*Carassius auratus*), black crappie (*Pomoxis nigro-maculatus*) and largemouth bass (*Micropterus salmoides*) and channel catfish (*Ictalurus punctatus*) were refractory to infection. Cook & Loften (1975) investigated the pathogenicity of the *Streptococcus* species initially isolated by Plumb *et al.* (1974) towards five species of fish. They found that the Gulf menhaden, spot, striped mullet and Atlantic croaker were highly susceptible, whereas the sea catfish (*Rinus felis*) was less so. Ohnishi & Jo (1981) found that beta-haemolytic *Streptococcus* species isolated from ayu in Japan were very pathogenic for tilapia, yellowtail and seabream (*Pagrus major*), but not for either carp (*Cyprinus carpio*) or black seabream (*Acanthopagrus schlegel*).

## Control

### Chemotherapy

There are reports that erythromycin is effective against streptococcal infections in cultured yellowtails (Shiomitsu *et al.* 1980, Katae *et al.* 1980) and rainbow trout (Kitao *et al.* 1987) at doses of 25−50 mg/kg body weight of fish/day for 4−7 days. Other antibiotics, like doxycycline (Kitao & Aoki 1979), kitasamycin, alkyl-trimethyl-ammonium-calcium-oxytetracycline, josamycin, oleandomycin and lincomycin have also been used to control streptococcosis in cultured yellowtail in Japan. Recently Aoki *et al.* (1990) reported resistance to these antibiotics among strains of *Streptococcus* species isolated in Japan.

### Preventive measures

If causative streptococci are present in mud and water throughout the aquatic environment, avoidance is not an easy or practical means of disease prevention. However, reducing overcrowding, overfeeding, unnecessary handling or trans-portation, and the prompt removal and slaughter of all moribund fish in ponds or net cages at an early stage of infection may prevent outbreaks or at least reduce their severity.

### Vaccine

Iida *et al.* (1982) and Sakai *et al.* (1987) reported that experimental vaccination provided protection against an artificial infection. However, commercial vaccines have not yet been developed.

# References

Aoki, T., Takami, K. & Kitao, T. (1990) Drug resistance in a non-hemolytic *Streptococcus* sp. isolated from cultured yellowtail, *Seriola quinqueradiata. Diseases of Aquatic Organisms*, **8**, 171–7.

Baya, A.M., Lupiana, B., Hetrick, F.M., Roberson, B.S., Luckacovic, R. & Poukish, C. (1990) Association of *Streptococcus* sp. with fish mortalities in Cheasapeake Bay and its tributaries. *Journal of Fish Diseases*, **13**, 251–3.

Boomker, J., Imes, G.D., Jr., Cameron, C.M., Naude, T.W. & Schoonbee, H.J. (1979) Trout mortalities as a result of *Streptococcus* infection. *Onderstepoort Journal of Veterinary Research*, **46**, 71–8.

Cars, O., Forsum, V. & Hjelm, E. (1975) New immunofluorescence method for identification of Group A, B, C, E, F and G streptococci. *Acta Pathologica Microbiologica Scandinavica*, Series B, **83**, 145–52.

Christensen, P., Kahlmeter, G., Jonsson, S., and Kronvall, G. (1973) New method for the serological grouping of streptococci with specific antibodies absorbed to Protein A-containing staphylococci. *Infection and Immunity*, **7**, 881–5.

Cook, D.W. & Lofton, S.R. (1975) Pathogenicity studies with a *Streptococcus* sp. isolated from fishes in an Alabama-Florida fish kill. *Transactions of the American Fisheries Society*, **104**, 286–8.

Dajani, A.S. (1973) Rapid identification of beta-hemolytic streptococci by counter-immunoelectrophoresis. *Journal of Immunology*, **110**, 1702–5.

Foo, J.T.W., Ho, B. & Lam, T.J. (1985) Mass mortality in *Siganus canaliculatus* due to streptococcal infection. *Aquaculture*, **49**, 185–95.

Fuller, A.T. (1938) The formamide method for the extraction of polysaccharides from hemolytic streptococci. *British Journal of Experimental Pathology*, **19**, 130–9.

Hardie, J.M. (1986) Genus Streptococcus Rosenbach 1884, 22[AL]. In *Bergey's Manual of Systematic Bacteriology*, Vol., 2. (Ed. by P.H.A. Sneath, N.S. Mair, M.E. Sharpe & J.G. Holt), pp. 1043–71. Williams and Wilkins, Baltimore.

Hoshina, T., Sano, T. & Morimoto, Y. (1958) A *Streptococcus* pathogenic to fish. *Journal of Tokyo University of Fisheries*, **44**, 57–68.

Iida, T., Wakabayashi, H. & Egusa, S. (1982) Vaccination for control of streptococcal disease in cultured yellowtail. *Fish Pathology*, **16**, 201–6.

Iida, T., Furukawa, K., Sakai, M. & Wakabayashi, H. (1986) Non-hemolytic *Streptococcus* isolated from the brain of the vertebral deformed yellowtail. *Fish Pathology*, **21**, 33–8.

Jo, Y. (1982) Streptococcal infections of cultured freshwater fish. *Fish Pathology*, **17**, 33–7.

Kaige, N., Miyazaki, T. & Kubota, S. (1984) The pathogen and histopathology of vertebral deformity in cultured yellowtail. *Fish Pathology*, **19**, 173–9.

Katae, H. (1982) The application to streptococcal infection in yellowtails. *Fish Pathology*, **17**, 77–85.

Katae, H., Kouno, K., Shimizu, M., Kusuda, R., Taniguchi, M., Shiomitsu, K. & Hasegawa, H. (1980) Studies on chemotherapy of fish disease with erythromycin-I. Absorbtion, distribution, excretion and residue of erythromycin in cultured yellowtails. *Fish Pathology*, **15**, 7–16.

Kawahara, E. & Kusuda, R. (1987) Direct fluorescent antibody technique for differentiation between alpha and beta-hemolytic *Streptococcus* spp. *Fish Pathology*, **22**(2), 77–82.

Kawahara, E., Nelson, J.S. & Kusuda, R. (1986) Fluorescent antibody technique compared to standard media culture for detection of pathogenic bacteria for yellowtail and amberjack. *Fish Pathology*, **21**(1), 39–45.

Kimura, H. & Kusuda, R. (1979) Studies on the pathogenesis of streptococcal infection in cultured yellowtail *Seriola* spp.: effect of the cell free culture on experimental streptococcal infection. *Journal of Fish Diseases*, **2**, 501–10.

Kimura, H. & Kusuda, R. (1982) Studies on the pathogenesis of streptococcal infection in cultured yellowtail, *Seriola* spp.: effect of crude exotoxin fraction from cell-free culture on experimental streptococcal infection. *Journal of Fish Diseases*, **5**, 471–8.

Kitao, T. (1982) The methods for detection of *Streptococcus* sp., causative bacteria of streptococcal disease of cultured yellowtail (*Seriola quinqueradiata*). Especially, their cultural, biochemical and serological properties. *Fish Pathology*, **17**, 17–26.

Kitao, T. (1983) Strain variation associated with pathogenesis of *Streptococcus* sp., the causative agent of streptococciosis in cultured yellowtail (*Seriola quinqueradiata*). Proceedings of the Second North Pacific Aquaculture Symposium, pp. 231−42. Tokai University, Japan.

Kitao, T. & Aoki, T. (1979) Therapeutic studies of doxycycline of streptococciosis of cultured yellowtail (*Seriola quinqueradiata*). *Bulletin of the Faculty of Agriculture, Miyazaki University*, **26**, 357−63.

Kitao, T., Aoki, T. & Iwata, K. (1979) Epidemiological study on streptococciosis of cultured yellowtail (*Seriola quinqueradiata*) − I. Distribution of *Streptococcus* sp. in seawater and muds around yellowtail farms. *Bulletin of the Japanese Society of Scientific Fisheries*, **45**, 567−72.

Kitao, T., Aoki, T. & Sakoh, R. (1981) Epizootic caused by β-haemolytic *Streptococcus* species in cultured freshwater fish. *Fish Pathology*, **15**, 301−7.

Kitao, T., Iwata, K. & Ohta, H. (1987) Therapeutic attempt to control of streptococciosis in cultured rainbow trout, *Salmo gairdneri*, by using erythromycin. *Fish Pathology*, **22**, 25−8.

Kusuda, R. & Hamaguchi, M. (1988) Extracellular and intracellular toxins of *Streptococcus* sp. isolated from yellowtail. *Bulletin of the European Association of Fish Pathologists*, **8**, 9−10.

Kusuda, R. & Hamaguchi, M. (1989) Determination of the median lethal dose of cell-associated toxins from *Streptococcus* sp. in the yellowtail, *Seriola quinqueradiata*. *Bulletin of the European Association of Fish Pathologists*, **9**, 117−18.

Kusuda, R. & Kimura, H. (1978) Studies on the pathogenesis of streptococcal infection in cultured yellowtails, *Seriola* spp.: the fate of *Streptococcus* sp. bacteria after inoculation. *Journal of Fish Diseases*, **1**, 109−14.

Kusuda, R. & Komatsu, I. (1978) A comparative study of fish pathogenic *Streptococcus* isolated from saltwater and freshwater fishes. *Bulletin of the Japanese Society of Scientific Fisheries*, **44**, 1073−8.

Kusuda, R., Kawai, K., Toyoshima, T. & Komatsu, I. (1976) A new pathogenic bacterium belonging to the genus *Streptococcus*, isolated from an epizootic of cultured yellowtail. *Bulletin of the Japanese Society of Scientific Fisheries*, **42**, 1345−52.

Kusuda, R., Komatsu, I. & Kawai, K. (1978) *Streptococcus* sp. isolated from an epizootic of cultured eels. *Bulletin of the Japanese Society of Scientific Fisheries*, **44**, 295.

Kusuda, R., Kawai, K., Salati, F., Banner, C.R. & Fryer, I.L. (1992) *Enterococcus seriolicida* sp. nov., a fish pathogen. *International Journal of Systematic Bacteriology*, **41**(3), 406−9.

Lancefield, R.C. (1933) A serological differentiation of human and other groups of hemolytic streptococci. *Journal of Experimental Medicine*, **57**, 571−95.

Maxted, W.R. (1948) Preparation of streptococcal extracts for Lancefield grouping. *Lancet*, August, **14**, 255−6.

Minami, T. (1979) *Streptococcus* sp., pathogenic to cultured yellowtail, isolated from fishes for diets. *Fish Pathology*, **14**, 15−19.

Minami, T., Nakamura, Y., Ikeda, Y. & Ozaki, H. (1979) A beta-hemolytic *Streptococcus* isolated from cultured yellowtail. *Fish Pathology*, **14**, 33−8.

Miyazaki, T. (1982) Pathological study on streptococciosis. Histopathology of infected fishes. *Fish Pathology*, **17**, 39−47.

Nagatsugawa, T. (1983) A streptococcal disease of cultured flounder. *Fish Pathology*, **17**, 281−5.

Ohnishi, K. & Jo, Y. (1981) Studies on streptococcal infection in pond-cultured fishes − I. Characteristics of a beta-hemolytic *Streptococcus* isolated from cultured ayu and amago in 1977−1978. *Fish Pathology*, **16**, 63−7.

Pier, G.B. & Madin, S.H. (1976) *Streptococcus iniae* sp. nov., a beta-hemolytic Streptococcus isolated from an Amazon freshwater dolphin, *Inia geoffrensis*. *International Journal of Systematic Bacteriology*, **26**, 545−53.

Pier, G.B., Madin, S.H. & Al-Nakeeb, S. (1978) Isolation and characterization of a second isolate of *Streptococcus iniae*. *International Journal of Systematic Bacteriology*, **28**, 311−14.

Plumb, J.A., Schachte, J.H., Gaines, J.L., Peltier, W. & Carroll, B. (1974) *Streptococcus* sp. from marine fishes along the Alabama and northwest Florida coast of the Gulf of Mexico. *Transactions of the American Fisheries Society*, **103**, 358−61.

Rantz, L.A. & Randall, E. (1955) Use of autoclaved extracts of hemolytic streptococci for serological grouping. *Stanford Medical Bulletin*, **13**, 290−1.

Rasheed, V. & Plumb, J.A. (1984) Pathogenicity of a non-haemolytic group B *Streptococcus* sp. in gulf killifish (*Findulus grandis* Baird & Girard). *Aquaculture*, **37**, 97−105.

Robinson, J.A. & Meyer, F.P. (1966) Streptococcal fish pathogen. *Journal of Bacteriology*, **92**, 512.

Rotta, J., Kraus, R.M., Lancefield, R.C., Everly, W. & Lackland, H. (1971) New approaches for the laboratory recognition of M types of group A streptococci. *Journal of Experimental Medicine*, **134**, 1298–315.

Sakai, M., Atsuta, S. & Kobayashi, M. (1986) A streptococcal disease of cultured jacopever, *Sebastes schlegeli. Suisanzoshoku*, **34**, 171–7.

Sakai, M., Kubota, R., Atsuta, S. & Kobayashi, M. (1987) Vaccination of rainbow trout, *Salmo gairdneri* against beta-hemolytic streptococcal disease. *Bulletin of the Japanese Society of Scientific Fisheries*, **53**, 1373–6.

Shiomitsu, K., Kusuda, R., Osuga, H. & Munekiyo, M. (1980) Studies on chemotherapy of fish disease with erythromycin — II. Its clinical studies against streptococcal infection in cultured yellowtails. *Fish Pathology*, **15**, 17–23.

Sugiyama, A., Kusuda, R., Kawai, K., Inada, Y. & Yoneda, M. (1981) The behavior of *Streptococcus* sp. bacteria in the organs of infected ayu. *Bulletin of the Japanese Society of Scientific Fisheries*, **47**, 1003–7.

Taniguchi, M. (1982) Influence of food condition on artificial peroral infection of yellowtail streptococciosis. *Bulletin of the Japanese Society of Scientific Fisheries*, **48**(12), 1721–3.

Watson, D.W. (1960) Host–parasite factors in group A streptococcal infections. Pyrogenic and other effects of immunologic distinct exotoxins related to scarlet fever toxins. *Journal of Experimental Medicine*, **111**, 255–84.

Yasunaga, N. (1982) Occurrence of *Streptococcus* sp., a pathogen of cultured yellowtail, in muscle of sardine for diets. *Fish Pathology*, **17**, 195–8.

# Chapter 13:
# Clostridial Infections

The genus *Clostridium*, which is grouped with other endospore forming bacteria, comprises Gram-positive anaerobic bacilli which may form oval or spherical endospores often distending the cell. In ageing cultures the Gram-positive staining reaction may be lost, and in a few species Gram-negative cells only have been seen. When motile, flagella are peritrichous. Species are chemo-organotrophic and may be saccharolytic, proteolytic, or both, producing a mixture of organic acids, alcohols and toxins. They grow well at pH 6.5−7.0, with a temperature range for optimal growth of 15−69°C. Although most are obligate anaerobes, tolerance to oxygen does vary. The mol % G + C of the DNA is 22−25.

Clostridia occur commonly where oxygen levels are restricted, in soil, sewage, marine sediment, decaying vegetable and animal products. They are numerous in the intestinal tract of man and animals. Some are opportunist pathogens of man and animals, causing wound and soft tissue infection and food poisoning and their pathogenicity is associated with potent exotoxins. Botulism, due to *Clostridium botulinum*, has been recorded in farmed salmonids, but the incidence is low. It is best controlled by improving hygiene and general environmental conditions.

## Introduction

Anaerobic bacteriology of fish is less well developed than other aspects of the discipline, owing in part to the more demanding cultural methods involved, requiring exclusion of free oxygen. This can be achieved by removing atmospheric oxygen and replacing it with an inert gas, by inoculating deeply into a solid medium such as agar, or by using a cooked meat medium (see Chapter 16) in which sterilized muscle tissue containing reducing substances is able to maintain anaerobic conditions in the depth of the tube. A range of media was evaluated (Sugita & Deguchi 1985) for the isolation of anaerobes from fresh water and it was found that no single medium gave maximum viable counts for all species tested. There is no doubt that anaerobes are often missed owing to insufficiently stringent cultural methods, although even if isolated they may be no more than commensals or secondary invaders. *Clostridium botulinum* remains the single accredited and serious pathogen of fish.

## *Clostridium botulinum*

Gram-positive, straight rods $0.8−1.6 \times 1.7−15.7\,\mu m$, occurring singly and in pairs, motile with peritrichous flagella. Oval or subterminal spores are formed which often distend the cell. It is a strict anaerobe and grows well on ordinary media between 25 and 37°C. Colonies of toxigenic strains are irregular, transparent, and haemolytic on horse blood agar. There are seven toxin types of *C. botulinum* (A−G), producing very potent neurotoxins which can be differentiated by their serological specificity and to some extent by their biochemical reactions (Holdeman & Brooks 1970, Smith & Hobbs 1974). The spores are very heat resistant. They can withstand moist heat at 100°C for several hours but are destroyed in 5 min at 120°C. The spores of type E, the fish pathogen, are the least heat resistant and may be inactivated by exposure to 80°C wet heat for 30 min.

   *C. botulinum* type E is saccharolytic; it ferments glucose, fructose and maltose, is non- or weakly proteolytic (Dolman 1957), indole-negative and catalase-negative. Phospholipase and lipase are produced giving zones of opacity and a pearly layer effect on egg yolk media (Duguid *et al.* 1975). Although *C. botulinum* grows best between 25 and 37°C, growth and toxin production can occur as low as 1−5°C.

## Laboratory diagnosis

*C. botulinum* is a strict anaerobe which can grow on a solid medium, such as Willis and Hobbs' selective medium, in the absence of air, or Robertson's cooked-meat broth. Pieces of excised tissue are inoculated into cooked meat broth and incubated for 6 days at 30°C (see Chapter 16). Culture filtrates may be tested for toxicity by injecting intraperitoneally into mice with and without the protection of type-specific antitoxins. Alternatively mixtures of culture filtrate and type-specific antitoxin may be injected subcutaneously into mice. Definitive diagnosis depends on isolating the organism and identifying specific toxin in the tissue of the fish affected.

## Epizootiology

Botulism has been diagnosed only in farmed salmonids reared in fresh water, but because *C. botulinum* is widespread in marine and freshwater sediments (Licciardello 1983) and in salmonid fish (Cann *et al.* 1975, Houghtby & Kaysner 1969) botulism must be considered during a disease outbreak where fish display characteristic signs. It is caused by fish ingesting the potent neurotoxin from contaminated feed or from the tissue of dead fish on which the bacterium has grown. Outbreaks have been recorded in trout (*Oncorhynchus mykiss*) in Denmark (Huss & Eskildsen 1974) and Britain (Cann & Taylor 1982) and in coho salmon (*Oncorhynchus kisutch*) in the USA (Eklund *et al.* 1982). *C. botulinum* type E has been incriminated in each case.

## Clinical signs

The neurotoxin causes progressive muscular paralysis affecting all but the caudal fin. This results in erratic swimming and loss of equilibrium. Affected fish float on the surface, sink to the bottom, apparently recover and repeat this cycle until death ensues (Frerichs & Roberts 1989).

**Control**

The incidence of botulism is low and associated with bad husbandry.
*C. botulinum*, which may be present even in the absence of disease, can be
inhibited by treatment with oxytetracycline at a dose of 8.8 g per 100 kg fish per
day for 10 days (Schiewe *et al.* 1988). The major reservoir of toxin and cause
of disease is fish which have died or are dying from the disease. Stock in
contaminated systems must be slaughtered, pond detritus removed and all
buried in quicklime. Ponds can be brought back into use within a month but
with additional improvement in water flow rates and reduced stocking densities
(Frerichs & Roberts 1989).

**Public health hazards**

The risk to human health of botulism associated with seafood is real but not
great. In a review of 1784 outbreaks of botulism in the USA (Centre for
Disease Control 1974), fish or fish products were implicated in 4.4% of outbreaks.
Most of these involved canned, smoked or vacuum packed seafood of the kind
usually consumed without the further cooking which might have inactivated the
toxin. Factors affecting the level of risk and the essential components of a safe
commercial process are considered in Chapter 17 and are well reviewed by
Licciardello (1983).

## Other anaerobes

*Eubacterium tarantellus* has been incriminated as the causative agent of a
neurological infection of striped mullet (*Mugil cephalus*) (Udney *et al.* 1976).
The genus *Eubacterium* comprises Gram-positive rods which may be pleomorphic
and are obligate anaerobes but do not form endospores. They are found in the
body cavities of man and animals and in plants where the oxygen concentration
is restricted. Some species are pathogenic. The mol % G + C of the DNA is
30−55. Bacteria demonstrated in sections of brain tissue of infected striped
mullet were isolated and characterized. They were long and slender, $1.3-1.6 \times 10.0-17.0 \mu m$, and non-motile. Colonies on solid medium were translucent,
rhizoid and slightly mucoid with a large zone of β-haemolysis when grown on
sheep blood agar. Although mol % G + C of the DNA was not determined,
other characteristics justified location within this genus and the species was
named *Eubacterium tarantellus* (Udney *et al.* 1977).

Infected fish displayed erratic swimming behaviour, twisting and spinning
until death occurred. Although *Eubacterium tarantellus* was isolated from the
brain of infected fish it was not proved with certainty that this was the primary
pathogen.

It is possible that other anaerobes also may be secondary pathogens in fish.

Anaerobes and microaerophilic bacteria are ubiquitous. They have been found in soil, aquatic sediments and the gastrointestinal tract of many animals including fish. Microorganisms are largely responsible for the development of anoxic conditions in these situations, allowing the microaerophils and strict anaerobes to become established (Jones 1986). Although aerobes and facultative anaerobes predominated, bottom muds from rivers and bays in Japan were found to contain $10^2-10^5$ cfu per g obligate anaerobes (Takano *et al.* 1984). Similarly several species of anaerobes were found in the intestine of many fish from both fresh and coastal waters, but again outnumbered by other bacteria (Sakata *et al.* 1984). *Bacteroides, Clostridium* species and microaerophilic cocci were found in the intestines of coastal fish (Sugita *et al.* 1988) and *Bacteroides* type A and type B were found to be the major anaerobic component of the gastrointestinal flora of freshwater fish (Sugita *et al.* 1983). These also were found in aquatic plants and the water sediment and it was suggested that the intestinal flora originated from the environment. The presence of certain anaerobes may confer benefit to the host. *Bacteroides* type A produces significant amounts of vitamin B, an essential requirement for some fish (Sugita *et al.* 1986). Alternatively they may become opportunist pathogens when tissue is damaged and becomes anoxic as, for example, in *Bacteroides* infections in soft tissue wounds in other animals (Holdeman *et al.* 1984).

# References

Cann, D.C. & Taylor, L.Y. (1982) An outbreak of botulism in rainbow trout, *Salmo gairdneri* Richardson, farmed in Britain. *Journal of Fish Diseases*, **5**, 393–9.

Cann, D.C., Taylor, L.Y. & Hobbs, G. (1975) The incidence of *Clostridium botulinum* in farmed rainbow trout raised in Great Britain. *Journal of Applied Bacteriology*, **39**, 331–6.

Center for Disease Control (1974) Botulism in the United States 1899–1973. In *Handbook for Epidemiologists, Clinicians and Laboratory Workers*. US Department of Health, Education & Welfare, Atlanta.

Dolman, C.E. (1957) Type E (fish borne) botulism: a review. *Japanese Journal of Medicine, Science and Biology*, **10**, 383–395.

Duguid, J.P., Marmion, B.P. & Swain, R.H.A. (1979) Growth and nutrition of bacteria. In *Medical Microbiology* 13th edn, Vol. 1., pp. 377–85. Churchill Livingstone, Edinburgh.

Eklund, M.W., Peterson, M.E., Poysky, F.T., Peck, L.W. & Conrad, J.F. (1982) Botulism in juvenile coho salmon, *Oncorhynchus kisutch* in the United States. *Aquaculture*, **27**, 1–11.

Frerichs, G.N. & Roberts, R.J. (1989) The bacteriology of teleosts. In *Fish Pathology*, 2nd edn (Ed. by R.J. Roberts), pp. 289–319. Ballière Tindall, London.

Holdeman, L.V. & Brooks, J.B. (1970) Variation among strains of *Clostridium botulinum* and related clostridia. Proceedings of the 1st Japan Conference on Toxic Micro-organisms 1968. US Government Printing Office, Washington DC, 278–86.

Holdeman, L.V., Kelley, R.W. & Moore, W.E.C. (1984) Genus 1. *Bacteriodes*, Castellani and Chalmers 1919, 959. In *Bergey's Manual of Systematic Bacteriology*, Vol. 1 (Ed. by N.R. Kreig & J.G. Holt), pp. 604–31. Williams & Wilkins, Baltimore.

Houghtby, G.A. & Kaysner, C.A. (1969) Incidence of *Clostridium botulinum* type E in Alaskan salmon. *Applied Microbiology*, **18**, 950–1.

Huss, H.H. & Eskildsen, U. (1974) Botulism in farmed trout caused by *Clostridium botulinum* type E. *Nordic Journal of Veterinary Medicine*, **26**, 733–8.

Jones, J.G. (1986) Anaerobic aquatic environments. Society of Applied Bacteriology Symposium Series, Number 13, pp. 101–13.

Licciardello, J.J. (1983) Botulism and heat-processed seafoods. *Marine Fisheries Review*, **45**(2), 1–7.

Sakata, T., Toda, S. & Kakimoto, D. (1984) Variation in the intestinal microflora of grey mullet, *Mugil cephalus*. Mini review data file Fisheries Research, Kagoshima University, 3, 59–62.

Schiewe, M.H., Novotny, A.J. & Harrell, L.W. (1988) Botulism of salmonids. In *Disease Diagnosis and Control in North American Marine Aquaculture. Developments in Aquaculture and Fisheries Science*, Vol. 17, 2nd edition (Ed. by C.J. Sindermann & D.V. Lightner), pp. 336–8. Elsevier, Oxford.

Smith, L.D.S. & Hobbs, G. (1974) Genus III *Clostridium* Prazmowski 1880, 23. In *Bergey's Manual of Determinative Bacteriology*, 8th edn Part 1 (Ed. by R.E. Buchanan & N.E. Gibbons), pp. 551–72. Williams and Wilkins.

Sugita, H. & Duguchi, Y. (1985) Evaluation of media for isolation of anaerobic bacteria from freshwater environments. *Bulletin of the Japanese Society of Scientific Fisheries*, **51**(12), 2081–7.

Sugita, H., Oshima, K., Tamura, M. & Deguchi, Y. (1983) Bacterial flora in the gastrointestine of freshwater fish. *Bulletin of the Japanese Society of Scientific Fisheries*, **49**(9), 1387–95.

Sugita, H., Miyajima, C. & Deguchi, Y. (1986) Vitamin B producing bacteria in the intestine of freshwater fishes. Program of the first international marine biotechnology conference, 60.

Sugita, H., Miyajima, C., Iwata, J., Arai, S., Kubo, T., Igarashi, S. & Deguchi, Y. (1988) Intestinal microflora of Japanese coastal fishes. *Bulletin of the Japanese Society of Scientific Fisheries*, **54**(5), 875–82.

Takano, M., Sakata, T. & Kakimoto, D. (1984) Microflora of the bottom muds in the Kotsuki River and Kinko Bay. Mini review data file Fisheries Research, Kagoshima University, 3, 63–6.

Udney, L.R., Young, E. & Sallman, B. (1976) *Eubacterium* spp. ATCC 29255: An anaerobic bacterial pathogen of marine fish. *Fish Health News*, **5**, 3–4.

Udney, L.R., Young, R. & Sallman, B. (1977) Isolation and characterization of an anaerobic bacterium *Eubacterium tarantellus* sp. nov., associated with striped mullet (*Mugil cephalus*) mortality in Biscayne Bay, Florida. *Journal of the Fisheries Research Board of Canada*, **34**, 402–9.

# Part 7:
# Acid-Fast Fish Pathogens

The property of acid-fastness, due to waxy substances in the cell walls, is present to a marked degree in the genus *Mycobacterium*, stained preparations of which can withstand decolorization by acidified alcohol and strong acids. *Nocardia*, a genus similar to *Mycobacterium*, is partially acid-fast and may be decolorized by alcohol. Mycobacteria are aerobic and grow slowly, forming rods and occasionally filaments. *Nocardia* grow more quickly, producing mycelia which fragment into rods and cocci. Both genera are Gram-positive but mycobacteria can be stained by this method only with difficulty. Mycobacteria and *Nocardia* both cause infections of fish.

# Chapter 14:
# Mycobacteriosis: Nocardiosis

The family Mycobacteriaceae, comprising the single genus *Mycobacterium*, consists at present of some 54 recognised species of aerobic, non-motile, non-spore-forming, rod-shaped bacteria which are characteristically acid-alcohol-fast at some stage of growth (Wayne & Kubica 1986). The common property of acid-alcohol-fastness is due to the presence of waxy substances in the cell wall which enable the carbo-fuchsin stained organisms to resist decolorization by acidified alcohol (Ziehl-Neelsen staining method) as well as strong mineral acids. Mycobacteria are also considered to be Gram-positive, although most species are not readily stainable by this method. They form straight or slightly curved rods $0.2-0.6 \times 1.0 - 10.0\,\mu m$ and branching or filamentous growth may occur, which fragments easily. Mol % G + C of the DNA is $62-70$.

Most are free living in the soil and water and some cause disease in man and animals. The species pathogenic for fish are *M. marinum*, *M. fortuitum* and *M. chelonae*. Because they are slow-growing, when attempting isolation from mixed flora, it may be necessary to destroy non-acid-fast contaminants with dilute acid or alkali before inoculating on to enriched medium containing selective antibiotics.

Mycobacteriosis is a piscine tuberculosis and affects a wide range of freshwater and marine species but particularly aquarium fish. It is a chronic systemic disease with granulomas forming both externally and scattered throughout the internal organs. Treatment is unsatisfactory and diseased stock should be destroyed, particularly since these pathogens are capable of affecting man as well as fish.

The term 'nocardioform' informally groups together a number of genera of organisms exhibiting the basic morphological feature of forming a filamentous mycelium, which breaks up into rod-shaped or coccoid elements as the culture ages (Lechevalier 1986). The currently recognised fish pathogens have been assigned to the genus *Nocardia* on the basis of morphological and cultural features, although the present-day classification of nocardioforms would also require chemical analysis to make a firm identification at genus level. Morphologically, *Nocardia* species are Gram-positive, although this reaction may be weak, and weakly acid-fast. They are aerobic, non-motile, and form branching rods $0.5-1.2\,\mu m$ diameter, and most form aerial hyphae on culture. The branching rods form a rudimentary to extensive substrate mycelium which usually fragments into bacillary and coccoid elements but a wide range of morphological complexity from unfragmented mycelia to chains of conidia or spores on vegetative and aerial hyphae may be found within the genus. Chemically, the cell wall contains major amounts of *meso*-diaminopimelic acid, arabinose and galactose characteristic of cell wall chemotype IV. Mol % G + C of the DNA is $64-72$ (Goodfellow & Lechevalier 1986). Nocardia are widely distributed and abundant in the soil, *Nocardia asteroides* has been implicated in fish disease and *N. kampachi* is an important pathogen of yellowtail (*Seriola quinqueradiata*).

## Fish mycobacterial pathogens

Mycobacterial infections of fish are invariably referred to as (piscine) tuberculosis or mycobacteriosis, irrespective of the specific identity of the causal organism. The first accounts of infection in both freshwater and marine fish reported histologically typical tuberculosis lesions containing acid-fast bacilli, and the descriptive term 'tuberculosis' subsequently became firmly established in all the early literature. Some decades later, however, Parisot & Wood (1960) observed that the typical tubercular inflammatory response of higher vertebrates was absent in mycobacterial infections of salmon, and suggested that 'mycobacteriosis' was a more appropriate descriptive term for the disease in fish. Since this atypical tissue reaction is not true for fishes in general, both tuberculosis and mycobacteriosis may be considered valid descriptions for piscine mycobacterial infections. Nowadays, the two terms tend to be used interchangeably, and often with less precise meanings than were perhaps originally intended. There is, however, an inherent connotational disadvantage with the word tuberculosis, which could be avoided by general acceptance of the more non-specific and aesthetically appealing term mycobacteriosis.

### Classification of fish mycobacterial pathogens

The aetiological agents of piscine mycobacteriosis have, over the years, been classified and re-classified into a wide variety of species, which is more a reflection of the evolvement of taxonomy than the isolation of different species of micro-organism. The first report of a mycobacterial infection in fish has always been attributed to Bataillon *et al.* (1897), who isolated acid-fast bacilli from a tuberculous lesion in a common carp (*Cyprinus carpio*). As the water had been contaminated with material from tuberculous persons, it was initially speculated that the human tubercle bacillus might have become adapted to fish, but the carp isolate was subsequently identified as a distinct species and named *Mycobacterium piscium* on the basis of its derivation (Bataillon, *et al.* 1902). The type culture of this organism (ATCC 9819) is, however, no longer available and *M. piscium* is not recognised as a valid species in *Bergey's Manual of Systematic Bacteriology*.

Aronson (1926) described the first now well-established fish pathogen, *Mycobacterium marinum*, following isolation of the organism from the viscera of a number of tropical marine fish species in the Philadelphia Aquarium. *M. marinum* was initially thought to infect marine fishes only, and was named accordingly, but is now known to be an ubiquitous species. Indeed, comparative sugar fermentation reactions (Ross 1960), together with published morphological, cultural and pathogenicity data, suggest that the original freshwater isolate of *M. piscium* was quite possibly a variant of *M. marinum*. Although *Mycobacterium platypoecilus*, isolated from a Mexican platyfish (*Platypoecilus maculatus*) by Baker & Hagan (1942), was formerly recognized as a valid species, it is now regarded as synonymous with *M. marinum*. The organism designated *Mycobacterium anabanti*, after the family name of the Siamese fighting fish from which it was isolated by Besse (1949), has never been accepted as a valid species and is also believed to be synonymous with *M. marinum*.

The second fish mycobacterial pathogen to be recognised was first isolated from neon tetra fish (*Hyphessobrycon innesi*) by Nigrelli (1953) and identified some years later by Ross & Brancato (1959) as *Mycobacterium fortuitum*. This appellation has been accorded precedence over *Mycobacterium ranae*, which holds chronological priority and may be encountered in the literature.

Mycobacteriosis of Pacific salmonids was first identified by Earp *et al.* (1953) and shown by subsequent surveys in 1957–1959 to be widely distributed in waters from Alaska to California (Ross *et al.* 1959, Ross 1963). Despite the presence of large numbers of acid-fast bacilli in the tissues of infected fish, the organisms proved extremely difficult to recover. Ross (1960) managed to obtain a number of cultures, however, and showed that although there was a close resemblance to *M. fortuitum*, three strains did not grow at 37°C and were non-pathogenic for mice. These isolates were named *Mycobacterium salmoniphilum* in recognition of their affinity with salmonid fish. Gordon & Mihm (1959) regarded all three strains as variants of *M. fortuitum*, but Grange (1981) has since reported the re-classification of the isolates as *Mycobacterium chelonei*. Ashburner (1977) first reported a *bona fide* incident of *M. chelonei* infection in chinook salmon (*Oncorhynchus tschawytscha*) in Australia, and noted the similarity of the organism to the CC and OR strains of *M. salmoniphilum*. Arakawa & Fryer (1984) subsequently identified six Pacific salmonid myco-bacterial isolates recovered between 1964 and 1982 as *M. chelonei* subsp. *piscarium*. These later strains were considered to be different from the earlier *M. salmoniphilum* isolates, although both sets of organisms had a common geographical origin, failed to grow at 37°C and were non-pathogenic for mice. Following an additional study in which subsp. *Piscarium* could not be sero-logically differentiated from either of the recognized subspecies *chelonei* or *abscessus*, it was suggested that the epithet *piscarium* be withdrawn and the strains be taxonomically regarded as *M. chelonei* (Arakawa *et al.* 1986). *M. chelonei* has now been linguistically corrected to *M. chelonae* (Wayne & Kubica 1986).

In summary, *M. marinum*, *M. fortuitum* and *M. chelonae* are the only three currently recognized species of fish pathogenic mycobacteria.

### Fish species susceptibility

It is almost 30 years since Nigrelli & Vogel (1963) published their now repeatedly quoted list of 151 species of freshwater and marine fishes in which mycobacterial disease had been diagnosed. In the intervening time, the recorded range of susceptible species has continued to increase, supporting the view expressed by Dulin (1979) that probably any species of fish may be infected. In practice, disease is most frequently recognised in aquarium fish, probably because such specimens are maintained under a degree of captivity stress for long periods of time, so allowing the slowly progressive infection to develop into a clinically diagnostic condition. With many cases of mycobacteriosis, diagnosis is based solely on the identification of acid-fast bacilli in histological sections of tissue lesions (Plate 34), and little or no attempt is made to isolate and identify the species of organism. From available evidence, however, the pathogenicity spectra of the three recognised species of mycobacteria appear to be as follows.

*M. marinum* forms the largest proportion of all mycobacteria isolated from fish. Tropical freshwater and tropical marine water fish may be infected but no authenticated case of natural infection in a temperate water fish has been reported. The identity of the organisms associated with the early accounts of disease in cod (*Gadus morhua*) (Alexander 1913) and halibut (*Hippoglossus hippoglossus*) (Sutherland 1922) has never been established.

The isolation of *M. fortuitum* has been less frequently documented than that of *M. marinum*, but the prevalence of infection is probably more widespread than generally suspected. Fish from both tropical and temperate waters may be infected. *M. fortuitum* is most commonly a pathogen of freshwater fish, although infection is also recognised to occur in marine species.

Infection with *M. chelonae* has so far been identified only in cold water salmonid species of fish. Published reports have specifically linked infection with the freshwater hatchery environment, but once established it appears to persist throughout the fresh- and saltwater phases of the life cycle.

## Characteristics of disease

Piscine mycobacteriosis is a systemic, chronic, progressive disease presenting various clinical features depending upon species and ecological conditions. The major accounts and reviews of the disease in tropical freshwater and marine aquarium environments all cite permutations of listlessness, anorexia, emaciation, dyspnoea, exophthalmia, skin discolouration and external lesions ranging from scale loss to nodules, ulcers and fin necrosis as signs of advancing infection (Wolke & Stroud 1978, Dulin 1979, Giavenni et al. 1980, van Duijn 1981) (Figs 14.1, 14.2). In cold water salmonids there may be no external signs of disease other than mortality, or else variable degrees of skin coloration, stunted growth and retarded sexual development (Parisot 1958, Ashburner 1977, Abernethy & Lund 1978). Internally, the nature and distribution of lesions which may develop is similar in both tropical and cold water fish species. Gross or microscopic greyish-white miliary granulomas may be found scattered or grouped in virtually any parenchymatous tissue, but especially the spleen, kidney and liver. Enlarged organs, peritonitis and oedema may all be apparent. Skeletal involvement with resulting deformity may also occur in long-standing cases in aquaria where fish are protected from natural predation.

The histopathology of the naturally developing granulomas characteristic of mycobacterial infections in fish has been the subject of more detailed study than any other aspect of the disease (Fig. 14.3), and reference should be made to the reviews of Conroy (1970), Ross (1970), Wolke & Stroud (1978) and van Duijn (1981) for comprehensive descriptions of these lesions. The pathogenesis of focal tubercular lesions has also been studied experimentally (Timur et al. 1977).

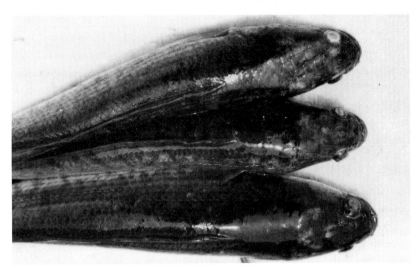

**Fig. 14.1**  Striped snakeheads with systemic mycobacteriosis showing the exophthalmia which characterizes the disease in this species (Courtesy of Dr S. Chinabut).

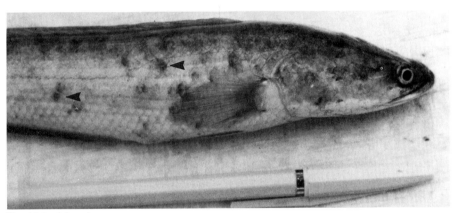

**Fig. 14.2**  (above) Haemorrhagic lesions on the body surface (arrowed) of snakeheads with severe mycobacteriosis (Courtesy of Dr S. Chinabut).

**Fig. 14.3**  (right) Tubercle granulomata in the haemopoietic tissue (G) of striped snakehead. Normal tubules (T) have been displaced by the inflammatory tissue (H&E ×500) (Courtesy of Dr S. Chinabut).

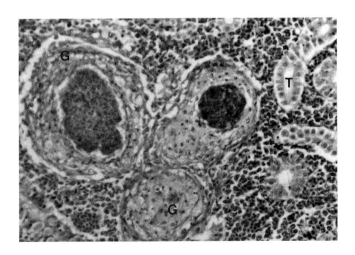

**Immune response to infection**

Bartos & Sommer (1981) have shown that rainbow trout (*Oncorhynchus mykiss*) produce typical delayed hypersensitivity reactions to experimental immunisation with *M. tuberculosis*, supporting the existence of T-cell-like mediated immune functions in teleost fish. The significance of these findings in the epizootiology and possible control of mycobacterial infections in fish has not been determined.

**Transmission of infection**

Mycobacterial infections of fish are probably transmitted naturally by ingestion of contaminated food or aquatic detritus, although bacterial invasion through damaged skin or gill tissue may also be possible. Potential sources of infective material are numerous and include the soil and water in which the fish pathogenic species are ubiquitous and remain viable for 2 years or more (Reichenbach-Klinke 1972). Organisms may be released into the environment from lesions in diseased fish or from a wide range of amphibians and reptiles also known to be susceptible to mycobacterial disease (Nigrelli & Vogel 1963). The feeding of infected trash fish has been circumstantially shown to have disseminated disease in cultured Pacific salmon (Ross *et al.* 1959) and snakehead fish (*Ophicephalus striatus*) (Chinabut *et al.* 1990). Infection via the ovarian route has also been demonstrated for the viviparous Mexican platyfish (*Xiphophorus maculatus*) (Conroy 1966) but discounted as a means of spreading the disease in salmon (Ross & Johnson 1962).

**Isolation and culture of mycobacteria**

The early primary isolations of fish mycobacteria were achieved using Dorset and Petroff egg agar media (Aronson 1926, Nigrelli & Vogel 1963), and inspissated egg or oleic acid-albumin agar formulations such as Dorset egg, Lowenstein-Jensen, Petragnani and Middlebrook 7H10 have since become the standard recommended isolation media (Dulin 1979, Austin & Austin 1987, Shotts & Teska 1989). Dubos agar, Sauton's agar and Ogawa egg formulations are similarly based media which have also been used successfully (Ashburner 1977, Arakawa & Fryer 1984). Cultures may not always be obtained, however, even from fish showing unequivocal evidence of infection (Abernethy & Lund 1978, Arakawa & Fryer 1984, Chinabut *et al.* 1990). Mycobacteria may also occasionally be isolated on general purpose bacteriological media such as tryptone soy agar (TSA) or brain-heart infusion agar (BHIA), provided that a large inoculum is used (Sanders & Fryer 1988), and Shotts & Teska (1989) have reported the successful use of MacConkey agar for the initial isolation of rapid growing species.

   All fish mycobacteria have been cultured at 20–30°C, and incubation in this temperature range for 2–30 days is suitable for isolation of all species. *M. fortuitum* and *M. chelonae* are classified as rapid growers, which are defined as species which produce easily seen growth from dilute inocula in less than 7 days' incubation under optimal conditions, although *M. chelonae*, paradoxically, may require several weeks' incubation for primary isolation (Grange 1981). *M. marinum* is a slow grower, which characteristically requires 7 or more days' incubation for visible growth. Once isolated, growth times may be reduced, and the fish pathogens, in common with many other species of mycobacteria, readily adapt to growth on simple substrates, using ammonia or amino acids as nitrogen sources and glycerol as carbon source in the presence of mineral salts (Wayne & Kubica 1984).

## Identification of fish pathogens

The cell morphology of the fish mycobacteria is not distinctive, and all species are encompassed within the general description of Gram-positive, acid-alcohol-fast, non-motile, non-sporing, pleomorphic rods $1.0-4.0 \times 0.2-0.6 \mu m$ with filamentous and coccoid forms also occurring.

Culturally, *M. marinum* is a slow grower requiring 2–3 weeks incubation for colonies to develop at an optimum growth temparature of 25°C. Primary isolation is not normally possible at 37°C but the organism may adapt to growth at this temperature on sub-culture. Colonies may be smooth and moist, rough and dry, flat or raised, depending on the culture medium used and length of incubation. Colonies grown in the dark are non-pigmented, but *M. marinum* is photochromogenic and when exposed to light develops a bright lemon yellow colour becoming orange with ageing. Biochemically, *M. marinum* does not reduce nitrate, whereas the slow growing, mammalian, photochromogenic *M. kansasii* can be isolated at 37°C and is nitratase positive.

*M. fortuitum* and *M. chelonae* are closely related rapid growers requiring less than 7 days incubation at 25°C for visible growth to develop. *M. fortuitum* also grows readily at 37°C, but none of the psychrophilic fish strains of *M. chelonae* have been cultured at this temperature. Both species of organism are non-chromogenic and normally produce cream to buff coloured colonies of variable consistency, depending upon culture medium and incubation time. Older cultures of *M. chelonae* may develop a purple colour (Grange 1981). Most other rapid growers produce yellow/orange pigmented colonies. *M. fortuitum* and *M. chelonae* may also be differentiated from all other mycobacteria by their ability to grow on MacConkey agar. Sanders & Fryer (1988) suggest iron uptake, sucrose utilization and nitrate reduction tests for the differentiation of *M. fortuitum* (positive reactions) and *M. chelonae* (negative reactions). The diagnostic characteristics of the fish pathogens are summarised in Table 14.1.

## Antigenic relationships

Results from a number of serological and dermal hypersensitivity studies have shown *M. marinum* to be antigenically distinct from all other mycobacterial species examined, and to form a very homogeneous grouping of organisms

**Table 14.1**  Diagnostic characteristics of fish pathogenic mycobacteria

|  | M. marinum | M. fortuitum | M. chelonae |
|---|---|---|---|
| Isolation at 25°C | + | + | + |
| 37°C | − | + | − |
| Rate of growth | slow | rapid | rapid |
| Pigmentation | photochromogen | − | − |
| Growth on MacConkey | − | + | + |
| Nitrate reduction | − | + | − |
| Iron uptake | ○ | + | − |
| Sucrose utilisation | ○ | + | − |

○ Not known

comprising only one or possibly two serotypes (Wayne & Kubica 1978). Although no serological studies specifically relating to fish isolates of *M. fortuitum* have been reported, this species of mycobacteria is also recognised as a unique taxon of organisms antigenically distinct from all other species, including the phenotypically similar *M. chelonae*. Two variants of *M. chelonae*, subsp. *chelonae* and subsp. *abscessus*, are at present identified on the basis of biochemical characters, although this subdivision has not been supported by chemical and serological analysis of cell surface antigens (Tsang *et al.* 1984). Arakawa *et al.* (1986) were similarly unable to differentiate serologically between a representative salmonid isolate of *M. chelonae* and type cultures of the two existing subspecies, indicating a high level of antigenic homology within the species despite marked phenotypic variations.

**Treatment and control**

The desirability as well as feasibility of treating mycobacterial infections of fish is an emotive and controversial issue. Frerichs & Roberts (1989) unequivocally express the view that there is no suitable treatment for affected fish, and that diseased stock should be destroyed and comprehensive disinfection of holding facilities undertaken before restocking. Dulin (1979) also considers that it is impractical and ill-advised to treat food fish reared commercially, but notes that isoniazid and rifampicin have been recommended for treating mycobacteriosis in valuable exotic marine species. Van Duijn (1981) is of the opinion that the health hazard to man has been exaggerated and describes a number of strategies for treating diseased fish, in particular the parenteral and oral administration of sulphisoxazole together with doxycycline or minocycline, and/or the addition of tetracycline to the water for fish which are too small to inject or are not feeding.

Natural spread of infection within a closed environment may be controlled by the addition to the tank of chloramine B or T at 10 mg/litre for 24 h, after which the water should be changed (van Duijn 1981). Feeding of contaminated fish products should be avoided but, if this doubtful practice is followed, the food must be pasteurised before use. Freezing does not kill the bacteria within a stored carcase (Ross *et al.* 1959).

No vaccines are available against fish mycobacteria, but the fact that fish are able to develop a cell-mediated immune response to mycobacterial antigens (Bartos & Sommer 1981) indicates a potential for the development of BCG-like vaccines. Such products might find particular application in the immunization of valuable, long-lived specimens but are unlikely to be commercially justifiable for farmed food fish.

## Public health considerations

*M. marinum*, *M. fortuitum* and *M. chelonae* are all capable of infecting warm-blooded vertebrates, including man. *M. marinum* is the most frequently encountered of the three species and causes cutaneous granulomas in man, usually of the elbow but also of the knee, fingers and feet, resulting from abrasions incurred in swimming pools ('swimming pool granuloma') or tropical fish aquaria. Lesions, which may ulcerate, usually heal spontaneously over a period of months. Early isolations of *M. marinum* from swimming pools and human wounds were initially thought to be a separate species and named *M. balnei* (Linell & Norden 1954). *M. fortuitum* is a relatively uncommon opportunist pathogen of man. Infection usually involves the skin following superficial trauma, but the organism has also been isolated from lungs, lymph nodes and other internal organs. *M. chelonae* has been isolated from a knee joint infection, injection abscesses and post-operative wound infections in man, but these strains were capable of growth at 37°C and are phenotypically distinct from the fish isolates identified to date. The human health risk from fish strains of *M. chelonae* is therefore probably extremely low.

# Fish *Nocardia* pathogens

Nocardiosis was first identified as a disease of tropical freshwater fish by Valdez & Conroy (1963). The same condition was described shortly afterwards in fingerling rainbow trout by Snieszko *et al.* (1964) and subsequently in brook trout (*Salvelinus fontinalis*) by Campbell & MacKelvie (1968). Despite differences in acid-fast staining reactions, colony pigmentation and growth temparature range, all these early freshwater isolates were considered to be *Nocardia asteroides*. A second proposed species, *Nocardia kampachi*, associated with mortality of cultured yellowtail in Japan, was initially isolated by Kariya *et al.* (1968) and Kubota *et al.* (1968). This organism has since become established as one of the most important pathogens of cultured yellowtail (Kawatsu *et al.* 1976).

## Fish species susceptibility

*Nocardia asteroides* infections have reportedly been observed in many freshwater species (van Duijn 1981), but too few disease outbreaks have been detailed in the literature to define the host or geographical range of the condition. The first fish isolate of *N. asteroides*, from neon tetra fish, was experimentally found to be pathogenic for paradise fish and three-spot gouramis but not for goldfish (*Carassius auratus*) (Conroy & Valdez 1962), suggesting that nocardiosis may be problematical in a range of tropical aquarium fish. Rainbow trout are undoubtedly also susceptible to infection, but information with regard to other temperate freshwater species is very limited. *N. kampachi* is recognised as an important marine pathogen of yellowtail but does not appear to have been identified in other species of fish.

### Characteristics of disease

Nocardiosis shares many clinical features with mycobacteriosis and, not surprisingly, some cases of nocardiosis have been mistakenly attributed to a mycobacterial infection. Nocardiosis is a chronic disease which usually occurs sporadically, involves only a small percentage of fish in a population and causes light mortalities, except in *N. kampachi* infections involving cultured yellowtail where mortalities can be high. Young fish are most often affected, but all age groups appear to be vulnerable, especially in late summer and early autumn.

Early signs of infection may include anorexia, inactivity, skin discoloration and emaciation. In later stages, nodular, caseous skin lesions which may ulcerate and abdominal distension due to the development of internal granulomata may be observed. In yellowtails, the appearance of cream-coloured nodules on the gills has led to the description 'gill tuberculosis' (Kusuda *et al.* 1974). Internally, nodular or diffuse granulomatous lesions may be found in skeletal muscle and any of the visceral organs or mesentery. Histologically the lesions are tuberculoid, with a distinctive fibrous capsule and an abundance of bacterial filaments which are obvious within the centre of the lesion, irrespective of the stain used (Frerichs & Roberts 1989). *N. asteroides* is usually acid-fast in ZN-stained tissue sections but *N. kampachi* is less likely to show this characteristic.

### Immune response to infection

No studies on the immune response of fish to infection with nocardioform organisms have been reported. Kusuda & Nakagawa (1978) however, found that yellowtails inoculated with heat or formalin killed *N. kampachi* developed high serum agglutinating antibody levels within 6 weeks, indicating that vaccination may be possible as a means of disease control.

### Transmission of infection

The route of infection with *Nocardia* sp. is not known, but as these organisms are widely distributed in nature in the soil, it would seem very possible that fish could be infected directly from the natural environment. Contaminated food and already diseased fish may also act as sources of infection.

### Isolation and culture of *Nocardia*

Most nocardiae will grow on a variety of media containing simple carbon and nitrogen sources, and can be readily isolated on standard bacteriological media including brain heart infusion agar (BHIA), tryptone soya agar (TSA) and nutrient agar (NA) incubated at 20–30°C. In practice, *Nocardia* spp. have probably been more often isolated on media such as Lowenstein-Jensen and Ogawa's egg formulation, as the clinical condition usually indicates a myco-bacterial infection.

Growth of *N. asteroides* appears in 4–5 days as ridged and folded, irregular, pinkish-white to yellow-orange colonies with aerial hyphae most prevalent along the colony margin. *N. kampachi* produces flat, wrinkled colonies after 10 days at 25°C.

### Identification of fish *Nocardia*

Colonial morphology together with the microscopic observation of Gram-positive, branching and often fragmenting, filamentous bacilli with aerial hyphae have historically sufficed to identify a bacterial isolate as *Nocardia* sp. (Fig. 14.4) although this would probably be considered inadequate by present-day taxonomists. The property of acid-fastness is not present in all strains and is, in any case, often difficult to demonstrate in culture.

Speciation of isolates as *N. asteroides* has generally been based on reactions in 25 selected physiological and biochemical tests proposed by Gordon & Mihm (1962). Acid is produced from glucose and glycerol but not from adonitol, arabinose, erythritol, inositol, lactose, maltose, mannitol, raffinose, sorbitol or xylose. Acetate, malate, propionate, pyruvate and succinate, but not benzoate, can be utilized as carbon sources. Casein, hypoxanthine, tyrosine and xanthine are not attacked. Although ability to grow at 35°C is also regarded as a key characteristic of *N. asteroides*, not all fish isolates have been cultivable at this temperature (Campbell & MacKelvie 1968).

*N. kampachi* is biochemically very similar to *N. asteroides*, with only a minor divergence in sugar fermentation and organic acid utilization patterns being noted by Kusuda & Taki (1973) and Kusuda *et al.* (1974). *N. kampachi* does not grow at 37°C but, as noted above, this characteristic will not necessarily differentiate this proposed species from all fish strains of *N. asteroides*.

### Treatment and control

Early investigators experienced considerable difficulty in inducing progressive nocardiosis in experimentally infected trout (Snieszko *et al.* 1964, Campbell &

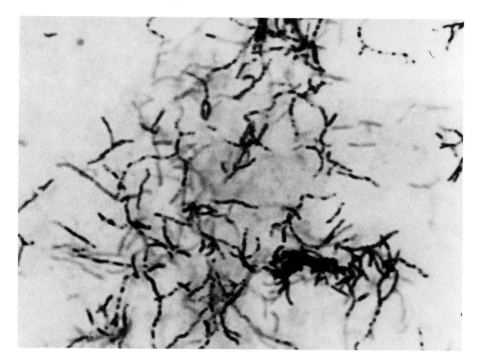

**Fig. 14.4** *Nocardia asteroides*: 3 days old culture on TSA. Gram stained showing branching rods and fragmented mycelium with characteristic patchy staining.

MacKelvie 1968) indicating that nocardiae are pathogenic only under certain environmental conditions. The only successful treatment of clinical disease reported is the oral or parenteral administration of a combination of sulphisoxazole and doxycycline or minocycline as advocated for the treatment of mycobacteriosis (van Duijn 1981). An improvement in condition should be noticed within 10 days, but continued medication for 3 weeks is advisable. A clean environment is probably the most important factor in the prevention of disease, particularly as it has been shown that *N. kampachi* is only able to survive for 2 days in open seawater but for more than 90 days in the presence of 100 ppm fish extracts (Kusuda & Nakagawa 1978). Vaccination has been investigated as a means of control but has not yet become commercially established.

## References

Abernethy, C.S. & Lund, J.E. (1978) Mycobacteriosis in mountain whitefish (*Prosopium williamsoni*) from the Yakima River, Washington. *Journal of Wildlife Diseases*, **14**, 333–6.

Alexander, D.M. (1913) A review of piscine tuberculosis, with a description of an acid-fast bacillus found in the cod. *Report of the Lancashire Sea Fish Laboratory*, **21**, 43–9.

Arakawa, C.K. & Fryer, J.L. (1984) Isolation and characterization of a new subspecies of *Mycobacterium chelonei* infectious for salmonid fish. *Helgolander Meeresuntersuchungen*, **37**, 329–42.

Arakawa, C.K., Fryer, J.L. & Sanders, J.E. (1986) Serology of *Mycobacterium chelonei* isolated from salmonid fish. *Journal of Fish Diseases*, **9**, 269−71.

Aronson, J.D. (1926) Spontaneous tuberculosis in salt water fish. *Journal of Infectious Diseases*, **39**, 315−20.

Ashburner, L.D. (1977) Mycobacteriosis in hatchery-confined chinook salmon (*Oncorhynchus tschawytscha* Walbaum) in Australia. *Journal of Fish Biology*, **10**, 523−8.

Austin, B. & Austin, D.A. (1987) *Bacterial Fish Pathogens: Disease in Farmed and Wild Fish*. Ellis Horwood Ltd, Chichester.

Baker, J.A. & Hagan, W.A. (1942) Tuberculosis of the Mexican platyfish (*Platypoecilus maculatus*). *Journal of Infectious Diseases*, **70**, 248−52.

Bartos, J.M. & Sommer, C.V. (1981) *In vivo* cell mediated immune response to *M. tuberculosis* and *M. salmoniphilum* in rainbow trout (*Salmo gairdneri*). *Developmental and Comparative Immunology*, **5**, 75−83.

Bataillon, E., Dubard, . & Terre, L. (1897) Un nouveau type de tuberculose. *Comptes rendus des Séances de la Societe Biologie*, **49**, 446−9.

Bataillon, E., Moeller, A. & Terre, L. (1902) Über die Identitat des Bacillus des Karpfens (Bataillon, Dubard und Terre) und des Bacillus der Blindsschleuche (Moeller). *Zentralblatt für Tuberkulose*, **3**, 467−8.

Besse, P. (1949) Epizootie à bacilles acido-resistants chez des poissons exotique. *Bulletin de l'Académie Vétérinaire de France*, **23**, 151−4.

Campbell, G. & MacKelvie, R.M. (1968) Infection of brook trout (*Salvelinus fontinalis*) by nocardiae. *Journal of the Fisheries Research Board of Canada*, **25**, 423−5.

Chinabut, S., Limsuwan, C. & Chanratchakool, P. (1990) Mycobacteriosis in the snakehead, *Channa striatus* (Fowler). *Journal of Fish Diseases*, **13**, 531−5.

Conroy, D.A. (1966) Observaciones sobre casos espontaneos de tuberculosis ictica. *Microbiologia espanola*, **19**, 93−113.

Conroy, D.A. (1970) Piscine tuberculosis in the sea water environment. In *Symposium on Diseases of Fishes and Shellfishes* (Ed. by S.F. Snieszko), pp. 273−8. Special Publication No. 5, American Fisheries Society, Washington DC.

Conroy, D.A. & Valdez, I.E. (1962) Un casos de tuberculosis en peces tropicales. *Revista Latinoamericana de Microbiologia*, **75**, 9−16.

Duijn, C. van (1981) Tuberculosis in fishes. *Journal of Small Animal Practice*, **22**, 391−411.

Dulin, M.P. (1979) A review of tuberculosis (mycobacteriosis) in fish. *Veterinary Medicine/Small Animal Clinician*, **74**, 731−5.

Earp, B.J., Ellis, C.H. & Ordal, E.J. (1953) Kidney disease in young salmon. Washington State Department of Fisheries, Special Report No. 1, 74pp.

Frerichs, G.N. & Roberts, R.J. (1989) The bacteriology of teleosts. In *Fish Pathology*, 2nd edn (Ed. by R.J. Roberts), pp. 289−319. Baillière Tindall, London.

Giavenni, R., Finazzi, M., Poli, G. & Grimaldi, C.N.R. (1980) Tuberculosis in marine tropical fishes in an aquarium. *Journal of Wildlife Diseases*, **16**, 161−8.

Goodfellow, M. & Lechevalier, M. (1986) Genus *Nocardia*. In *Bergey's Manual of Systematic Bacteriology*, Vol. 2 (Ed. by P.H.A. Sneath, N.S. Mair & M.E. Sharpe), pp. 1459−71. Williams and Wilkins, Baltimore.

Gordon, R.E. & Mihm, J.M. (1959) A comparison of four species of mycobacteria. *Journal of General Microbiology*, **21**, 736−48.

Gordon, R.E. & Mihm, J.M. (1962) The type species of the genus *Nocardia*. *Journal of General Microbiology*, **27**, 1−10.

Grange, J.M. (1981) *Mycobacterium chelonei*. *Tubercle*, **62**, 273−6.

Kariya, T., Kubota, S., Nakamura, Y. & Kira, K. (1968) Nocardial infection in cultured yellowtail (*Seriola quinqueradiata* and *S. purpurascens*) I. Bacteriological study. *Fish Pathology*, **3**, 16−23.

Kawatsu, H., Homma, A. & Kawaguchi, K. (1976) Epidemic fish diseases and their control in Japan. In *Advances in Aquaculture* (Ed. by T.V.R. Pillay & W.A. Dill), pp. 197−201. Fishing News Books Ltd, Farnham, Surrey.

Kubota, S., Kariya, T., Nakamura, Y. & Kira, K. (1968) Nocardial infection in cultured yellowtail (*Seriola quinqueradiata* and *S. purpurascens*) II. Histological study. *Fish Pathology*, **3**, 24−33.

Kusuda, R. & Nakagawa, A. (1978) Nocardial infection of cultured yellowtail. *Fish Pathology*, **13**, 25–31.

Kusuda, R. & Taki, H. (1973) Studies on a nocardial infection of cultured yellowtail I. Morphological and biochemical characteristics of *Nocardia* isolated from diseased fishes. *Bulletin of the Japanese Society of Scientific Fisheries*, **39**, 937–43.

Kusuda, R., Taki, H. & Takeuchi, T. (1974) Studies on a nocardia infection of cultured yellowtail II. Characteristics of *Nocardia kampachi* isolated from a gill-tuberculosis of yellowtail. *Bulletin of the Japanese Society of Scientific Fisheries*, **40**, 369–73.

Lechevalier, H.A. (1986) Nocardioforms. In *Bergey's Manual of Systematic Bacteriology*, Vol. 2 (Ed. by P.H.A. Sneath, N.S. Mair & M.E. Sharpe), pp. 1458–9. Williams and Wilkins, Baltimore.

Linell, F. & Norden, A. (1954) *Mycobacterium balnei*. A new acid-fast bacillus occurring in swimming pools and capable of producing skin lesions in humans. *Acta Tuberculosea Scandinavica* (supplement), **33**, 1–85.

Nigrelli, R.F. (1953) Two diseases of the Neon Tetra, *Hyphessobrycon innesi*. *Aquarium Journal (San Francisco)*, **24**, 203–8.

Nigrelli, R.F. & Vogel, H. (1963) Spontaneous tuberculosis in fishes and other cold-blooded vertebrates with special reference to *Mycobacterium fortuitum* Cruz from fish and human lesions. *Zoologica*, **48**, 131–44.

Parisot, T.J. (1958) Tuberculosis of fish. *Bacteriological Reviews*, **22**, 240–5.

Parisot, T.J. & Wood, E.M. (1960) A comparative study of the causative agent of a mycobacterial disease of salmonid fishes II. A description of the histopathology of the disease in chinook salmon (*Oncorhynchus tschawytscha*) and a comparison of the staining characteristics of the fish disease with leprosy and human tuberculosis. *American Review of Respiratory Diseases*, **82**, 212–22.

Reichenbach-Klinke, H.H. (1972) Some aspects of mycobacterial infections in fish. Symposium of the Zoological Society of London No. 30, 17–24.

Ross, A.J. (1960) *Mycobacterium salmoniphilum* sp. nov. from salmonid fishes. *American Review of Respiratory Diseases*, **81**, 241–50.

Ross, A.J. (1963) Mycobacteria in adult salmonid fishes returning to National fish hatcheries in Washington, Oregon and California in 1958–59. US Fish and Wildlife Services, Special Scientific Report on Fisheries 462, 5pp.

Ross, A.J. (1970) Mycobacteriosis among Pacific salmonid fishes. In *Symposium on Diseases of Fishes and Shellfishes* (Ed. by S.F. Snieszko), pp. 279–83. Special Publication No. 5, American Fisheries Society, Washington DC.

Ross, A.J. & Brancato, F.P. (1959) *Mycobacterium fortuitum* Cruz from the tropical fish *Hyphessobrycon innesi*. *Journal of Bacteriology*, **78**, 392–5.

Ross, A.J. & Johnson, H.E. (1962) Studies of transmission of mycobacterial infections in chinook salmon. *Progressive Fish Culturist*, **24**, 147–9.

Ross, A.J., Earp, B.J. & Wood, J.W. (1959) Mycobacterial infections in adult salmon and steelhead trout returning to the Columbia River Basin and other areas in 1957. US Fish and Wildlife Services, Special Scientific Report on Fisheries 332, 34pp.

Sanders, J.E. & Fryer, J.L. (1988) Bacteria of fish. In *Methods in Aquatic Bacteriology* (Ed. by B. Austin), pp. 115–42. John Wiley & Sons Ltd, Chichester.

Shotts, E.B. & Teska, J.D. (1989) Bacterial pathogens of aquatic vertebrates. In *Methods for the Microbiological Examination of Fish and Shellfish* (Ed. by B. Austin & D.A. Austin), pp. 164–86. Ellis Horwood Ltd, Chichester.

Snieszko, S.F., Bullock, G.L., Dunbar, C.E. & Pettijohn, L.L. (1964) Nocardial infection in hatchery-reared fingerling rainbow trout (*Salmo gairdneri*). *Journal of Bacteriology*, **88**, 1809–10.

Sutherland, P.L. (1922) A tuberculosis-like disease in a saltwater fish (halibut) associated with the presence of an acid-fast tubercle-like bacillus. *Journal of Pathology and Bacteriology*, **25**, 31–5.

Timur, G., Roberts, R.J. & McQueen, A. (1977) The experimental pathogenesis of focal tuberculosis in the plaice (*Pleuronectes platessa* L.). *Journal of Comparative Pathology*, **87**, 83–7.

Tsang, A.Y., Barr, V.L., McClatchy, J.K., Goldberg, M., Drupa, I. & Brennan, P.J. (1984)

Antigenic relationships of the *Mycobacterium fortuitum* — *Mycobacterium chelonae* complex. *International Journal of Systematic Bacteriology*, **34**, 35–44.

Valdez, I.E. & Conroy, D.A. (1963) The study of a tuberculosis-like condition in neon tetras (*Hyphessobrycon innesi*) II. Characteristics of the bacterium isolated. *Microbiologia espanola*, **16**, 245–53.

Wayne, L.G. & Kubica, G.P. (1986) Family Mycobacteriaceae. In *Bergey's Manual of Systematic Bacteriology*, Vol. 2 (Ed. by P.H.A. Sneath, N.S. Mair & M.E. Sharpe), pp. 1436–57. Williams & Wilkins, Baltimore.

Wolke, R.E. & Stroud, R.K. (1978) Piscine mycobacteriosis. In *Mycobacterial Infections of Zoo Animals*. (Ed. by R.J. Montali), pp. 269–75. Smithsonian Institute Press, Washington, DC.

# Part 8:
# Rickettsias and Chlamydias

The order Rickettsiales comprises small cocco-bacilliary or pleomorphic Gram-negative micro-organisms with typical bacterial cell walls but capable of multiplication only within host cells. All undergo binary fission but display wide variation in other characteristics. They are parasitic or mutualistic and many can cause diseases in vertebrate and invertebrate hosts.

The Chlamydiales likewise are small coccoid microorganisms with an obligately intracellular mode of multiplication. They are distinguished from the Rickettsiales by having a developmental cycle of morphologically distinct specialised cell types, including elementary bodies and larger reticulate bodies which undergo binary fission. They differ also in the composition of the cell wall and in metabolism.

# Chapter 15:
# Epitheliocystis and Salmonid Rickettsial Septicaemia

There are few examples of prokaryotic obligate intracellular parasites in fin fish. The only significant example until recently was epitheliocystis caused by an organism placed in a new taxon within the Order Chlamydiales. This Order comprises coccoid obligate intracellular micro-organisms which multiply within cytoplasmic vacuoles and change from small rigid-walled infectious forms to larger flexible non-infectious forms that divide by fission. These develop into a new generation of daughter cells which can survive extracellularly and infect new host cells. They are metabolically limited and are Gram-negative, although more usually stained by one of the Romanowsky stains such as Giemsa or Machiavello. The single genus within the Chlamydiales is *Chlamydia*.

Since 1989 reports have been published of rickettsial-like organisms associated with a serious disease affecting coho salmon (*Oncorhynchus kisutch*) in Chile. These have been tentatively characterized classified as *Piscirickettsia salmonis* within the Order Rickettsiales. However, insufficient information is yet available to allow a completely satisfactory classification of either the Order or rickettsia-like organisms. Their morphology is coccoid, often pleomorphic, and they multiply only inside the host cell. While all members undergo binary fission there is great variation in shape, staining reactivity and other characteristics within the Order.

## Epitheliocystis

### Species specificity

Host specificity has yet to be adequately investigated. It appears that horizontal transmission occurs readily within a species (Plehn 1920, Hoffmann *et al.* 1969). The evidence for transmission between species is largely based on morphological studies with their attendant limitations. Similar morphological forms have been observed within families, e.g. Salmonidae (Rourke *et al.* 1984, Bradley *et al.* 1988). There is also substantial evidence to suggest that different families of host are affected by different morphological forms of epitheliocystis organisms, and circumstantial evidence of resistance to transmission between families (Hoffman *et al.* 1969). This led Paperna *et al.* (1981) to suggest that cross infection between families of fish is unlikely.

### Clinical signs

Despite being most frequently observed on the gills, epitheliocystis has also been detected on the skin (Hoffman *et al.* 1969) and on the pseudobranch (Crespo *et al.* 1990). The fresh cysts usually appear transparent or white, although Wolf (1981) reported occasionally detecting a yellow coloration.

The relationship between epitheliocystis and disease is based primarily on circumstantial evidence. No one has managed to fulfil Koch's Postulates for this condition. Therefore the clinical signs are assigned by association rather than by demonstration of a causal relationship. The signs are primarily associated with damage to the gills and include excessive mucus production and respiratory distress. Others have been reported, including renal and alimentary pathology (Miyazaki *et al.* 1986, Bradley *et al.* 1988).

## *Pathology*

Epitheliocystis appears in several forms. These are related to the number of cysts present and the hosts' response to them. The number of cysts can range from one or two up to massive infections, which have been referred to as hyperinfections. The host response to cysts can be benign, where there is no reaction, or a limited localised epithelial hyperplasia. Alternatively the host can develop a proliferative response involving a widespread severe epithelial hyperplasia. Although the proliferative response is usually associated with a hyperinfection, it has been seen in the presence of only a few cysts in *common carp* (Miyazaki *et al.* 1986). Similarly there have been cases of hyperinfection in the absence of pathological proliferation (Paperna *et al.* 1981).

## *Development of the affected cell*

The earliest form of epitheliocystis reported is a small number of membrane-bound basophilic organisms within the cytoplasm of the host cell. As the inclusion expands, initially there is enlargement of the host cell nucleus, which develops a distinct nucleolus. Subsequently the nucleus is distorted, displaced to the margin of the cell and eventually lost. The remnants of the host cell membrane and cytoplasm are retained as an eosinophilic hyaline capsule surrounding the cysts.

In the early stages the host cell may be spindle shaped, usually enlarging into a spherical cyst. This cyst may subsequently be distorted into an ellipsoid by the pressure of surrounding tissue. The affected cell can reach a size of 400 μm diameter (Herman & Wolf 1987), but is usually smaller than this. In some species the cyst is quite robust and in the later stages of development can be expressed from the host tissues with light pressure (Molnár & Boros 1981). However, in other species the cyst is more fragile (Fig. 15.1). It has been suggested that the cysts may be made up from a number of host cells. This opinion has not been supported by subsequent evidence (Plate 35).

## *Reaction surrounding the host cell*

Benign reaction
The benign reaction to the epitheliocystis-affected cell varies between species. In some cases there is little or no reaction in the surrounding cells, for example

in salmonids. In other species there is a distinct but limited epithelial hyperplastic response, enclosing the infected cell in a capsule of cuboidal to squamous epithelial cells. This hyperplastic response may take some time to develop (Zachary & Paperna 1977). The cyst and surrounding hyperplastic tissue may fill the interlamellar space and develop a surrounding blood lacuna. The hyperplastic tissue may undergo necrosis and even elicit a mild leucocytic response. This process eventually results in release of the mature epitheliocystis cysts.

### Proliferative reaction

The proliferative reaction is associated with massive hyperplasia of the epithelial tissue, distorting or even obliterating the normal architecture of the gills (Fig. 15.2). Large blood lacunae may develop and areas of necrosis with leucocyte infiltration are common in the advanced stages.

### EM appearance of host cells

Electron microscopy demonstrates degeneration of the cytoplasmic organelles of the infected host cell. There is an electron-dense layer close to the inclusion, with swollen mitochondria and cisternae of the endoplasmic reticulum. Microfibril and hyaline-like bodies, indicating degeneration, have been observed both in the affected cell and in those surrounding it. The membrane separating the parasite from the host cell cytoplasm may be convoluted. In salmonids it is less convoluted, but small, membrane-bound, cytoplasmic vesicles, extending into the parasitic cyst, have been observed. These may be clathrin-coated vesicles which have a transport related function (Bradley *et al.* 1988).

It has been suggested that the organisms affect a range of different host cell types. Histologically the host cells of *Cyprinus carpio* would appear to be mucus cells (this view is supported by their positive staining reaction with PAS), whereas in Atlantic salmon (*Salmo salar*) the affected cells bear a strong resemblance to epithelial cells. On electron microscopic evidence it has been claimed that epitheliocystis can affect epithelial, chloride and mucus cells (Paperna & Alves de Matos 1984). Other reports based on the position of the cells (Miyazaki *et al.* 1986) have suggested that endothelial cells are involved. Desser *et al.* (1988) hypothesized that the host cell in some cases might be a macrophage transformed into an epithelioid cell. As the host cell can be transformed by the effect of the parasite (Kordova 1978, Morrison & Sprague 1981, Hase 1985), the affected cell cannot be definitively identified on morphological evidence.

## Bacterium

### Staining

Histological sections stain positive with Giemsa and Macchiavello, basophilic with H & E and negative with Gram, periodic acid Schiff (PAS) and Gimenez.

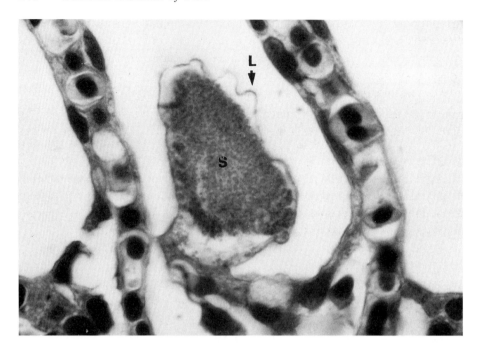

**Fig. 15.1**  Epitheliocystis infected epithelial cell on the gill of an Atlantic salmon. L = limiting membrane of the cell. S = swollen cytoplasm, almost entirely replaced by epitheliocystis organisms (H&E × 1000).

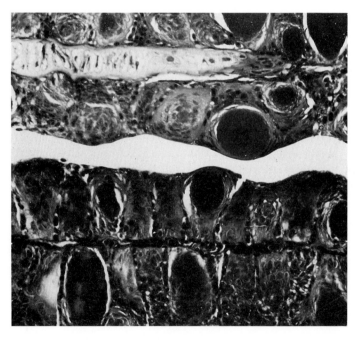

**Fig. 15.2**  Proliferative reaction to epitheliocystis in the gill of a gilthead bream (H&E × 150) (Courtesy of Dr I. Paperna).

## *Morphology*

Because of technical difficulties, most existing studies are based on transmission electron microscopy (TEM) of naturally infected fish. Definitive information will require comparison of identically propagated and processed sequential samples. The existing studies have faced several obstacles when investigating epitheliocystis organisms. First, the TEM picture provides a view of the organisms at only one point in their development, with limited information regarding their subsequent development. Second, there appear to be morphologically distinct organisms in different families of host. Until cross infection is thoroughly investigated the effect of the host on the morphology of the parasite cannot be defined. However, it is known that such an effect has been demonstrated in mammals (Kordova 1978).

Five main morphological types of epitheliocystis have been described. These are the initial body, elongated cells, round cells, small cells and the head and tail cells. The other types described appear to be due, at least in part, to artefacts. The forms of epitheliocystis observed in different species of host are summarized in Table 15.1. All stages or forms of epitheliocystis have some common features. They are surrounded by a trilaminar membrane consisting of two electron-dense layers separated by a lucent band. The cytoplasm contains ribosome-like particles and nucleoid material of variable density.

### The initial body (or reticulate body)

These terms are used to describe the early stages of chlamidial development and have been applied to some forms of epitheliocysts owing to morphological similarities. The cells are irregularly shaped with electron-lucent cytoplasm containing many ribosome-like particles and dense bits of punctate chromatin. They range in size from 0.7 to 1.25 µm in diameter.

### Elongated cells

There are two forms of these cells, the so called Primary Long Cells (PLC) and the Intermediate Long Cells (ILC). These forms resemble in structure and mode of division the giant or initial bodies of the Rickettsiella genus (Paperna *et al.* 1981). The PLC range in size from a maximum of 7.5 µm in length by 0.3−0.6 µm in diameter. They have electron-lucent cytoplasm with loose fibrilar nucleoid material and peripheral ribosome-like particles. The PLC might be considered another form of initial body. The ILC are produced from the PLC by binary fission and budding. They are generally shorter ($1-2 \times 0.3-0.6$ µm) with a more dense nucleoid. Estimating the length of these cells has proved difficult but it has been suggested that there may be different mean sizes in different species of host (Paperna *et al.* 1981).

### Round/oval cells

These cells have also been referred to as intermediate bodies, the form between

**Table 15.1** The forms of epitheliocystis observed in different species of host

| Host | Epitheliocystis cell type observed | | References |
|---|---|---|---|
| *Acanthopagrus schlegeli* (Bream, Australia) | | | Egusa (1987) |
| *Aristichthys nobilis* (Bighead carp) | | + | Molnár & Boros (1981) |
| *Ctenopharyngon idella* (Grass carp) | | + | Molnár & Boros (1981) |
| *Cyprinus carpio* (Common carp) | RC(D)/SC | * | Plehn (1920) |
| | | + | Molnár & Boros (1981) |
| *Dicentrarchus labrax* (Sea bass) | EC(D) | | Paperna & Baudin-Laurencin (1979) |
| | | + | Paperna et al. (1981) |
| *Hippoglossoides platessoides* (American plaice) | RC | | Morrison & Shum (1983) |
| *Hypophthalmichthys molitrix* (Silver carp) | | + | Molnár & Boros (1981) |
| *Ictalurus nebulosus* (Brown bullhead) | IB(D)/RC(D)/SC or small RC | + | Desser et al. (1988) |
| *Ictalurus punctatus* (Channel catfish) | RC(D) | | Zimmer et al. (1984) |
| *Lepomis macrochirus* (Blue gill) | RC | + | Hoffman et al. (1969) |
| *Liza aurata* (Long finned grey mullet) | RC | | Paperna & Sabnai (1980) |
| *Liza ramada* (Grey mullet) | EC(D)/SC | * | Paperna (1977) |
| *Liza subviridis* | | + | Paperna et al. (1978) |
| | | | Paperna & Sabnai (1980) |
| *Morone americanus* (White perch) | RC(D) | | Wolke et al. (1970) |
| *Morone saxatilis* (Striped bass) | RC(D)/EC(D) | * | Wolke et al. (1970) |
| | | | Herman (1984) |
| *Mugil cephalus* (Common grey mullet) | | * | Paperna & Sabnai (1980) |
| | | + | Paperna et al. (1981) |
| *Oncorhynchus mykiss* (Rainbow trout) | IB(D)/RC(D)/HTC | | Rourke et al. (1984) |
| | | * + | Herman & Wolf (1987) |
| *Oreochromis aureus* × *niloticus* (Tilapia) | EC(D)/SC | | Paperna et al. (1981) |
| *Oreochromis mossambicus* (Tilapia) | EC(D)/SC | | Paperna et al. (1981) |
| *Pagrus major* (Red Sea bream) | RC(D) | * + | Miyazaki et al. (1986) |
| *Salmo salar* (Atlantic salmon) | | | Turnbull et al. (1989) |
| *Salmo trutta* (Brown trout) | | | Turnbull (unpublished data) |
| *Salvelinus namaycush* (Lake trout) | IB(D)/RC(D)/HTC | * + | Bradley et al. (1986) |
| *Seriola dumerili* (Amberjack) | RC(D) | * + | Crespo et al. (1990) |
| *Sparus aurata* (Gilthead sea bream) | EC(D)/RC(D)/SC | * + | Paperna (1977) |
| | | | Paperna et al. (1981) |
| *Takifugu rubripes* (Tiger puffer) | RC | | Miyazaki et al. (1986) |
| *Upensus mollucensis* | | | Paperna & Sabnai (1980) |

+ = Proliferative from reported    * Associated with mortalities    (D) = Dividing    HTC = Head and tail cell
IB = Initial body    EC = Elongated cell    RC = Round cell    SC = Small cell

the initial and elementary bodies of *Chlamydia* species. The cells, usually round or oval but occasionally irregular-shaped, conform to the basic epithelio-cystis structure. Size ranges of 0.3–1 µm in diameter have been reported. They have never been detected in a cyst containing elongated cells. In many species they have been observed in the stages of division, from initial division of the nucleoid to large chains of connected organisms. They have also been seen as the only form of epitheliocystis within a cyst with no evidence of division. Paperna *et al.* (1981) observed these non-dividing forms only in cells with the EM appearance of chloride cells (in *Sparus aurata*, *Liza aurata* and *Mugil cephalus*). They suggested that this might be evidence for arrested development as a result of the host cells' influence.

The role of this form of the organism within different families of host is far from clear. It is possible that forms of epitheliocystis with different development cycles may produce a round cell form at different stages.

Small cells
These are assumed to be the infective final stage of development, equivalent to the elementary bodies of *Chlamydia* species. Some workers have described what appear to be small round cells as elementary bodies. However, there are a number of reports of a form with a distinct morphology in addition to relatively small size. These distinct small cells can be either round or bullet-shaped. They have the trilaminar membrane and dense cytoplasm, and the nucleoid is compact dense and surrounded by an electron-lucent halo. In some species of host the nucleoid is more dense than the cytoplasm (e.g. *M. cephalus*); in others it is less dense (e.g. *S. aurata*) (Paperna *et al.* 1981). These small cells are also characterized by electron lucent vacuoles in the cytoplasm. In *C. carpio* it would appear that small cells of two different sizes (0.5–0.7 × 0.3–0.5 µm or 0.9–1.3 × 0.5–0.7 µm) can be produced by separate routes of division (Paperna & Alves de Matos 1984). In other species, e.g. *S. aurata*, the small cells are of relatively consistent size (0.46–0.48 µm diameter) and produced by only one route. Although small cells have been observed connected to earlier forms, eventually they separate into individual units.

Head and tail cells
These cells, first reported by Rourke *et al.* (1984), have been observed in two species of salmonids. They have all the common epitheliocystis features and a shape consisting of an eliptical head (0.3 × 0.4 µm) containing a dense nucleoid and tail (up to 0.3 µm in length) with a small round expansion on the end (0.125 µm diameter). It is not clear what, if any, role, this form fulfills. It may represent a failed attempted division, an artefact or a normal form of the epitheliocystis in this species of host. It does bear a remarkable resemblance to a degenerating form of *Coxiella burnetii*, an organism resembling members of the *Rickettsia* genus (Weiss & Moulder 1984).

Other features

Two other features have been reported. The first is the presence of fine fibrils bridging the two electron dense portions of the trilaminate membrane in later stages of the organism. The filaments were arranged in a hexagonal configuration (Paperna & Alves de Matos 1984, Desser *et al.* 1988). These filaments are similar to those described in the elementary body of *Chlamydia psittaci* (Matsumoto & Manire 1970). The second is the presence of a small inclusion in the cytoplasm of the organisms in the process of division (Paperna *et al.* 1978).

As already mentioned the interpretation of this area of study presents considerable problems. However at present a pleomorphic development cycle would appear to be normal for epitheliocystis in all hosts. There is evidence of production of the final component at different stages of development in *common carp* (Paperna & Alves de Matos 1984). There seems to be arrested development in some cases (Paperna *et al.* 1981). Finally there is considerable evidence to support the view that there are different morphological forms of epitheliocystis in different families of fish.

Classification

Attempts to classify these organisms based on EM morphology have so far been unsuccessful. It has been suggested that they may be a species of *Rickettsia* (Paperna *et al.* 1981) or *Chlamydia* (Wolf 1981). In some hosts (e.g. *Ictaluris nebulosus*) the morphology of the parasite bears a striking resemblance to *Chlamydia* species. However, there is less of a resemblance in other species. In addition, two studies (Turnbull 1987, Bradley *et al.* 1988) have failed to detect the lipopolysaccharide Chlamydial genus-specific antigen. It is probable that these organisms represent a new taxon or group of new related taxa within the Chlamydiales.

**Epizootiology**

The benign form is a chronic condition that has been observed in fish of all ages from farmed and wild stocks. The proliferative condition has usually been observed in young (0+) farmed stock but was reported in wild caught *Liza ramada* (Paperna 1977). It has been suggested that a benign infection can progress to a proliferative response as a result of adverse cultural conditions or other forms of stress (Paperna & Sabnai 1980), including an association with low temperature (e.g. Plehn 1920, Crespo *et al.* 1990).

It is difficult to ascribe a definite role to epitheliocystis with relation to disease, and indeed in most cases the proliferative response could have been caused by concurrent factors.

There are reports of synchronous infection in individuals and groups of fish from the same area (Paperna & Alves de Matos 1984). Herman (1984) also observed such release of cysts from *M. saxatilis*. Although spread within the fish following ingestion has been proposed (Zachary & Paperna 1977) as the method of synchronisation, there is as yet little evidence to support this view.

### Geographical distribution

Epitheliocystis is widely distributed and has already been reported from North America, South-East Asia, the Middle East, Europe and South Africa. There is every possibility that it may be present in other parts of the world but has yet to be reported.

### Transmission

There is evidence of horizontal transmission within a species by cohabitation (Plehn 1920, Hoffman *et al.* 1969) and via fomites (Paperna *et al.* 1977). Evidence of transmission between species is very limited, Hoffman *et al.* (1969) found no direct evidence for such transmission.

### Significance

With the exception of Paperna (1977) there are no systematic surveys, and so it is impossible to speculate on incidence or distribution. In addition it is often difficult to define the relationship between epitheliocystis and observed pathology and mortalities and it is important to stress that this organism has only been 'associated' with the mortalities recorded in the species listed in Table 15.1, namely *Sparus aurata*, *Liza ramada*, *Cyprinus carpio*, *Oncorhynchus mykiss*, *Morone saxatilis*, *Pagrus major*, *Salvelinus namaycush*, *Mugil cephalus*, and *Seriola dumerili*.

### Control

In the absence of systematic study of chemotherapeutics the information available is purely anecdotal. Paperna *et al.* (1978) found that the condition resolved following in-feed treatment with chloramphenicol. Hoffman *et al.* (1969) suggested that their failure to cultivate the organism might have resulted from the presence of penicillin in the culture medium. So far avoidance is the only known method of control and even this has to be based on the limited knowledge of transmission.

## Salmonid Rickettsial septicaemia (SRS)

This septicaemic condition of salmonids, also known as coho salmon syndrome or huito disease, was first reported in Chile in 1989 by Bravo & Campos, though it may have been observed as early as 1981. Since then the incidence and associated mortalities have increased dramatically. As a result there has been a considerable research effort which has improved our understanding of the condition rapidly over a short period of time. Most of the information regarding this condition is contained within five publications: Bravo & Campos (1989), Fryer *et al.* (1990), Cvitanich *et al.* (1991), Branson & Diaz-Munoz (1991) and Fryer *et al.* (1992).

### Species specificity

The disease was thought to affect only farmed coho salmon. However, since January 1990 it has also been reported in Atlantic salmon, chinook salmon (*Oncorhynchus tschawytscha*) and rainbow trout. All these fish were sampled from Chilean salt water sites (Cvitanich *et al.* 1991).

### Clinical signs

#### Gross

Predictably the clinical signs vary between outbreaks and individual fish. The fish may show the classical signs of ill health, i.e. dark colour, lethargy, and swimming near the surface or at the side of the net. Alternatively, some fish die with very few signs of abnormality. External lesions include pale gills and skin lesions (Fig. 15.3). The latter range from small areas of raised scales through white raised plaques to shallow ulcers (Branson & Diaz-Munoz 1991). Internally the fish may have evidence of ascites, peritonitis and pallor. The gastrointestinal tract, swimbladder and visceral fat may have petechial haemorrhages. The spleen, liver and kidney are often swollen, with pale discolouration of the last two named organs. Occasionally the liver may be haemorrhagic or have yellow multifocal subcapsular nodules (Fig. 15.4). Pericarditis has also been reported from a small proportion of the terminally ill fish.

#### Histological

The most significant finding is the presence of small (0.4−1.5 µm diameter) basophilic Rickettsia-like Organisms (RLO) usually in the cytoplasm of host cells although they may be observed free in the tissue (Fig. 15.5). They have been observed in most tissues of the body, especially in association with lesions.

There is necrosis and oedema of the haematopoietic tissue with a granulomatous response. The condition is characterized by disseminated intravascular coagulation with necrosis of the thrombi and vascular endothelium (Fig. 15.6). There may also be some perivascular cellular inflammation. These vascular changes, which occur in all tissues, are similar to those in other animals affected by rickettsial organism (Pinkerton 1971, Jones & Hunt 1983, Valli

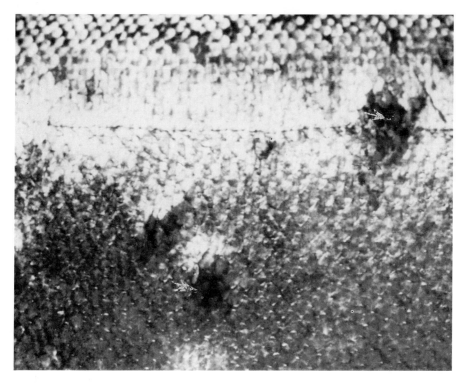

**Fig. 15.3** Skin lesions (on coho salmon) (arrowed) associated with *Piscirickettsia salmonis*. Small areas of raised scales are accompanied by larger more haemorrhagic lesions (Courtesy of Mr E. Branson).

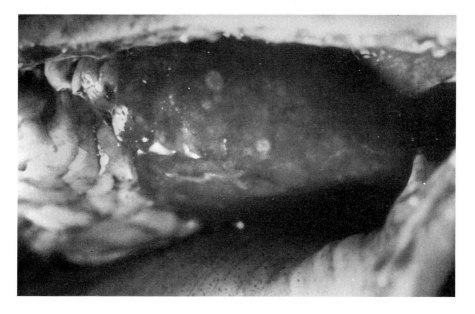

**Fig. 15.4** Nodular lesions in the liver of coho salmon infected with *Piscirickettsia salmonis* (Courtesy of Dr J.D. Cvitanich).

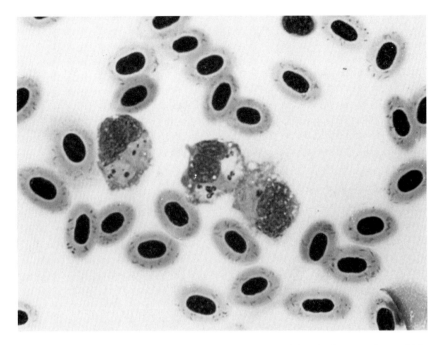

**Fig. 15.5** Macrophages in a peripheral blood smear showing rickettsia-like organisms within the cytoplasm (Giemsa × 1200) (Courtesy of Dr J.D. Cvitanich).

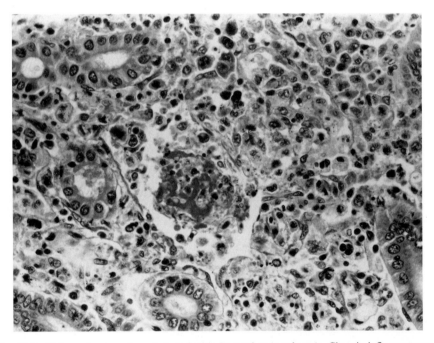

**Fig. 15.6** Kidney of coho salmon infected with *Piscirickettsia salmonis*. Chronic inflammatory tissue is in the process of replacing haemopoietic tissue and there is a mural thrombus of fibrin and infected macrophages, with red blood cells, in the central vascular channel (H&E × 400) (Courtesy of Dr J.D. Cvitanich).

1985). The liver can suffer focal to diffuse necrosis. The RLO have been reported within cytoplasmic vacuoles, free in the cytoplasm and outside host cells. The kidney and spleen both show generalized haematopoietic and vascular pathology. Additionally, in the kidney there may be oedema of the capsule, mild glomerular nephritis and limited tubular degeneration.

Endocarditis, variable pericarditis and focal hyaline necrosis of the myocardium have been detected in the heart. In the intestine there is often infection resulting in a granulomatous response and necrosis and sloughing of the mucosa. The gills have been described as suffering multifocal epithelial hyperplasia with more severe consolidation in some cases.

The skin lesions consist to varying degrees of necrosis of the epidermis, dermis and underlying musculature. The associated cellular inflammatory response can spread along the intra-muscular septa.

The remaining tissues of the body may all suffer from vascular pathology and the associated presence of the RLO. In some fish large dark-staining basophilic cells (20 × 10 μm) may be present in the haematopoietic tissue (Branson & Diaz-Munoz 1991). These cells consist of a large nucleus with very little cytoplasm. Occasionally they are the only intact cells in areas of necrosis. The origin and function of these cells is not known.

### Haematology

The pale coloration of affected fish is a reflection of the low haematocrit. The normal value is in the region of 35–50%, whereas in fish with SRS it was between 2 and 35%. A simultaneous neutrophilia (10–20 × normal) was demonstrated by Branson & Diaz-Munoz (1991) and Cvitanich *et al.* (1991) observed an increase in circulating macrophages, often containing RLO or cell debris. It has been suggested that fish showing skin lesions often have more severe histopathological changes (Branson & Diaz-Munoz 1991).

The clinical and histological signs have been observed in the absence of significant losses. This may indicate that SRS is yet another fish disease that requires some additional factors to precipitate severe losses.

## Bacterium

### Morphology

This pleomorphic/coccoid organism is an obligate intracellular parasite which usually develops within a cytoplasmic vacuole. The RLO can occur singly in diffuse groups or dense morula-like masses. They have also been seen in the process of binary fission. Under TEM they have a cell wall which occasionally has a rippled appearance. Beneath the cell wall is a plasma membrane closely applied to the cytoplasm. The cell contains numerous ribosome-like particles, single or multiple fibrilar nucleoid regions and small electron lucent vacuoles.

The vacuoles are not bound by a membrane and are of variable size and number.

The RLO stain positively with Giemsa, methyline blue, Pinkerton's adaption of Gimenez and basophilic with haematoxylin and eosin. They are Gram-negative and do not stain with PAS, Zeil Neilson, Gimenez or Macchiavello.

## Cultural characteristics

Attempts to culture the RLO on 41 artificial media failed. However, they have been grown on a number of cell lines of salmonid and non-salmonid origin, i.e. CHSE-214, CHH-1 CSE-119, TRG-2, EPC and FHM (Cvitanich *et al.* 1991, Fryer *et al.* 1990, 1992). The organism is capable of replication between 10−21°C but the optimal temperature is 15−18°C. The RLO produced a cytopathic effect causing cytoplasmic vacuolation and rounding up of the infected cells.

Following three successive passes through cell culture the washed RLO were still capable of reproducing the disease when injected into coho salmon at 15°C.

Antigenic studies have so far been limited. However, the RLO did not react with a monoclonal antibody raised against the Chlamydial genus-specific lipo-polysacchoride antigen. Therefore they are probably not a member of the *Chlamydia* genus. Fryer *et al.* (1990) and Cvitanich *et al.* (1991) concluded that the RLO may be a member of the family Rickettsiaceae and the tribe Ehrlichieae, but subsequent studies of its RNA composition led Fryer *et al.* (1992) to the conclusion that the pathogen was a gamma proteobacterium for which they proposed the new genus and species appelation *Piscirickettsia salmonis* gen. nov. sp. nov.

## Diagnosis

At present diagnosis is based on gross and histological signs and demonstration of the RLO.

## Pathogenesis

The vascular pathology observed in SRS is similar to that associated with intravascular spread of mammalian rickettsia. Therefore this infection may also develop from a haematogenous spread (Branson & Diaz-Munoz 1991).

## Epizootiology

### Geographical distribution

SRS was first reported from the Gulf of Ancud, between the island of Chiloe and the mainland south of Puerto Montt, in the south of Chile. So far it has been reported only from sea water sites. There are no indigenous salmonids on the Pacific coast of South America. All those present have been introduced for sport or commercial aquaculture. The epidemiology suggests that the RLO originated from a local marine source and subsequently infected the imported salmonids.

*Transmission*

Initially SRS was observed in fish 6−12 weeks after transfer to salt water, starting in April and lasting until August (Autumn and mid-winter in Chile). Outbreaks have now also occurred in December (Spring). The original cases were associated with a period of fluctuating temperature and a non-toxic algal bloom. However, the losses continued after the bloom dispersed and the temperature stabilized. In subsequent outbreaks there has been no strong correlation with environmental conditions.

Experimentally the condition has been transmitted by injection. Subsequently it passed horizontally to cohabiting fish. It has been proposed that the source of infection may be the faeces of affected fish. The horizontal transfer occurred both in fresh and salt water, although the time to death was longer in fresh water. Experimental transmission took place in the absence of vectors, but vectors may still play a role in natural transmission. At present there is no evidence of vertical transmission, but since the RLO have been detected in both ovaries and testes this route is also possible.

**Significance**

In a short time this condition has had a dramatic effect on the Chilean aquaculture industry. SRS was reported on four farms in April 1989 and in 32 farms 1 year later. The monthly mortalities generally range from 1 to 20% but can reach 40%. The average cumulative losses are 60% but have exceeded 90% on some sites. An estimated 1.5 million coho salmon (0.2−2 kg) died from SRS in 1989. The severity of the condition encouraged some farms to cultivate other salmonid species. However, recent outbreaks in a number of salmonid species may render this strategy ineffective. Risk of SRS being accidentally exported from Chile must be taken most seriously.

**Prevention**

There is no known method of preventing spread within sea water. At present, fish tissues from broodstock are Gram-stained and screened for the presence of RLO. The fertilized eggs are then routinely disinfected with iodophores. Whether as a result of these precautions or not there have as yet been no outbreaks in freshwater fish from Chilean salmonid broodstock.

Therapy is in the very early stages of investigation. In vitro trials have been conducted and the cytopathic effect has been prevented by the addition of clarithomycin, sarafloxacin, erythromycin, oxytetracycline, tetracycline and chloramphenicol, but not by spectinomycin or penicillin G. This finding was unexpected since most species of *Chlamydia* and *Rickettsia* are sensitive to penicillin (Moulder 1984). Despite the rapid advances already achieved, far more information will be required if the Chilean salmonid aquaculture industry is not to be permanently damaged by this condition.

### Other rickettsia-like organisms in fish

There are two other isolated reports of rickettsia-like organisms in fish (Mohamed 1939, Davis 1986) and reports of a canine pathogen (*Neorickettsia helminthoeca*) which is transmitted by the metacercaria of a small fluke (*Nanophyetus salmincola*) via the tissues of salmonids in North America (Jones & Hunt 1983).

## References

Bradley, T.M., Newcomer, C.E. & Maxwell, K.O. (1988) Epitheliocystis associated with massive mortalities of cultured lake trout *Salvelinus namaycush*. *Diseases of Aquatic Organisms*, **4**, 9–18.

Branson, E.J. & Diaz-Munoz, D.N. (1991) Description of a new disease condition occurring in farmed coho salmon, *Oncorhynchus kisutch* (Walbaum), in South America. *Journal of Fish Diseases*, **14**(2), 147–56.

Bravo, S. & Campos, M. (1989) Coho salmon syndrome in Chile. Fish Health Section, *American Fisheries Newsletter*, **17**(2), 3.

Crespo, S., Grau, A. & Padrós, F. (1990) Epitheliocystis disease in the cultured amberjack. *Seriola dumerili* Risso (Carangidae). *Aquaculture*, **90**, 197–207.

Cvitanich, J.D., Garate, N.O. & Smith, C.E. (1991) The isolation of a rickettsia-like organism causing disease and mortality in Chilean salmonids and its confirmation by Koch's postulate. *Journal of Fish Diseases*, **14**(2), 121–45.

Davis, A.J. (1986) A Rickettsia-like organism from dragonets, *Callionymus lyra* L. (Teleostei: Callionymidae) in Wales. *Bulletin of the European Association of Fish Pathologists*, **6**(4), 103–4.

Desser, S., Paterson, W. & Steinhagen, D. (1988) Ultrastructural observations on the causative agent of epitheliocystis in brown bullhead, *Ictalurus nebulosus* Lesueur, from Ontario and a comparison with the chlamydiae of higher vertebrates. *Journal of Fish Diseases*, **11**, 453–60.

Egusa, S. (1987) Epitheliocystis disease a review. *Fish Pathology*, **22**, 165–72.

Fryer, J.L., Lannan, C.N., Garcés, L.H., Larenas, J.J. & Smith, P.A. (1990) Isolation of a Rickettsiales-like organism from diseased coho salmon (*Oncorhynchus kisutch*) in Chile. *Fish Pathology*, **25**(2), 107–14.

Fryer, J.L., Lannan, C.N., Giovannoni, J.J. & Wood, N.D. (1992) *Piscirickettsia Salmonis* gen. nov., sp. nov., the causative agent of an epizootic disease in salmonid fishes. *International Journal of Systematic Bacteriology*, **42**, 120–6.

Hase, T. (1985) Developmental sequence and surface membrane assembly of rickettsiae. *Annual Reviews of Microbiology*, **39**, 69–88.

Herman, R.L. (1984) Striped bass fingerling mortality involves multiple factors. *Fish Health News*, **14**, III–V.

Herman, R.L. & Wolf, K. (1987) Epitheliocystis infection of fishes. US Fisheries & Wildlife Services Fish Disease leaflet No. 75, 1–4.

Hoffman, G.L., Dunbar, C.E., Wolf, K. & Zwillenberg, L.O. (1969) Epitheliocystis, a new infectious disease of bluegill (*Lepomis macrochirus*). *Antonie van Leeuwenhoek Journal of Microbiology and Serology*, **35**, 146−56.

Jones, T.C. & Hunt, R.D. (1983) *Veterinary Pathology*, Diseases caused by Mycoplasmatales, Rickettsiales and Spirochaeteales. pp. 511−73. Lea & Febiger, Philadelphia.

Kordova, N. (1978) *Chlamydia, Rickettsia*, and their cell wall defective varients. *Canadian Journal of Microbiology*, **24**, 339−52.

Matsumoto, A. & Manire, G.P. (1970) Electron microscopic observations on the fine structure of cell walls of *Chlamydia psittaci. Journal of Bacteriology*, **104**, 1332−7.

Miyazaki, T., Fujimaki, Y. & Hatai, K. (1986) A light and electron microscopic study on epitheliocystis disease in cultured fishes. *Bulletin of the Japanese Society of Scientific Fisheries*, **52**, 199−202.

Mohamed, Z. (1939) The discovery of rickettsia in a fish. Ministry of Agriculture, Egypt. Technical and Scientific Service. Veterinary Section. Bulletin No. 214, 6pp.

Molnár, K. & Boros, G. (1981) A light and electron microscopic study of the agent of carp mucophilosis. *Journal of Fish Diseases*, **4**, 325−34.

Morrison, C. & Shum, G. (1983) Epitheliocystis in American plaice *Hippoglossoides platessoides. Journal of Fish Diseases*, **6**, 303−8.

Morrison, C.M. & Sprague, V. (1981) Electronmicroscope study of a new genus and new species of microsporida in the gill of Atlantic cod *Gadus Morhua* L. *Journal of Fish Diseases*, **4**, 15−32.

Moulder, J.W. (1984) Looking at chlamydia without looking at their hosts. *American Society of Microbiology*, **50**, 353−62.

Paperna, I. (1977) Epitheliocystis infection in wild and cultured sea bream (*Sparus aurata*, Sparidae) and grey mullets (*Liza ramada*, Mugilidae). *Aquaculture*, **10**, 169−76.

Paperna, I. & Alves de Matos, A.P. (1984) The development cycle of epitheliocystis in carp, *Cyprinus carpio* L. *Journal of Fish Diseases*, **7**, 137−47.

Paperna, I. & Baudin-Laurencin, F. (1979) Parasitic infections of sea bass, *Dicentrarchus labrax*, and gilt head sea bream, *Sparus aurata*, in mariculture facilities in France. *Aquaculture*, **16**, 173−5.

Paperna, I. & Sabnai, I. (1980) Epitheliocystis diseases in fishes. In *Fish Diseases* (Ed. by W. Ahne), pp. 228−34. Springer Verlag, Berlin.

Paperna, I., Sabnai, I. & Castel, M. (1978) Ultrastructural study of epitheliocystis organisms from gill epithelium of the fish *Sparus aurata* (L.) and *Liza ramada* (Risso) and their relation to the host cell. *Journal of Fish Diseases*, **1**, 181−9.

Paperna, I., Sabnai, I. & Zachary, A. (1981) Ultrastructural studies in piscine epitheliocystis: evidence for a pleomorphic development cycle. *Journal of Fish Diseases*, **4**, 459−72.

Pinkerton, H. (1971) Rickettsial, chlamydial, and viral diseases. In *Pathology*, Vol. 1 (Ed. by W.A.D. Anderson), pp. 365−408. The C.V. Mosby Co., St Louis.

Plehn, M. (1920) New parasites in the skin and gills of fish. *Ichthyochtrium* and *Mucophilus*). (Neue Parasiten in Haut und Kiemen von Fischen. *Ichthyochytrium* und *Mucophilus*. Centralblatt für bakteriologie, Parasitenkunde, Infektionskranilheiten und Hygiene I. Abteilung Originale, **85**, 275−81.

Rourke, A.W., Davis, R.W. & Bradley, T.M. (1984) A light and electron microscope study of epitheliocystis in juvenile steelhead trout, *Salmo gairdneri* Richardson. *Journal of Fish Diseases*, **7**, 1−9.

Turnbull, J.F. (1987) *An Investigation into a Possible Carrier State of Furunculosis*. M.Sc. Thesis, Institute of Aquaculture, University of Stirling.

Turnbull, J.F., Richards, R.H. & Tatner, M.F. (1989) Evidence that superficial branchial colonies on the gills of *Salmo salar* L. are not *Aeromonas salmonicida. Journal of Fish Diseases*, **12**, 449−58.

Valli, V.E.O. (1985) The haematopoietic system. In *Pathology of Domestic Animals*, Vol. 3 (Ed. by K.V.F. Jubb, P.C. Kennedy & N. Palmer), pp. 84−216. Academic Press Inc., New York.

Weiss, E. & Moulder, J.W. (1984) The Rickettsias and Chlamydias. In *Bergey's Manual of Determinative Bacteriology*, Vol. 1 (Ed. by N.R. Kreig & J.G. Holt), pp. 687−739. Williams & Wilkins, Baltimore/London.

Wolf, K. (1981) Report. Chlamydia and rickettsia of fish. *Fish Health News*, **10**, 1−4.

Wolke, R.E., Wyand, D.S. & Khairallah, L.H. (1970) A light and electron microscopic study of epitheliocystis disease in the gills of Connecticut striped bass (*Morone saxatilis*) and white perch (*Morone americanus*). *Journal of Comparative Pathology*, **80**, 559−63.

Zachary, A. & Paperna, I. (1977) Epitheliocystis disease in the striped bass *Morone saxatilis* from Chesapeake Bay. *Canadian Journal of Microbiology*, **23**, 1404−14.

Zimmer, M.A., Ewing, M.S. & Kocan, K.M. (1984) Epitheliocystis disease in the channel catfish *Ictalurus punctatus* (Rafinesque). *Journal of Fish Diseases*, **7**, 407−10.

# Part 9:
# The Practice of Fish Bacteriology

The two chapters in this final part deal firstly with the laboratory procedures needed to investigate bacteria isolated from fish and secondly
with the impact of fish bacterial pathogens on human health.

Practical aspects of isolation, purification and identification of bacterial
fish pathogens are considered in the final chapter. Standard bacteriological
techniques are employed with special modifications to meet the needs of
different aquatic species, e.g. lower optimum temperatures for growth,
adaptation to a low nutrient environment and slow growth rate out-paced
by competitors. The methods given have been selected on the experience
of a general diagnostic service and are well suited to such laboratories.

Human health may be affected both directly by the pathogen, and
indirectly as a result of antibacterial therapy of the fish population. Illness
caused by infection occurs rarely, by intoxication somewhat more commonly, and although the potential hazards of antibacterial therapy are
well recognized there is little evidence of actual occurrence from this
source. Legislation is already in place and being developed further in
many countries to ensure the safety of fish as a food source.

# Chapter 16:
# Isolation and Identification of Fish Bacterial Pathogens

The principles and procedures followed for the laboratory isolation and identification of fish bacterial pathogens are essentially the same as those applied to the investigation of bacterial infections in man and other animals, except that a meaningful microbiological examination of fish almost invariably requires destruction of the host. Lower incubation temperatures are indicated for the isolation of fish bacteria, but the aseptic sampling techniques, culture media and biochemical characterization tests are basically the same as those used in mammalian bacteriology. Modifications to the mineral content of the substrates must be made when material from marine or estuarine fish is to be examined, and a few special media are needed for the growth of certain organisms with specific nutritional requirements. Bacteria from poikilothermic animals are generally slower growing than those from homeothermic species, so that the time intervals specified for the interpretation of metabolic tests with mammalian bacteria may also require extension for the phenotypic characterization of fish isolates.

## Sampling for bacteriological examination

Bacteriological examinations of fish are generally carried out either for diagnostic purposes on overtly diseased specimens or as part of a health certification procedure on clinically normal stock, and the sampling procedure will vary according to the requirements of these two situations.

### Disease diagnosis

Whenever possible, a number of affected fish should be examined, ranging from those showing only minimal evidence of disease to moribund specimens, as the recovery of the same organism from different fish facilitates assessment of the clinical significance of any isolate. Freshly dead specimens may also be examined, particularly if no moribund fish are available.

Opinions vary as to precisely how many fish should be sampled, but ten is the most commonly recommended number. However, the disease history of the stock, nature of the clinical condition, availability of suitable specimens, value of the individual fish or pressure on laboratory facilities may justify or dictate the sampling of fewer numbers. Moribund specimens provide the most useful samples since it is these which normally harbour large numbers of pathogens. Similar specimens are also preferred for virological and histopathological examinations. It is difficult to define 'freshly dead' as the rate of post-mortem tissue decomposition and invasion with commensal micro-organisms will vary, depending upon environmental conditions, particularly temperature. A cold-water fish kept on ice may still provide satisfactory bacteriological samples 24 h later, whereas a warm-water fish left in its natural habitat may be wholly unsatisfactory within 1 hour of death. The pathologist must exercise personal judgement based upon experience to decide whether or not a particular dead specimen is worth sampling, and interpret any results in the context of the condition of the fish at the time of examination.

**Health certification**

The number of fish to be sampled for health certification purposes will depend upon the size of the population to be examined and the requirements of any statutory regulations relating to the issue of such a certificate. Many countries now have disease control and certification regulations which, although broadly similar in intent, may differ considerably in detail and it is imperative that the pathologist is fully conversant with the relevant requirements before carrying out a testing programme. As the primary purpose of certification testing is to identify the presence of specified latent infections in asymptomatic carrier fish, the sample size is usually based on obtaining a 95% probability of detecting at least one infected fish in a population with an assumed prevalence of 2, 5 or 10% of carriers. The computer generated table of Ossiander & Wedemeyer (1973) is generally used to determine the required sample size (Table 16.1). It cannot be over-emphasized that failure to isolate a particular pathogen from a population sample, no matter how large, of clinically healthy fish is no guarantee of the absence of the agent either from the specimens examined or from the remaining stock.

# Examination of fish

A comprehensive bacteriological investigation of fish can be carried out only on sacrificed specimens. Ideally, the fish should be killed immediately prior to examination by decapitation, severance of the spinal cord behind the head, or anaesthetic overdose. The use of anaesthetic agents is contra-indicated if a parasitological examination is also required, as any live parasites on the specimen will be killed. It may sometimes be necessary, as in the case of particularly rare or valuable fish, to avoid sacrificing the specimen. In such instances, examination will be limited to the external body surface and biopsy or tissue fluid material obtained from the anaesthetized fish.

A visual examination of the body surface and gills will reveal any gross external lesions. Many disease processes, including both acute and chronic forms of many septicaemic conditions, can give rise to ulcers, furuncles or granulomas. Fins, tail and gills may show proliferative or necrotic changes. Wet mounts of lesion material should be made if a 'myxobacterial' infection of skin, fins, tail or gills is indicated. Scrapings from lesions or small pieces of excised tissue are transferred to a microscope slide, mounted in water under a coverslip and examined with a high-power dry objective. Cytophagaceae are

**Table 16.1** Sample size required to detect at least one infected fish in populations with 2, 5 or 10% carrier fish (95% confidence level)

| Population size* | Assumed carrier prevalence | | |
|:---:|:---:|:---:|:---:|
| | 2% | 5% | 10% |
| 50 | 46 | 29 | 20 |
| 100 | 76 | 43 | 23 |
| 250 | 110 | 49 | 25 |
| 500 | 127 | 54 | 26 |
| 1 000 | 136 | 55 | 27 |
| 2 500 | 142 | 56 | 27 |
| 5 000 | 145 | 57 | 27 |
| 10 000 | 146 | 57 | 27 |
| 100 000 | 147 | 57 | 27 |
| > 100 000 | 150 | 60 | 30 |

\* For intermediate population sizes, use sample size for next larger population listed.

seen as long, slender rods which may or may not exhibit flexing movements. Identification should be confirmed by examination of stained smears and isolation of the organism in culture. Wet mounts and stained smears of skin lesion material not attributable to infection with filamentous bacteria are of more limited value, as damaged fish tissue is invariably invaded by opportunistic bacteria or fungi which cannot be distinguished from other possible primary pathogens on the basis of cell morphology and staining reaction alone. Culture of organisms from external lesions presents similar diagnostic problems, as growth of secondary organisms may mask or even completely displace the initial causative agent. Searing the surface of the lesion with a heated scalpel blade prior to sampling with an inoculating loop or pasteur pipette does not always overcome the problem, as secondary invaders may be established throughout the lesion.

Following external examination of the fish, the body cavity is opened to expose the internal organs. Disinfection of the surface of the fish by swabbing with 70% alcohol is often recommended, but experience has shown that this makes little practical difference in the examination of overtly diseased specimens. It should, however, be adhered to in health certification procedures, where the greatest care must be taken to avoid environmental contamination. Dissecting instruments are conveniently sterilized by dipping in 70% alcohol and flaming before use. An incision is made through the body wall in the mid-ventral line opposite the base of the pectoral fins. Using blunt-ended scissors, the incision is extended anteriorly to the symphysis of the mandible and posteriorly to just short of the vent, taking care not to puncture the intestine. Any adhesions between the body wall and underlying viscera are carefully separated and the two sides of the body wall pinned back to the dissecting surface. Alternatively, one side of the body wall may be removed by making a roughly semi-circular incision along the boundary of the cavity from the vent to the base of the pectoral fin. This alternative procedure is appropriate for the examination of flat fish and may be found more suitable for exposing the viscera of many round fish species.

The history and clinical appearance of diseased fish will normally indicate the appropriate tissues for bacteriological examination. The kidney should always be sampled, as this often provides the most satisfactory and significant isolation of pathogens in pure culture, together with other tissues showing discrete or diffuse lesions. Where a septicaemic condition is suspected, liver, spleen and heart blood sampling is also indicated. For health certification purposes, the tissues to be sampled are specified in the relevant requirements, which should be consulted before testing commences. Although tissue material should ideally be aseptically sampled using a bacterial loop or straight wire, this is often virtually impossible with very small fish. In such instances, as much care as possible should be taken to minimize the risk of contamination from contiguous tissues.

As with external lesions, Gram stained smears of internal tissue material are of limited bacteriological value except for the rapid, presumptive diagnosis of bacterial kidney disease (BKD). This procedure is particularly useful in the case of clinically diseased fish, in which the presence of large numbers of small $(0.3-1.0 \times 1.0-1.5\,\mu m)$, strongly Gram-positive bacilli in smears from grossly abnormal kidney is highly indicative of infection with *Renibacterium salmoninarum*. The method is much less satisfactory in the early stages of the disease, or for the identification of the carrier state in clinically healthy fish, where only very few organisms may be scattered throughout macroscopically normal kidney tissue, and are not readily distinguishable from melanin granules and other morphologically similar bacteria such as lactobacilli. Ziehl-Neelsen (ZN) stained smears of nodular or granulomatous visceral lesions suggestive of a mycobacterial or nocardial infection may reveal the presence of acid-fast organisms.

Although disease history and clinical signs will provide valuable clues as to the likely cause of a pathological condition, many taxonomically related and unrelated bacteria induce similar clinical signs and pathological features. Thus, with the possible exception of clinical *R. salmoninarum* infections, the essential prerequisite for the definitive diagnosis of bacterial diseases of fish is the isolation of the causal organism in pure culture.

## Isolation of bacteria

Almost all the recognized fish bacterial pathogens are aerobic and the direct inoculation of solid media is routinely used for the initial isolation of these organisms. Preliminary broth enrichment before plating out is not usually required but has been found useful to enhance the recovery of *Yersinia ruckeri* (see Chapter 5). Bacteria are often recovered as pure culture growth, but as mixed infections are not infrequent and sample contamination is an ever-present hazard, it is important that culture plates should be inoculated and streaked out to obtain isolated colonies directly from the sample. Fluid media are appropriate for the isolation of anaerobes.

A selective or a non-selective approach may be adopted in the choice of media for isolation purposes. The first approach uses specifically designed media to selectively support the growth of, and provisionally identify, certain groups or species of pathogens. The second approach uses non-inhibitory media which will support the growth of a wide range of organisms. The use of selective media is particularly indicated for the relatively rapid screening of specimens for the presence of one or more specified pathogens, whereas the use of non-selective media provides a broader measure of the bacteriological status of the fish. Both approaches have obvious advantages and disadvantages and the microbiologist will need to be guided by experience and the requirements of the examination in the choice of media.

**Non-selective general purpose media**

Most fish pathogens are naturally occurring saprophytes which normally utilize organic and mineral matter in the aquatic environment for their growth and multiplication. It is therefore not surprising that these organisms are relatively non-fastidious in their nutrient requirements and can be isolated on a range of general purpose bacteriological media. Commercially available formulations of tryptone or trypticase soya agar (TSA) and brain heart infusion agar (BHIA) have now become almost universally accepted as the standard non-selective media for freshwater fish bacteriology. Nutrient agar (NA) is a very satisfactory alternative medium. All three media may be supplemented with 5%(v/v) mammalian blood, which improves the growth of streptococci and certain other organisms and also allows determination of haemolytic activity.

Although TSA, BHIA and some NA formulations contain 0.5%(w/v) NaCl, certain marine organisms, particularly *Vibrio* spp., require a higher salt concentration for primary isolation. For the examination of marine or estuarine fish, TSA, BHIA or NA should therefore be supplemented to contain 2% (w/v) NaCl or be prepared using filtered sea water. Alternatively, marine agar 2216 (MA) (Difco), a relatively low nutrient medium which contains a supplement duplicating the major mineral components of sea water, may be used. Once isolated, the high salt requirement may be lost and subculturing can often be carried out on standard TSA or BHIA medium. The range of recognized fish pathogens which may be isolated on these general purpose media is given in Table 16.2.

Low-nutrient — low agar formulations are required for the isolation in culture of the long, slender, non-motile or motile-by-gliding group of Gram-negative, chromogenic 'myxobacteria' taxonomically ascribable to the *Flavobacterium*, *Cytophaga*, *Flexibacter* or *Sporocytophaga* genera. Cytophaga agar (Anacker & Ordal 1959) has been the most widely used non-selective medium for freshwater

**Table 16.2**  Fish pathogens which may be isolated aerobically on non-selective TSA, BHIA or NA media

| | |
|---|---|
| *Aeromonas hydrophila* | *Pseudomonas fluorescens* |
| *Aeromonas salmonicida* | *Pseudomonas (Alteromonas) piscicida* |
| *Edwardsiella ictaluri* | *Streptococcus* spp. |
| *Edwardsiella tarda* | *Vibrio alginolyticus* |
| *Flavobacterium* spp. | *Vibrio anguillarum* |
| *Lactobacillus piscicola* | *Vibrio carchariae* |
| *Nocardia asteroides* | *Vibrio cholerae (non-01)* |
| *Nocardia kampachi* | *Vibrio damsela* |
| *Pasteurella piscicida* | *Vibrio ordalii* |
| *Plesiomonas shigelloides* | *Vibrio salmonicida* |
| *Providencia rettgeri* | *Vibrio vulnificus* |
| *Pseudomonas anguilliseptica* | *Yersinia ruckeri* |
| *Pseudomonas chloraphis* | |

isolates, but good growth has also been obtained with several modifications of this medium such as those described by Wakabayashi & Egusa (1974) and Shieh (1980).

*Cytophaga* agar (Anacker & Ordal 1959)

| | |
|---|---|
| Tryptone | 0.5 g |
| Yeast extract | 0.5 g |
| Beef extract | 0.2 g |
| Sodium acetate | 0.2 g |
| Agar | 9.0 g |
| Distilled water to | 1000 ml |

Mix and dissolve ingredients by heating, adjust to pH 7.2−7.4 and sterilize by autoclaving.

Few marine strains of Cytophagaceae tolerate transfer to fresh water and, furthermore, the salt requirement cannot always be met by the addition of NaCl alone (Wakabayashi *et al.* 1986). Cytophaga agar, or one of the modified formulations, prepared in 50−70% sea water, is therefore advocated for recovery from estuarine and marine fish. Marine agar 2216 has also been found suitable for the isolation of seawater-dependent strains (G.N. Frerichs, unpublished data).

The use of fluid media is indicated for the isolation of anaerobic fish pathogens. Although *Clostridium botulinum* and *Eubacterium tarantellus* are the only two species which have so far been implicated as causal agents of disease, routine examinations for anaerobic organisms are seldom undertaken and such infections may be more widespread than hitherto realized. Robertson's cooked meat medium, containing a fermentable sugar, is a suitable general purpose isolation medium which will support the growth of all anaerobes, including the strictly anaerobic *Cl. botulinum*, but other standard anaerobic techniques and media have also been successfully used (Udey *et al.* 1977).

**Selective media**

In addition to the use of certain commercially available selective media developed initially for mammalian bacteriology, a number of formulations have been described for the culture and identification of specific aquatic micro-organisms of fish.

Rimler-Shotts medium contains specific amino acids, maltose and novobiocin to facilitate the rapid identification of *Aeromonas hydrophila*. This organism forms yellow colonies (maltose fermentation) without black centres (no $H_2S$ production) following incubation at 37°C. Incubation at this high temperature is required to prevent growth of *Aeromonas salmonicida*, which will produce similarly pigmented colonies at lower temperatures. Certain Enterobacteriaceae, notably *Yersinia ruckeri*, will also produce yellow colonies, and an oxidase test is necessary to differentiate the isolates. This should be carried out on a subculture made on a general purpose medium as the oxidase reaction is inhibited by the presence of acid.

Rimler–Shotts medium (Shotts & Rimler 1973)

| | |
|---|---|
| L-lysine HCl | 5.0 g |
| L-ornithine HCl | 6.5 g |
| L-cysteine HCl | 0.3 g |
| Maltose | 3.5 g |
| Sodium thiosulphate | 6.8 g |
| Ferric ammonium citrate | 0.8 g |
| Sodium deoxycholate | 1.0 g |
| Sodium chloride | 5.0 g |
| Yeast extract | 3.0 g |
| Novobiocin | 0.005 g |
| Bromothymol blue | 0.03 g |
| Agar | 13.5 g |
| Distilled water to | 1000 ml |

Mix and dissolve ingredients by stirring, adjust pH to 7.0 and boil for 1 min. Cool to 45°C and dispense.

*Edwardsiella ictaluri* isolation medium has been developed to permit the primary isolation and presumptive identification of this slow growing organism in the presence of more rapidly growing bacteria such as *Aeromonas* sp.

*Edwardsiella ictaluri* agar (Shotts & Waltman 1990)

| | |
|---|---|
| Tryptone | 10 g |
| Yeast extract | 10 g |
| Phenylalanine | 1.25 g |
| Ferric ammonium citrate | 1.2 g |

| Bile salts | 1.0 g |
| Bromothymol blue | 0.003 g |
| Agar | 15 g |
| Distilled water | 980 ml |

Mix and dissolve ingredients by heating, adjust pH to 7.0 and sterilize by autoclaving. After cooling to 50°C, add filter sterilized mannitol to 0.35% (v/v) and colistin sulphate to 10 µg/ml.

Hsu−Shotts medium is a modified cytophaga agar containing neomycin for the selective isolation of gliding bacteria.

Hsu−Shotts medium (Bullock *et al.* 1986)

| Tryptone | 2.0 g |
| Yeast extract | 0.5 g |
| Gelatin | 3.0 g |
| Agar | 15 g |
| Water to | 1000 ml |

Use distilled fresh water or filtered sea water as appropriate. Mix and dissolve by heating and sterilize by autoclaving. After cooling to 45°C, add filter sterilized neomycin sulphate to 0.0004% (w/v).

Commercially available media containing cetrimide, which inhibits the growth of most Gram-negative organisms, may be used for the selective isolation of *Pseudomonas* spp. These formulations also contain $MgCl_2$ and $K_2SO_4$, which enhance pigment production by these organisms.

Thiosulphate−citrate−bile salt−sucrose agar (TCBS) was developed for the isolation of certain *Vibrio* spp. of medical importance, but has since proved useful for the selective recovery of many fish pathogenic species. It is not an ideal selective medium, however, as the growth of some vibrios, particularly *V. ordalii*, is also inhibited (Lee & Donovan 1985). Sucrose-fermenting species (yellow colonies) are differentiated from non-sucrose-fermenters (green colonies). Slight growth of other bacteria may occur but the colonies are usually easily distinguished from *Vibrio* spp.

Shotts−Waltman (SW) selective medium containing Tween 80, sucrose and bromothymol blue indicator has been formulated for the isolation and presumptive identification of *Yersinia ruckeri*. Colonies of *Y. ruckeri* appear green, with surrounding opaque haloes due to a zone of Tween 80 hydrolysis. The value of SW medium is limited by the occurrence of Tween 80 negative strains of *Y. ruckeri* (Davies & Frerichs 1989).

Shotts−Waltman medium (Waltman & Shotts 1984)

| Tryptone | 2.0 g |
| Yeast extract | 2.0 g |

| | |
|---|---|
| Sodium chloride | 5.0 g |
| Calcium chloride (hydrated) | 0.1 g |
| Bromothymol blue | 0.003 g |
| Tween 80 | 10 ml |
| Agar | 15 g |
| Distilled water | 980 ml |

Mix and dissolve ingredients by heating, adjust pH to 7.4 and sterilize by autoclaving. After cooling to 50°C, add 10 ml filter sterilized sucrose (0.5 g/ml).

**Special media**

The great majority of fish pathogens are non-fastidious in their nutritional requirements and only *Renibacterium salmoninarum* and certain *Mycobacteria* spp. need specifically enriched media for isolation. Infection with these agents is usually suspected on clinical and pathological evidence or following examination of stained smears, and isolation is not normally attempted in the absence of such indications.

 *R. salmoninarum* has an absolute requirement for L-cysteine. Serum also enhances growth and a number of media containing 10–20% serum or blood and 0.1% (w/v) L-cysteine have been developed to isolate the organism directly from fish tissue. The formulation known as KDM 2 or Evelyn's medium is most widely used.

 KDM 2 medium (Evelyn 1977)

| | |
|---|---|
| Peptone | 10 g |
| Yeast extract | 0.5 g |
| L-cysteine HCl | 1.0 g |
| Agar | 15 g |
| Distilled water to | 900 ml |

Mix and dissolve ingredients by heating, adjust pH to 6.5 and sterilize by autoclaving. Allow to cool to 45°C and add 100 ml foetal calf serum. The medium gradually deteriorates with time and the base medium should not be stored longer than 3 months. Complete medium should be used within 1–2 weeks of preparation.

 Good growth has also been obtained by replacing the serum component with 1 g/l activated charcoal, which acts as a detoxifying agent (Daly & Stevenson 1985). Other serum-free media such as cysteine-supplemented Mueller Hinton agar have been used successfully for the maintenance of stock cultures but less reliably for primary isolation. In addition to the requirement for L-cysteine, *R. salmoninarum* is a particularly slow growing organism, and although growth from heavily infected material usually occurs within 4–10 days, dilute inocula may require up to 6 weeks incubation before visible colonies develop. Cultures are thus prone to overgrowth with faster growing contaminants or other patho-gens, and a selective medium (SKDM) incorporating a number of antimicrobial compounds has been proved effective for the isolation of the pathogen from samples requiring extended incubation.

SKDM medium (Austin *et al*. 1983)

| | |
|---|---|
| Tryptone | 10 g |
| Yeast extract | 0.5 g |
| Cycloheximide | 0.05 g |
| Agar | 10 g |
| Distilled water | 900 ml |

Mix and dissolve ingredients by heating, adjust pH to 6.8 and sterilize by autoclaving. After cooling add 100 ml foetal calf serum and filter sterilized solutions of L-cysteine HCl (0.1% w/v), D-cycloserine (0.00125% w/v), poly-myxin B sulphate (0.0025% w/v) and oxolinic acid (0.00025% w/v).

*Mycobacterium marinum*, *Mycobacterium fortuitum* and *Mycobacterium chelonae* are the three recognized species causing mycobacteriosis of fish. Many other names appear in the literature but these are now considered to be synonymous with or variants of one of these three species. Isolation, when required, can be carried out using standard egg or glycerol based media such as Lowenstein–Jensen, Dorset egg or Middlebrook 7H10 agar slopes. Ogawa's egg medium has also been found satisfactory (Arakawa & Fryer 1984).

Ogawa's egg medium (Tsukamura 1967)

| | |
|---|---|
| Sodium glutamate | 1.0 g |
| KH$_2$PO$_4$ | 1.0 g |
| Distilled water | 100 ml |
| Whole eggs | 200 ml |
| Glycerol | 6 ml |
| Malachite green | 6 ml of 2%(w/v) solution |

Dissolve sodium glutamate and KH$_2$PO$_4$ in distilled water and mix in remaining ingredients. Adjust the pH to 6.8 and sterilize as culture slopes at 90°C for 1 h.

## Culture incubation

The optimum temperature for growth of the different fish pathogens varies considerably, but most can be cultured over a fairly wide range between 15° and 30°C. For practical purposes a single incubation temperature between 20° and 25°C is satisfactory for primary isolation. Two important exceptions are *Renibacterium salmoninarum* and *Vibrio salmonicida*, which have an optimum temperature of 15°C, and cultures should be incubated accordingly when infection with either of these pathogens is suspected. Incubation temperatures outside the 15−30°C range are required for certain subsequent characterization tests.

Colony growth will vary with the medium and incubation temperature used, but may be expected to appear within 3 days in most instances, except for *R. salmoninarum*, *Mycobacterium* spp. and *Nocardia* spp., in which incubation for several weeks may be required for colonies to develop. It is advisable to seal or tightly wrap plates for *R. salmoninarum* isolation to ensure moisture retention during prolonged incubation.

## Identification of bacterial isolates

The important principle of obtaining pure cultures prior to carrying out identification tests cannot be over-emphasized. Mixed cultures are commonly encountered on primary isolation, particularly when non-selective media are used, and purification by subculture is essential both for accurate identification and obtaining reference cultures of the organism.

Serological methods such as whole-cell or antibody-coated latex agglutination tests and the fluorescent antibody technique (FAT) have been widely used for the identification of fish pathogens. More recently, the enzyme-linked immuno-sorbent assay (ELISA), notably in the form of commercially available rapid diagnostic kits, has also been developed for the diagnosis of a variety of disease conditions. However, the sensitivity and specificity of any serological test depends on the variable quality of the antisera used and the diversity of expressed antigenic components of the agent under examination. The indications for the use of serodiagnostic methods are therefore the rapid, presumptive, identification of pathogens, the confirmation of an identification based on phenotypic characteristics and the serological typing of identified isolates. It is highly inadvisable to rely on serology alone for a definitive identification of an isolate.

The conventional procedures for the phenotypic identification of fish pathogens are adaptations of the step-by-step or progressive methods established for medical and veterinary pathogens, exemplified by *Cowan and Steel's Manual for the Identification of Medical Bacteria* (Cowan 1974). The first step aims to determine a few fundamental characters of the organism to assign it to a family, genus or other grouping. With the aid of diagnostic tables, further sets of selected tests are then carried out to provide an identification. The principle weakness of this methodology is that an organism may have an anomalous character which makes identification from a limited set of tests almost impossible. Among the fish pathogens, pigment production or non-production and motility are two heavily weighted characters for which strain variation is not infrequent.

As with all other step-by-step identification schemes in medical and veterinary bacteriology, the Gram reaction is the first characterization test applied to isolates from fish. The majority of fish pathogens are short, Gram-negative rods belonging to the Enterobacteriaceae, Pseudomonadaceae or Vibrionaceae families, which may all be responsible for acute septicaemias with few symptoms and high mortalities, chronic conditions with variable lesions and low mortalities, or asymptomatic latent infections. These three families are differentiated by the oxidase and glucose oxidation-fermentation (O–F) tests. The long, slender, Gram-negative Cytophagaceae may also cause heavy losses in fish stocks. Gram-positive organisms, including a few which are also acid-fast, are less frequently encountered but can be of major importance in certain fish species under particular conditions (Austin & Austin 1987, Frerichs & Roberts 1989).

Further phenotypic characterization may be carried out using 'conventional' or 'rapid' test methods or a combination of both. However, a choice has often to be made between alternative recognized methods for many of the conventional tests and also between the ever-increasing range of commercially available rapid diagnostic systems. The comprehensive and practical descriptions of conventional test media and methods set out in *Cowan and Steel's Manual for the Identification of Medical Bacteria* (Cowan 1974) are appropriate and widely used for the characterization of most fish pathogens, apart from the Cytophagaceae and *Renibacterium salmoninarum*, which have no medical counterpart species. For the examination of marine organisms the media should be supplemented to contain 2% NaCl or prepared in marine salts solution comprising NaCl (2.4% w/v), $MgSO_4.7H_2O$ (0.7% w/v) and KCl (0.075% w/v) (Austin & Austin 1987). The time and temperature of incubation must also be modified appropriately for aquatic organisms. As with the conventional test systems, the various rapid diagnostic kits for the identification of enteric and non-enteric Gram-negative bacteria and Gram-positive cocci have been designed primarily for human pathogens capable of metabolic activity at 37°C. The identification data bases for these systems are therefore limited in so far as fish pathogens are concerned, but with adaptations to incubation conditions and the bacterial suspension medium for marine organisms, some kits have nevertheless been found very useful in the examination of aquatic organisms. Discrepancies may occur between reactions obtained with conventional and rapid test methods, as illustrated by Davies & Frerichs (1989) for the citrate utilization, gelatin hydrolysis and Voges-Proskauer tests for *Yersinia ruckeri*, and this possibility together with strain variations should be borne in mind when determining the identification of an isolate.

Diagnostic tables are normally derived from many papers and monographs, often providing conflicting data which are difficult to reconcile in the form of a single tabulated symbol. The principal sources for the construction of the tables in the present text are *Bergey's Manual of Systematic Bacteriology*, Volumes 1 and 2 (Kreig & Holt 1984, Sneath *et al.* 1986) and the relatively recent publications by Frerichs & Hendrie (1985), Austin & Austin (1987), Sanders & Fryer (1988) and Shotts & Teska (1989), which provide the references for the relevant original papers.

# Gram-negative bacteria

### Cytophagaceae

Members of this family are best isolated on low nutrient media supplemented, where appropriate, with marine salts. Generally, growth is limited on richer general purpose media. All members contain yellow, orange or red carotenoid pigments, and the fish isolates, together with flavobacteria, are often collectively referred to as the yellow-pigmented bacteria (YPB) group of pathogens. Cytophagaceae characteristically form flat or raised, yellow or orange coloured colonies with a thin spreading irregular edge. All species exhibit gliding motility, which is best determined by placing a coverslip over the swarming edge of a colony on a moist, thinly poured agar plate and observing microscopically at $400-1000\times$ magnification. In stained smears the organisms are seen as long, slender rods, $0.5-0.8 \times 2-10\,\mu m$, but filamentous forms extending to $100\,\mu m$ or greater in length may also be observed. Flavobacteria, in contrast, grow on general purpose media, do not produce swarming colonies and are non-motile.

The taxonomic position of the Cytophagaceae associated with fish diseases has undergone many changes over the years and does not yet appear to be finally resolved. *Flexibacter columnaris*, *Flexibacter psychrophilus* (syn. *Flexibacter aurantiacus*; *Cytophaga psychrophila*) and *Flexibacter maritimus* are the three principal recognized pathogenic species.

*Flexibacter columnaris* causes columnaris disease in freshwater environments, normally at temperatures above 15°C, whereas *F. psychrophilus* is associated with cold water or peduncle disease in fresh water at temperatures below 12°C. This association with temperature is reflected in the laboratory, where *F. columnaris* will grow at 30°C or higher but *F. psychrophilus* has an upper limit of 25°C or lower, depending upon the strain. In cytophaga broth and similar fluid media *F. columnaris* will not tolerate the addition of more than 0.5%(w/v) NaCl, whereas *F. psychrophilus* will grow in the presence of 0.8% − 1.0%(w/v) NaCl. Few biochemical tests are of value to differentiate the two species, but *F. columnaris* is oxidase and $H_2S$ positive and *F. psychrophilus* oxidase and $H_2S$ negative. A slide agglutination test (Anacker & Ordal 1959) has been recommended for the confirmatory identification of both *F. columnaris* and *F. psychrophilus* (Amos 1985). All strains of *F. columnaris* have been found to possess at least one common antigen, and antisera prepared against this organism do not cross-react with *F. psychrophilus*, which similarly appears to form a relatively homogeneous group of organisms (Bullock 1972). *F. maritimus* causes a columnaris disease-like condition in marine fish. Like *F. columnaris*, growth occurs over a wide temperature range (15−34°C), but the organism has an obligate requirement for at least 30% natural or artificial sea water in the culture medium. *F. maritimus* is oxidase positive and $H_2S$ negative.

Cytophagaceae which are antigenically distinct from the three recognized species are frequently associated with bacterial gill disease, fin and tail rot and other ulcerative skin lesions of freshwater and marine fish, although the relationship of these organisms to primary aetiology remains uncertain. Most of these cytophagas remain unspeciated and may be variants of recognized species or representative of new unclassified groupings.

**Flavobacteria**

The genus *Flavobacterium* has a number of taxonomic similarities to the Cytophagaceae and, like the cytophagas, flavobacteria have been associated with outbreaks of bacterial gill disease (Wakabayashi *et al.* 1980). Flavobacteria may be isolated on cytophaga or standard nutrient agar media with the formation of yellow-orange pigmented, round, convex, entire colonies. The organisms are non-motile, slender rods $0.5 \times 3-8\,\mu m$ in size, often occurring in short chains. Flavobacteria are strict aerobes, giving an oxidative reaction in the glucose O$-$F test, and are oxidase positive. Acid is most frequently produced from glucose, fructose, maltose and trehalose but adonitol, dulcitol, inositol and sorbitol are not attacked. Most strains are proteolytic and hydrolyse casein, gelatin and Tween 80. Tests for arginine dihydrolase, lysine and ornithine decarboxylase and $H_2S$ production are invariably negative. Further research is needed on the speciation of fish flavobacteria and isolates are usually simply designated *Flavobacterium* sp.

**Enterobacteriaceae**

Three species of enterobacteria from two genera, *Edwardsiella* and *Yersinia*, are important pathogens of fish. *Edwardsiella ictaluri* and *Edwardsiella tarda* are principally associated with acute septicaemic and abscessive conditions, respectively, in cultured warm-water fish, particularly catfish and eels. *Yersinia ruckeri* is the specific causal agent of enteric redmouth (ERM) in salmonid fish and has also been isolated from a variety of non-salmonid species of freshwater feral fish. *Providencia (Proteus) rettgeri* has been documented as an opportunistic pathogen of traumatized silver carp (*Hypophthalmichthys molitrix*) (Bejerano *et al.* 1979) and *Citrobacter freundii* implicated as a pathogen of sunfish (*Mola mola*) (Sato *et al.* 1982).

Enterobacteriaceae are readily isolated on general purpose media although *E. ictaluri* is a relatively slow grower and may be masked by more rapidly growing organisms such as *Aeromonas*. All species produce similar smooth, round, raised, off-white colonies. The organisms are Gram-negative, straight rods $0.5-1.0 \times 1.0-3.0\,\mu m$ in size and classified as enterobacteria on the basis of fermentative glucose O$-$F test and negative oxidase reactions. The fish pathogens, apart from some strains of *Y. ruckeri*, are all motile by peritrichous flagellae. Enterobacteriaceae are biochemically fairly reactive and speciation may be determined from diagnostic tables (Table 16.3). Test kits such as the API 20E$^{(R)}$ system are well suited to the characterization of this family of micro-organisms.

## Pasteurellaceae

*Pasteurella piscicida* is the only recognized fish pathogen in this family of bacteria. The organism has been shown to be responsible for outbreaks of septicaemic and granulomatous conditions in a number of marine fish species. *P. piscicida* may be isolated on marine agar or general purpose media containing at least 0.5%(w/v) NaCl. Optimum growth is obtained on media containing 1.5%(w/v) NaCl. Colonies are round, raised, entire and greyish-yellow in colour. Morphologically the cells are Gram-negative, non-motile rods about 0.5 × 1.5 μm in size. Filamentous cells may be seen in young cultures and coccobacillary forms in older cultures. Bipolar staining is often seen. The organism is fermentative in the glucose O−F test and oxidase positive but is otherwise fairly unreactive. Positive arginine dihydrolase and weakly positive Voges−Proskauer and acid from glucose reactions are characteristic responses. *P. piscicida* is unusual in that it is also sensitive to 0/129 vibriostat, a characteristic normally only associated with *Vibrio* sp.

## Pseudomonadaceae

The Pseudomonadaceae comprises a vast number of species of bacteria, at present distributed between three genera possessing the basic properties of this family of organisms. Pseudomonads are widely distributed in nature, particularly the aquatic environment, and are frequently present on the body surface of healthy fish. Pseudomonads are probably also the most frequently isolated environmental contaminants in fish bacteriology. The genus *Pseudomonas* contains a number of important medical and veterinary pathogens and three species have been described at various times as the causal agents of disease in fish. *P. fluorescens* has been associated with septicaemic and ulcerative conditions in a wide range of fish species, *P. anguilliseptica* with red spot disease (Sekitenbyo) of eels and *P. chloraphis* with mortalities in Amago trout. Other species may also be implicated as secondary pathogens in different stress related disease problems. The organism referred to in the literature as *P. piscicida* (originally *Flavobacterium piscicida*) requires a sea-water or NaCl base for growth and has now been provisionally transferred to the genus *Alteromonas* as *A. piscicida* (Baumann *et al.* 1984).

Species of *Pseudomonas* are nutritionally non-fastidious and may be readily isolated on general purpose media. A variety of soluble and non-soluble pigments may be produced and the presence of the soluble yellow-green, fluorescent pigment fluorescein is a useful identification characteristic. Some strains may produce a reddish-brown diffusible pigment which can be mistaken for a

**Table 16.3**  Characteristics of fermentative, oxidase negative, Gram-negative rods

| | Edwardsiella ictaluri | Edwardsiella tarda | Yersinia ruckeri | Providencia rettgeri | Citrobacter freundii | Hafnia alvei |
|---|---|---|---|---|---|---|
| Motility (25°C) | +[1] | + | d | + | + | + |
| β-galactosidase | − | − | + | − | + | + |
| Arginine dihydrolase | − | − | − | − | d | − |
| Lysine decarboxylase | + | + | + | − | − | + |
| Ornithine decarboxylase | + | + | + | − | d | + |
| Simmon's citrate | − | −[2] | − | + | + | − |
| H₂S production | − | + | − | − | + | − |
| Urease | − | − | − | + | − | − |
| Tryptophane deaminase | − | − | − | + | − | − |
| Indole | − | + | − | + | − | − |
| Voges-Proskauer reaction | − | − | d | − | − | + |
| Gelatin hydrolysis | − | − | + | − | − | − |
| Acid from: | | | | | | |
| Glucose | + | + | + | + | + | + |
| Mannitol | − | − | + | + | + | + |
| Inositol | − | − | − | + | − | − |
| Sorbitol | − | − | d | − | + | − |
| Rhamnose | − | − | − | + | + | + |
| Sucrose | − | − | − | − | d | − |
| Melibiose | − | − | − | − | d | − |
| Arabinose | − | − | − | − | + | + |

[1] *E. ictaluri* is non-motile at 35°C
[2] *E. tarda* is Christensen's citrate positive
d = variable reaction

similar pigment associated with typical strains of *Aeromonas salmonicida*. *Pseudomonas* sp. are strictly aerobic, Gram-negative, motile rods $0.5-1.0 \times 1.5-5.0 \mu m$ in size. The organisms are oxidative or non-reactive in the glucose O−F test and most species are oxidase positive. Additional characterization tests are given in Table 16.4. The API 20E and similar enterobacteria test kits are of limited value for the speciation of pseudomonads as these organisms are relatively unreactive in sugar fermentation tests, and apart from arginine hydrolysis, citrate utilization and gelatin hydrolysis reactions, negative results are most likely to be obtained.

## Vibrionaceae

The family Vibrionaceae includes two genera, *Vibrio* and *Aeromonas*, which are distributed world-wide and together constitute the most frequently encountered and, arguably, the most important species of fish pathogens. Molecular studies have indicated two distinct lines of descent for *Vibrio* and *Aeromonas* and it has been proposed that the genus *Aeromonas* be elevated to the family status of Aeromonadaceae (Colwell 1986), but this re-classification awaits international acceptance and the long-recognized grouping is retained at present. *Plesiomonas shigelloides* has also been implicated as a fish pathogen (Cruz *et al.* 1986) within the Vibrionaceae. The re-classification of *Haemophilus piscium*, the causal agent of ulcer disease of trout, as an atypical form of *Aeromonas salmonicida* has been accepted in *Bergey's Manual of Systematic Bacteriology*.

All *Vibrio* species except *V. cholerae* and *V. metschnikovii* have an absolute requirement for Na$^+$ for growth, whereas *Aeromonas* and *Plesiomonas* species are non-halophilic. Vibrios are therefore principally found in marine and estuarine aquatic habitats and are predominantly pathogens of fish and other animals in these environments. Aeromonads, by contrast, are essentially freshwater organisms, and consequently potential pathogens of freshwater animals. This distinction is not absolute, however, and aeromonad infections of marine fish and vibriosis of freshwater species may both occur. The disease processes are similar for both groups of organisms and extend over a spectrum of conditions from acute septicaemia to chronic ulceration.

Vibrionaceae are nutritionally non-fastidious and the majority of species may be isolated on general purpose media containing 0.5% (w/v) NaCl. The growth of all species of *Vibrio*, however, is stimulated by NaCl, even if Na$^+$ is not an absolute requirement, and medium supplemented to contain 2% (w/v) NaCl is advantageous for the primary isolation of these organisms. Seawater based media provide an excellent alternative. Selective media such as TCBS for *Vibrio* sp. and Rimler−Shotts for motile *Aeromonas* sp. may also be used. On non-selective media colonies are white, cream or buff in colour, round, raised and entire. Typical strains of *A. salmonicida* isolated from salmonids aerobically break down tyrosine in the medium to produce a brown, diffusible pigment

**Table 16.4** Characteristics of oxidative, oxidase positive, Gram-negative rods

| | *Pseudomonas anguilliseptica* | *Pseudomonas chloraphis* | *Pseudomonas fluorescens* | *Pseudomonas putida* | *Alteromonas piscicida* |
|---|---|---|---|---|---|
| Motility | + | + | + | + | + |
| Fluorescin pigment | – | – | + | + | – |
| Other pigment | – | G | – | – | Y |
| Glucose O–F test | – | O | O | O | O |
| Growth at  5°C | + | + | + | + | – |
| 37°C | – | d | d | d | + |
| Growth in 0% NaCl | – | + | + | + | – |
| Nitrate reduction | – | + | d | d | – |
| Arginine dihydrolase | – | + | + | + | – |
| Gelatin hydrolysis | + | + | + | – | + |

G = green crystalline pigment  Y = yellow pigment

All species are lysine decarboxylase, ornithine decarboxylase, indole, methyl red and Voges–Proskauer reaction negative

d = variable result

which is generally regarded as an important diagnostic trait. Pigment production is suppressed under microaerophilic conditions. However, a similar diffusible pigment is known to be produced by some strains of *A. hydrophila* and melanogenic *Pseudomonas* species. A brown pigment producing strain of *V. anguillarum* has also been isolated from rainbow trout (*Oncorhynchus mykiss*) (G.N. Frerichs, unpublished) so identification of *A. salmonicida* should not be based on pigment production alone.

In stained smears *Vibrio*, *Aeromonas* and *Plesiomonas* are seen as Gram-negative, short-to-medium rods $0.5-1.0 \times 1.0-4.0\,\mu m$ in size. *Vibrio* species may be straight or curved in shape whereas species of the other genera are invariably straight. *A. salmonicida* usually appears coccobacillary, particularly when freshly isolated. The Vibrionaceae are facultative anaerobes and all species of *Vibrio*, *Aeromonas* and *Plesiomonas* characteristically give a fermentative reaction in the glucose O−F test. All species in each genus except *V. metschnikovii* and *V. gazogenes* are also oxidase positive. All species are motile with the important exception of *A. salmonicida*, which is always non-motile. *Vibrio* and *Plesiomonas* species are sensitive to the vibriostatic agent 0/129 (150 µg) and this test is used to distinguish these genera from the 0/129 resistant *Aeromonas* group. *Pasteurella piscicida* is the one other fermentative, oxidase positive fish pathogen also sensitive to 0/129.

Historically, vibriosis is one of the oldest recognized infectious diseases of fish and *V. anguillarum* was the first specific fish pathogen to be isolated in the laboratory. *V. anguillarum* remains the most frequently encountered fish vibrio but *V. alginolyticus*, *V. carchariae*, *V. cholerae* (non-01), *V. damsela*, *V. ordalii* (*V. anguillarum* biotype 2), *V. salmonicida* and *V. vulnificus* biogroup 2 are now additionally recognized pathogens. Yet further species have been identified in association with shellfish diseases. Species identification may be obtained from diagnostic tables using NaCl supplemented media (Table 16.5). Salt requirement and tolerance tests should be carried out using 1%(w/v) tryptone water (Lee & Donovan 1985) containing the required concentrations of NaCl and incubated for 72 h. Temperature tolerance tests may be done using NaCl supplemented 1%(w/v) tryptone broth incubated for 24 h at 37°C or 14 days at 4°C (Dawson & Sneath 1985). Visible turbidity is recorded as a positive growth in each instance. A slide or microtitre agglutination test is recommended for the confirmatory diagnosis of *V. anguillarum* and *V. ordalii* (Amos 1985).

The genus *Aeromonas* is naturally and conveniently divided into motile and non-motile groups of organisms. The mesophilic, motile group comprises *A. hydrophila* (syn. *A. liquefaciens*), *A. sobria* and *A. caviae* (syn. *A. hydrophila* subsp. *anaerogenes*). *A. punctata* is no longer a recognized species and isolates previously identified as *A. punctata* would now be classified as *A. hydrophila* or *A. sobria*. All three species of motile aeromonads have been recovered from fish, although *A. hydrophila* is the most frequently isolated and significant pathogen. Distinguishing phenotypic traits are summarized in Table 16.6.

The non-motile, psychrophilic group of aeromonads has been speciated as

**Table 16.5** Characteristics of fermentative, oxidase positive, 0/129 (150 µg) sensitive, Gram-negative, motile rods

| | Vibrio anguillarum | Vibrio ordalii | Vibrio salmonicida | Vibrio cholerae (non 01) | Vibrio carchariae | Vibrio damsela | Vibrio vulnificus gp2 | Vibrio alginolyticus | Plesiomonas shigelloides |
|---|---|---|---|---|---|---|---|---|---|
| Growth at 4°C | − | − | + | − | − | − | − | − | − |
| Growth at 37°C | + | − | − | + | + | + | + | + | + |
| Growth in 0% NaCl | − | − | − | + | − | − | − | − | + |
| Growth in 3% NaCl | + | + | + | + | + | + | + | + | + |
| Growth in 7% NaCl | − | − | − | − | + | − | − | + | − |
| 0/129 (10 µg) sensitivity | S | S | S | S | R | S | S | R | d |
| Growth on TCBS | Y | − | ● | Y | Y | G | G | Y | − |
| β-galactosidase | + | − | − | + | − | + | + | − | + |
| Arginine dihydrolase | + | − | − | − | − | + | − | − | + |
| Lysine decarboxylase | − | − | − | + | + | − | + | + | + |
| Ornithine decarboxylase | − | − | − | + | + | − | − | + | + |
| Citrate utilization | + | − | − | − | − | − | + | d | − |
| H₂S production | − | − | − | + | − | + | − | − | − |
| Urease | − | − | − | − | + | − | − | − | − |
| Indole | + | − | − | + | + | − | − | + | + |
| Voges–Proskauer reaction | + | − | − | + | − | + | − | + | − |
| Gelatin hydrolysis | + | + | + | + | + | − | + | + | − |
| Acid from: Glucose | + | + | + | + | + | + | + | + | + |
| Mannitol | + | − | d | − | + | − | − | + | − |
| Inositol | − | − | − | − | − | − | − | − | + |
| Sorbitol | + | − | − | − | ● | − | − | − | − |
| Sucrose | + | + | − | + | + | − | − | + | − |
| Arabinose | + | − | − | − | − | − | − | − | − |

Note: *V. salmonicida* tests carried out at 15°C
G = green colonies; Y = yellow colonies
d = variable reaction ● = not known

**Table 16.6** Characteristics of fermentative, oxidase positive, 0/129 (150 μg) resistant, Gram-negative rods

| | *Aeromonas hydrophila* | *Aeromonas sobria* | *Aeromonas caviae* | *Aeromonas salmonicida* | | | |
| --- | --- | --- | --- | --- | --- | --- | --- |
| | | | | subsp. *salmonicida* | subsp. *achromogenes* | subsp. *masoucida* | atypical |
| Motility | + | + | + | – | – | – | – |
| Growth at 37°C | + | + | + | – | – | – | d |
| Diffusible brown pigment | – | – | – | + | + | + | d |
| β-galactosidase | + | + | + | + | + | + | d |
| Arginine dihydrolase | + | + | + | + | + | + | – |
| Lysine decarboxylase | d | d | d | d | – | – | – |
| Ornithine decarboxylase | – | – | – | – | – | – | – |
| Simmon's citrate | d | d | d | – | – | – | d |
| H$_2$S production | + | + | – | – | – | + | – |
| Urease | – | – | – | – | – | – | – |
| Indole | + | + | + | – | d | + | d |
| Voges–Proskauer reaction | + | d | – | – | – | + | d |
| Gelatin hydrolysis | + | + | + | + | – | + | d |
| Aesculin hydrolysis | + | – | + | + | – | + | d |
| Growth in KCN | + | – | + | – | – | – | ● |
| Acid from:   Glucose | + | + | + | + | + | + | + |
| Mannitol | + | + | + | + | – | + | d |
| Inositol | – | – | – | – | – | – | – |
| Sorbitol | d | d | d | – | – | – | – |
| Sucrose | + | + | + | – | + | + | d |
| Arabinose | + | + | + | + | – | + | d |

d = variable reaction ● = not known

*A. salmonicida*. Three subspecies are at present recognized. Typical brown pigment producing, indole and sucrose fermentation negative strains isolated from salmonid fish are classified as *A. salmonicida* subsp. *salmonicida*. Subspecies *achromogenes* and *masoucida* are non-pigment-producing, indole and sucrose fermentation positive pathogens, also of salmonid fish, which can be differentiated by Voges−Proskauer, aesculin hydrolysis and mannitol fermentation reactions (Table 16.6). In addition to these three subspecies however, a considerable number of atypical strains have been isolated, mainly from ulcerative conditions of cyprinid fish but also from salmonids, which deviate from the described subspecies in a number of biochemical characteristics. This atypical group now includes *Haemophilus piscium*. The present classification scheme is patently less than ideal and it has been proposed by McCarthy & Roberts (1980) that there should be a regrouping of strains into three subspecies as follows: *A. salmonicida* subsp. *salmonicida*, typical isolates from salmonids; *A. salmonicida* subsp. *achromogenes* (incorporating subsp. *masoucida*), atypical isolates from salmonids; and *A. salmonicida* subsp. *nova*, atypical isolates from non-salmonid fish. This more easily understandable sub-division of the species has yet to be generally accepted.

Despite the high degree of phenotypic variation between the recognized subspecies and atypical isolates, *A. salmonicida* is a serologically homogeneous species and confirmatory identification by serological methods is an established procedure. The whole-cell slide agglutination test (Rabb *et al.* 1964) is quick and easy to perform but is suitable only for smooth, non-agglutinating strains, which unfortunately form the minority of isolates from clinical cases of disease. Reducing the electrolyte concentration of the suspending fluid to 0.05% will permit the examination of some rough strains, but otherwise techniques such as the latex agglutination test (McCarthy 1975) are indicated.

The genus *Plesiomonas* comprises only the single species *P. shigelloides*. The organism ferments inositol, which is a very rare trait in *Vibrio* and *Aeromonas*. Other phenotypic characters are included with the 0/129 sensitive vibrios in Table 16.5.

## Gram-positive bacteria

### *Lactobacillus* spp.

Lactobacilli have been identified as part of the normal bacterial flora of both freshwater and marine fish. There is some debate as to whether these organisms should also be regarded as potential fish pathogens, although they have been implicated in outbreaks of a post-spawning, stress related condition of salmonids known as pseudokidney disease. The name *Lactobacillus piscicola* has been proposed for a group of isolates specifically associated with this condition (Hiu *et al.* 1984). From the practical viewpoint of the disease diagnostician however, the greater significance of lactobacilli may be the possible mis-identification of the organisms as *Renibacterium salmoninarum* in Gram stained smears of kidney tissue.

*Lactobacillus* spp. are readily isolated as small, round, entire, opaque colonies on general purpose media incubated at 20−25°C for 48 h. Morphologically the organisms are Gram-positive, non-motile short rods or coccobacilli 0.5 × 1.0− 3.0 μm in size, which may be seen singly or in short chains reminiscent of streptococci. Lactobacilli are oxidase and catalase negative and do not reduce nitrates. Indole and $H_2S$ are not produced. Gelatin is not hydrolyzed. Metabolism is fermentative and acid is produced from a variety of sugars including glucose, maltose, mannitol and sucrose, but not from arabinose, inositol or rhamnose.

### *Renibacterium salmoninarum*

The single species of the relatively recently established genus *Renibacterium* is one of the few unequivocal obligate bacterial parasites of fish, and is the specific causative agent of bacterial kidney disease (BKD) of salmonids. A rapid, presumptive diagnosis of BKD may be made by the observation of the presence of small, strongly Gram-positive bacilli in smears from kidney or other affected tissues, but as these organisms may be confused with melanin granules or morphologically similar coryneform bacteria or lactobacilli, confirmatory identification tests are always indicated. The indirect FAT (Bullock & Stuckey 1975) and the direct FAT (Bullock *et al.* 1980), which may be applied to smears, formalin fixed or frozen tissues, have become widely accepted as serological confirmatory tests. The ELISA procedure has been applied to the specific detection of *R. salmoninarum* soluble antigen in fish tissue (Pascho & Mulcahy 1987).

Whenever possible, the diagnosis of BKD should include isolation of the causative organism in culture. *R. salmoninarum* has an absolute growth requirement for cysteine, and the use of specifically enriched media and prolonged incubation for up to 6 weeks at an optimum temperature of 15°C is necessary for successful cultivation. Colonies are characteristically round, raised, entire, creamy yellow in colour and of varying size. Morphologically the organisms are strongly Gram-positive, non-motile, very short rods 0.3−1.0 × 1.0−1.5 μm in size. *R. salmoninarum* is catalase positive, oxidase negative and has a distinguishing API−Zym$^{(R)}$ profile after 18 h at 15°C as follows:

− + − + − + − − + − + + − − − − + − − (+) − (Austin & Austin 1987).

### *Streptococcus* spp.

Streptococcal disease conditions have been described in a considerable variety of cultured and wild fish species from freshwater, estuarine and seawater environments. Streptococci may be isolated on standard general purpose media but growth is enhanced by blood, and supplementation of a basic agar medium with 5%(v/v) mammalian blood is recommended for recovery from clinical material. The addition of blood also allows the determination of haemolytic activity.

Small, white, translucent colonies develop within 48 h. In stained smears the Gram-positive cocci are seen to form chains and biochemically are catalase negative. In contrast, the *Micrococcus/Staphylococcus* group of organisms appear as pairs or clusters and are catalase positive. The taxonomic status of the fish pathogenic streptococci has not been satisfactorily resolved. Haemolytic activity is generally regarded as an important phenotypic trait of streptococci and α-haemolytic, β-haemolytic and non-haemolytic strains have all been isolated from fish. Selected *Streptococcus* characterization tests, including hydrolysis of sodium hippurate, growth at 10°C and 45°C, growth in 6.5%(w/v) NaCl and growth at pH 9.6 have given variable results. Some isolates have been identified as Lancefield serogroup B or D, but many others have proved to be serologically untypable. It seems possible from the available data that new *Streptococcus* species or subspecies will be defined among the fish pathogens.

## Anaerobic bacteria

*Clostridium botulinum* and *Eubacterium tarantellus* are the only two species of anaerobic bacteria which have so far been implicated as fish pathogens, although other anaerobes have been recovered from fish intestines and may be recognized as pathogens in the future.

*Cl. botulinum* may be isolated by strict anaerobic culture on egg-yolk or blood enriched media, although the more usually recommended procedure is the inoculation of intestinal contents and tissues into freshly prepared cooked meat medium and incubation for 6 days at 30°C. On lactose egg-yolk agar *Cl. botulinum* produces an iridescent film (pearly layer) over the surface of the colonies and a zone of opalescence in the surrounding medium (lecithovitellin reaction) but no fermentation of lactose, indicated by the absence of a red halo round the area of growth. The elaboration of neurotoxin by the organism is demonstrated by the inoculation of mice with liquid culture filtrates, and identification of the specific toxin by neutralization of the lethal effect with monovalent antisera (Cann *et al.* 1965). A definitive diagnosis of botulism also requires the demonstration of the toxin in the tissue of affected fish.

*Eubacterium tarantellus* has been isolated from brain tissue of estuarine fish displaying signs of meningitis using BHIA incubated anaerobically or Brewer's thioglycollate medium. Colonies are flat, translucent, colourless and rhizoid in appearance and are β-haemolytic on blood-supplemented BHIA plates. On primary isolation the organisms are filamentous ($>100\,\mu$m), asporogenous, Gram-positive rods which on subculture break up into smaller bacilli 1.5 ×

10−17 μm in size. *E. tarantellus* is non-motile, catalase negative and grows well at 37°C. Additional phenotypic traits have been described by Udey *et al.* (1977).

## Mycobacteriaceae

Mycobacteriosis has so far been reported in over 150 species of fish. At present, the recognized fish pathogens are speciated as *M. marinum*, *M. fortuitum* and *M. chelonae* (formerly *M. chelonei*), although many other names appear in the literature. Thus, *M. platypoecilus* and *M. anabanti* are synonymous with *M. marinum*. *M. ranae* is synonymous with *M. fortuitum*. The salmon pathogen *M. salmoniphilum* is on occasion referred to as a variant of *M. fortuitum*, but has now been more specifically classified as *M. chelonae* (Grange 1981) within the *M. fortuitum* complex.

The diagnosis of mycobacteriosis is more often than not based on the identification of acid-fast bacteria in histological sections of tubercular lesions, and little attempt is made to isolate the organism in culture. Standard media for mycobacteria are recommended for the isolation of the fish pathogens although many strains may also be cultivated on general purpose media. *M. marinum* is classified as a slow grower with visible growth appearing after 7 days incubation at 30°C. *M. fortuitum* and *M. chelonae* are rapid growers, with colonies developing within 5 days at 30°C. *M. fortuitum* grows well at 37°C but *M. marinum* and *M. chelonae* cannot be cultivated at this temperature. *M. marinum* is photochromogenic with the production of bright yellow colonies on exposure to light, whereas colonies of *M. fortuitum* and *M. chelonae* remain cream to buff in colour. Sanders & Fryer (1988) suggest iron uptake, sucrose utilization and nitrate reduction tests for the further differentiation of *M. fortuitum* (positive reactions) and *M. chelonae* (negative reactions).

## Nocardioforms

The nocardioforms are Gram-positive, aerobic, non-motile actinomycetes exhibiting a complete life cycle, including germination from resting microcysts, simple and complex fission, and branching. The organisms may thus appear in coccal, rod-shaped or long, branching, multiseptate filamentous forms. *Nocardia* spp. produce an aerial mycelium in culture. *Nocardia asteroides* and the proposed *Nocardia kampachi* have been isolated from fish.

Nocardias may be isolated on media used for mycobacteria or general purpose bacteriological media. Ridged and folded, irregular, white or yellow-orange colonies with aerial hyphae develop in 10−21 days. The characteristic of branched mycelia in stained smears distinguishes *Nocardia* from filamentous bacteria. *N. asteroides* and *N. kampachi* are biochemically very similar but *N. kampachi*, unlike *N. asteroides*, reportedly does not grow at 37°C.

# References

Amos, K.H. (Ed.) (1985) *Procedures for the Detection and Identification of Certain Fish Pathogens*, 3rd edn. Fish Health Section, American Fisheries Society. Corvallis, Oregon.

Anacker, R.L. & Ordal, E.J. (1959) Studies on the myxobacterium *Chondrococcus columnaris* I. Serological typing. *Journal of Bacteriology*, **78**, 25–32.

Arakawa, C.K. & Fryer, J.L. (1984) Isolation and characterization of a new subspecies of *Mycobacterium chelonei* infections for salmonid fish. *Helgoländer Meeresuntersuchungen*, **37**, 329–42.

Austin, B. & Austin, D.A. (1987) *Bacterial Fish Pathogens: Disease in Farmed and Wild Fish*. Ellis Horwood Ltd, Chichester.

Austin, B., Embley, T.M. & Goodfellow, M. (1983) Selective isolation of *Renibacterium salmoninarum*. *FEMS Microbiology Letters*, **17**, 111–14.

Baumann, P., Gauthier, M.J. and Baumann, L. (1984) Genus *Alteromonas*. In *Bergey's Manual of Systematic Bacteriology*, Vol. 1 (Ed. by N.R. Kreig & J.G. Holt), pp. 343–52. Williams & Wilkins, Baltimore.

Bejerano, Y., Sarig, S., Horne, M.T. & Roberts, R.J. (1979) Mass mortalities in silver carp *Hypophthalmichthys molitrix* (Valenciennes) associated with bacterial infection following handling. *Journal of Fish Diseases*, **2**, 49-56.

Bullock, G.L. (1972) Studies on selected myxobacteria pathogenic for fishes and on bacterial gill disease in hatchery-reared salmonids. *Technical Paper No. 60*. Bureau of Sport Fisheries and Wildlife, Fish and Wildlife Service. Washington, D.C.

Bullock, G.L. & Stuckey, H.M. (1975) Fluorescent antibody identification and detection of the *Corynebacterium* causing kidney disease of salmonids. *Journal of the Fisheries Research Board of Canada*, **32**, 2224–7.

Bullock, G.L., Griffin, B.R. & Stuckey, H.M. (1980) Detection of *Corynebacterium salmoninus* by direct fluorescent antibody test. *Canadian Journal of Fisheries and Aquatic Sciences*, **37**, 719–21.

Bullock, G.L., Hsu, T.C. & Shotts, E.B. (1986) Columnaris disease of fishes. *Fish Disease Leaflet No. 72*. US Department of the Interior, Fish and Wildlife Service, Washington DC.

Cann, D.C., Wilson, B.B., Hobbs, G., Shewan, J.M. & Johannsen, A. (1965) The incidence of *Clostridium botulinum* Type E in fish and bottom deposits in the North Sea and off the coast of Scandinavia. *Journal of Applied Bacteriology*, **28**, 426–30.

Colwell, R.R., MacDonnell, M.T. & DeLey, J. (1986) Proposal to recognize the family Aeromonadaceae fam. nov. *International Journal of Systematic Bacteriology*, **36**, 473–7.

Cowan, S.T. (1974) *Cowan & Steel's Manual for the Identification of Medical Bacteria*, 2nd edn. Cambridge University Press, Cambridge.

Cruz, J.M., Saraiva, A., Eiras, J.C., Branco, R. & Sousa, J.C. (1986) An outbreak of *Plesiomonas shigelloides* in farmed rainbow trout, *Salmo gairdneri* Richardson, in Portugal. *Bulletin of the European Association of Fish Pathologists*, **6**, 20–22.

Daly, J.G. & Stevenson, R.M.W. (1985) Charcoal agar, a new growth medium for the fish disease bacterium *Renibacterium salmoninarum*. *Applied and Environmental Microbiology*, **50**, 868–71.

Davies, R.L. & Frerichs, G.N. (1989) Morphological and biochemical differences among isolates of *Yersinia ruckeri* obtained from wide geographical areas. *Journal of Fish Diseases*, **12**, 357–65.

Dawson, C.A. & Sneath, P.H.A. (1985) A probability matrix for the identification of vibrios. *Journal of Applied Bacteriology*, **58**, 407–23.

Evelyn, T.P.T. (1977) An improved growth medium for the kidney disease bacterium and some notes on using the medium. *Bulletin de l'Office International des Epizooties*, **87**, 511–13.

Frerichs, G.N. & Hendrie, M.S. (1985) Bacteria associated with diseases of fish. In *Isolation and Identification of Micro-organisms of Medical and Veterinary Importance* (Ed. by C.H. Collins & J.M. Grange), pp. 355–71. Society for Applied Bacteriology Technical Series No. 21. Academic Press, London.

Frerichs, G.N. & Roberts, R.J. (1989) The bacteriology of teleosts. In *Fish Pathology*, 2nd edn. (Ed. by R.J. Roberts), pp. 289–319. Ballière Tindall, London.

Grange, J.M. (1981) *Myxobacterium chelonei*. *Tubercule*, **62**, 273–6.

Hiu, S.F., Holt, R.A., Sriranganathan, N., Seidler, R.J. & Fryer, J.L. (1984) *Lactobacillus piscicola*, a new species from salmonid fish. *International Journal of Systematic Bacteriology*, **34**, 393−400.

Kreig, N. & Holt, J.G. (Eds) (1984) *Bergey's Manual of Systematic Bacteriology*, Vol. 1. Williams & Wilkins, Baltimore.

Lee, J.V. & Donovan, T.J. (1985) *Vibrio, Aeromonas* and *Pleisiomonas*. In *Isolation and Identification of Micro-organisms of Medical and Veterinary Importance* (Ed. by C.H. Collins & J.M. Grange), pp. 13−33. Society for Applied Bacteriology Technical Series No. 21. Academic Press, London.

McCarthy, D.H. (1975) Detection of *Aeromonas salmonicida* antigen in diseased fish tissue. *Journal of General Microbiology*, **88**, 185−7.

McCarthy, D.H. & Roberts, R.J. (1980) Furunculosis of fish − the present state of our knowledge. In *Advances in Aquatic Microbiology* (Ed. by M.A. Droop & H.W. Jannasch), pp. 293−341. Academic Press, London.

Ossiander, F.J. & Wedemeyer, G. (1973) Computer program for sample sizes required to determine disease incidence in fish populations. *Journal of the Fisheries Research Board of Canada*, **30**, 1383−4.

Pascho, R.J. & Mulcahy, D. (1987) Enzyme-linked immunosorbent assay for a soluble antigen of *Renibacterium salmoninarum*, the causative agent of salmonid bacterial kidney disease. *Canadian Journal of Fisheries and Aquatic Sciences*, **44**, 183−91.

Rabb, L., Cornick, J.W. & McDermott, L.A. (1964) A macroscopic-slide agglutination test for the presumptive diagnosis of furunculosis in fish. *Progressive Fish Culturist*, **26**, 118−20.

Sanders, J.E. & Fryer, J.L. (1988) Bacteria of fish. In *Methods in Aquatic Bacteriology* (Ed. by B. Austin), pp. 115−42. John Wiley & Sons Ltd, Chichester.

Sato, N., Yamane, N. & Kawamura, T. (1982) Systemic *Citrobacter freundii* infection among sunfish *Mola mola* in Matsushima aquarium. *Bulletin of the Japanese Society of Scientific Fisheries*, **48**, 1551−7.

Shieh, H.S. (1980) Studies on the nutrition of a fish pathogen, *Flexibacter columnaris*. *Microbios Letters*, **13**, 129−33.

Shotts, E.B. & Teska, J.D. (1989) Bacterial pathogens of aquatic vertebrates. In *Methods for the Microbiological Examination of Fish and Shellfish* (Ed. by B. Austin & D.A. Austin), pp. 164−86. Ellis Horwood Ltd, Chichester.

Shotts, E.B. & Waltman, W.D. (1990) An isolation medium for *Edwardsiella ictaluri*. *Journal of Wildlife Diseases*, **26**, 214−18.

Shotts, E.B., Jr & Rimler, R. (1973) Medium for the isolation of *Aeromonas hydrophila*. *Applied Microbiology*, **26**, 550−3.

Sneath, P.H.A., Mair, N.S. & Sharpe, M.E. (Eds) (1986) *Bergey's Manual of Systematic Bacteriology*, Vol. 2. Williams & Wilkins, Baltimore.

Tsukamura, M. (1967) Identification of mycobacteria. *Tubercle*, **48**, 311−38.

Udey, L.R., Young, E. & Sallman, B. (1977) Isolation and characterization of an anaerobic bacterium, *Eubacterium tarantellus* sp. nov., associated with striped mullet (*Mugil cephalus*) mortality in Biscayne Bay, Florida. *Journal of the Fisheries Research Board of Canada*, **34**, 402−9.

Wakabayashi, H. & Egusa, S. (1974) Characteristics of myxobacteria associated with some freshwater fish diseases in Japan. *Bulletin of the Japanese Society of Scientific Fisheries*, **40**, 751−7.

Wakabayashi, H., Egusa, S. & Fryer, J.L. (1980) Characteristics of filamentous bacteria isolated from a gill disease of salmonids. *Canadian Journal of Fisheries and Aquatic Sciences*, **37**, 1499−504.

Wakabayashi, H., Hikida, M. & Masumura, K. (1986) *Flexibacter maritimus* sp. nov., a pathogen of marine fishes. *International Journal of Systematic Bacteriology*, **36**, 396−8.

Waltman, W.D. & Shotts, E.B. (1984) A medium for the isolation of *Yersinia ruckeri*. *Canadian Journal of Fisheries and Aquatic Sciences*, **41**, 804−6.

# Chapter 17:
# Public Health Aspects of Bacterial Infections of Fish

Fish is the primary source of animal protein in many countries, and for many millions, particularly in poorer sections of the community, it far exceeds meat or milk (Borgstrom 1962, Higgins & Kolbye 1984). In developing countries, inclusion of fish fundamentally improves the diet of the vast majority of the population, while in the western world it is increasingly seen as a health promoting food. A recent survey indicated that 25% of the population of the United States of America intended to reduce their consumption of red meat and increase intake of fish and poultry for health reasons (Gutting 1990). Fish, with less connective tissue than other animal flesh and no elastin (Fox 1978), is easily digestible. It contains less fat but a higher proportion (60−85%) of mono-unsaturated or polyunsaturated fatty acids and is thought to be associated with reducing the risk of human cardiovascular disease. The omega−3 fatty acids have been found to have cholesterol lowering properties as well as decreasing blood clotting activity (Browne 1990). With so much benefit accruing from fish as a human food source it is important to recognize potential health hazards with which it might be associated so that they can be reduced as far as possible. Bacterial infection of fish and fish products may influence human health either directly by inducing disease or indirectly through the effect on the human subject of residues of antimicrobial agents used to treat such infections in fish.

## Bacteria from fish affecting human health

Human infections that may be caused by bacteria in fish include food poisoning and gastroenteritis (due to *Salmonella, Vibrio* and *Clostridium* spp., *Campylobacter jejuni* and others), superficial conditions such as wound infections and mycobacteriosis. Pathogens which have been known to be transferred to man from fish or their aquatic environment are shown in Table 17.1. Scombrotic fish poisoning caused by excessive histamine production in the muscle of certain fish, mainly in the families Scombridae and Scomberosocidae, is the result of amino acid breakdown by bacteria including those shown in Table 17.2.

The range and frequency of fish-borne bacterial infections of man is relatively limited. This may be due in part to the fundamentally different bacterial flora affecting man and fish. Many commensal and pathogenic bacteria of fish are psychrophilic and fail to grow at human body temperature (37°C) (e.g. *Aeromonas salmonicida*), while others, although not strictly psychrophilic have lower temperature optima. Some do grow well in both fish and humans and are able to cause disease in both; *Vibrio parahaemolyticus* can cause vibriosis in fish and food poisoning in humans. Although there have been instances of localized infection, for example by pseudomonads entering through damaged skin and establishing wound infections, or erysipeloid due to *Erysipelothrix rhusiopathiae*, most infections are the result of consuming contaminated seafood.

**Table 17.1**  Bacteria of significance as human pathogens isolated from fish or their immediate environment

| | |
|---|---|
| *Salmonella* spp. | food poisoning |
| *Vibrio* spp. | food poisoning |
| *Campylobacter jejuni* | gastro-enteritis |
| *Plesiomonas shigelloides* | gastro-enteritis |
| *Edwardsiella tarda* | diarrhoea |
| *Aeromonas hydrophila* | diarrhoea, septicaemia |
| *Pseudomonas* spp. | wound infection |
| *Mycobacterium marinum* | mycobacteriosis |
| *Erysipelothrix rhusiopathiae* | erysipeloid |
| *Leptospira interrogans* | leptospirosis |
| *Clostridium botulinum* | botulism |

After Austin & Austin (1989)

**Table 17.2**  Histamine-producing bacteria isolated from marine fish

| | |
|---|---|
| *Citrobacter freundii* | *Klebsiella pneumoniae* |
| *Clostridium perfringens* | *Klebsiella* sp. |
| *Edwardsiella* sp. | *Proteus mirabilis* |
| *Enterobacter aerogenes* | *Proteus morganii* |
| *Enterobacter cloacae* | *Proteus vulgaris* |
| *Escherichia coli* | *Proteus* sp. |
| *Hafnia alvei* | *Vibrio alginolyticus* |
| | *Vibrio* sp. |

After Frank (1985)

Then the risk to public health arises if toxigenic strains multiply to high numbers during improper handling and storage (Hood *et al.* 1983, Colwell 1984). Fresh fish deteriorates quickly in storage owing to autoenzymatic action and bacterial degradation. It becomes unfit for consumption on these grounds, produces a strong odour and no longer poses a health risk. This is in contrast to foods such as eggs, poultry or dairy produce, which may contain hazardous numbers of bacterial pathogens such as *Salmonella* spp. without showing any obvious signs of spoilage.

## Incidence of fish-borne food poisoning

The proportion of food-borne disease due to fishery products varies between countries depending on climate, dietary customs and socio-economic factors, making direct international comparison difficult. Some countries, such as the United Kingdom and the United States of America, have centralized surveillance programmes on food-borne infection. Elsewhere this information is scarce, although there are many reports on the presence of human bacterial pathogens in fish and the potential hazard they represent but without epidemiological follow-up (Buck & Spotte 1986, Palumbo *et al.* 1989). It is not always possible to separate data on fish from seafood in total. Shellfish as filter feeders are much more vulnerable to acquiring and harbouring human pathogens typically derived from untreated or improperly treated sewage. They also may acquire species pathogenic for man, mainly *Vibrio* and *Aeromonas* spp., from the aquatic environment (Morris & Black 1985). Food poisoning due to eating contaminated shellfish is well reviewed by West (1989).

The proportion of food-borne outbreaks of disease due to fish was 12% in Australia (1967−71), 9.3% in the United States of America, 5.8% in Canada and 0.5% in England and Wales (1973−5) (Todd 1978). Incidence in the United States of America has been increasing. About 11% (233) of food-borne disease outbreaks reported between 1970 and 1978 were due to seafood including fish (Bryan 1980) and this rose to 24% (301) between 1979 and 1984 (Bryan 1986). Much of this upsurge was due to infections with *Vibrio* spp., attributed to the increased consumption of raw seafood and increased travel abroad (Janda & Bryant 1987) and fish were involved in 57% of the 301 cases. Distribution of outbreaks throughout the United States of America was very uneven; 81% were reported from only nine states or territories, 49% from four and 35% from Hawaii alone (Spencer-Garrett 1988). In Scotland the reports of the foodborne surveillance programme from 1980 to 1989 show that the incidence of outbreaks due to fish or shellfish was low compared with meat/meat products, chicken or milk (see Table 17.3): 0.9% of outbreaks and 0.6% of cases were due to fish (Communicable Disease Scotland Unit 1980−9). In contrast, the Food and Health Organisation recorded public health problems as acute in African countries, where waters were at risk of pollution by human faeces (FAO 1981). Staphylococcal intoxication or botulism due to *C. botulinum* or the milder non neurological poisoning due to *C. perfringens* were noted but no precise data were given.

## Bacterial growth on fish for human consumption

### Bacterial spoilage of fish

Fish spoilage is a complex process involving microbiological and non-microbiological processes (Herbert *et al.* 1971, Liston 1980, 1982, Huss 1983). Non-microbiological deterioration is caused by endogenous proteolytic enzymes which are concentrated particularly in the head and viscera (Backhoff 1976) and attack these organs and surrounding tissue after death. Activity is particularly great in fish which recently had been feeding heavily and it leads to early rupture of the gut with dissemination of general contents including enzymes and micro-organisms. Enzymatic spoilage may be compounded by deterioration due to oxygenation of unsaturated fatty substances causing loss of flavour and development of rancidity (Connell 1990).

During life, micro-organisms are present on the external surfaces of the fish and in the gut, but the flesh is normally sterile. After death of the fish, micro-

**Table 17.3** Outbreaks and cases of human food poisoning in Scotland by food vehicle

| | 1980 | | 1981 | | 1982 | | 1983 | | 1984 | | 1985 | | 1986 | | 1987 | | 1988 | |
|---|---|---|---|---|---|---|---|---|---|---|---|---|---|---|---|---|---|---|
| | o* | c* | o | c | o | c | o | c | o | c | o | c | o | c | o | c | o | c |
| Fish | 1 | 19 | 1 | 8 | 4 | 10 | 1 | 2 | 3 | 8 | 1 | 4 | 1 | 2 | 1 | 18 | 5 | 21 |
| Shellfish | 2 | 1 | 4 | 9 | 6 | 13 | 4 | 14 | NA | NA | NA | NA | 1 | 4 | 5 | 64 | 7 | 37 |
| Eggs | 1 | NA | 1 | NA | NA | NA | 3 | 4 | 1 | 11 | NA | NA | 2 | 33 | 2 | 9 | 8 | 40 |
| Milk | 5 | 75 | 9 | 812 | 15 | 541 | 16 | 27 | 4 | 25 | 8 | 84 | 2 | 10 | 5 | 30 | 1 | 4 |
| Chicken | 35 | 366 | 45 | 300 | 39 | 187 | 49 | 389 | 46 | 395 | 23 | 290 | 25 | 181 | 40 | 375 | 44 | 254 |
| Meat/meat products | 27 | 283 | 46 | 448 | 34 | 277 | 24 | 299 | 38 | 442 | 25 | 232 | 25 | 173 | 24 | 201 | 24 | 308 |
| Turkey | NA | NA | 6 | 45 | 8 | 252 | 7 | 25 | 4 | 9 | 3 | 268 | 1 | 2 | 2 | 5 | 2 | 8 |
| All causes | 147 | 1305 | 238 | 2077 | 276 | 2100 | 278 | 1643 | 256 | 1517 | 185 | 1485 | 184 | 987 | 234 | 1825 | 219 | 1646 |

o* outbreaks  c* cases

In 4 years *Salmonella* sp. were implicated in shellfish borne outbreaks and in two *Campylobacter* was isolated.

The fish-borne cases were due to an unspecified agent or toxin but not to the common food poisoning bacteria tested for, namely *Salmonella, Bacillus cereus, Campylobacter, Clostridium perfringens* or *Staphylococcus.*

In the 9 years from 1980 to 1988 there were 2017 outbreaks and 14 585 cases of food poisoning in Scotland, of which 18 outbreaks and 92 cases were associated with fish as the food vehicle.

organisms diffuse into the flesh and increase, slowly at first, and then more rapidly causing a sequence of changes in the odour and flavour. The rate of deterioration due to all processes can be slowed by storage at low temperature without delay and by removal of the viscera, skin and head.

Spoilage due to elevated temperature is an extensive problem in less well developed countries, particularly where refrigeration and other processing facilities are restricted. Over half the world's total catch of fish, crustaceans and molluscs is landed in the tropics, with 35% of this in Asia (FAO 1988). The situation with regard to aquaculture is even more critical, with 85% by volume and 78% by value of global production now occurring in Asia and the Pacific (FAO 1990). Several methods of preservation are practised to delay these effects, icing, canning, chemical preservation and others.

The bacterial flora of fish, derived essentially from the aqueous environment (Wood 1953), varies with seasonal and environmental factors (Shewan 1961, 1971) and is further affected by the type of storage and processing which follows catching. Fish from sub-tropical waters have a high percentage of mesophiles, such as *Bacillus* spp., coryneforms and micrococci, while in fish caught in cold waters, psychrophiles such as *Pseudomonas*, *Achromobacter* and *Flavobacterium* spp. predominate (Shewan 1961, 1962). With storage at low temperatures numbers of *Pseudomonas* spp. increase greatly and were found to reach 60−90% of the total bacterial count in cold-water fish (Shewan *et al.* 1960), while others decreased or stayed fairly constant in number. In brined fish micrococci and coryneforms were found to predominate (Shewan 1962) and micrococci composed over 90% of the flora in dry-salted fish (Dussault 1958).

*Pseudomonas*, *Alteromonas* and related species are considered to make up the major part of the spoilage flora (van Spreekins 1977). They are capable of growing actively at low temperatures, near 0°C, and attacking thioamino acids and thioamines to produce hydrogen sulphide and other volatile sulphides. The chemical changes during spoilage of fish by bacterial action has been the subject of much investigation (Shewan 1977, Martin *et al.* 1982, Connell 1990), with particular interest focused on substances that accumulate in the tissue and can be easily measured to provide practical methods of determining fish quality. Accumulation of trimethylamine from trimethylamine oxide as a result mainly of bacterial action has been used to assess the quality of many marine species (Hebard *et al.* 1982, Huss *et al.* 1986). Other more general microbiological methods are available to determine total bacterial counts or counts of specific indicator organisms to assess the extent of risk to public health (Connell 1990).

### Microbiological criteria for food quality

Below the extreme where fish is clearly aesthetically unacceptable for human consumption, neither a total bacterial count nor a count of sulphide producing bacteria alone can be taken as a guide of fitness as food. Guidelines setting microbiological criteria for foods were drawn up originally in the Codex Alimentarius (FAO 1977) and defined more precisely by the International Commission on Microbiological Specifications for Foods (ICMSF 1986). Micro-biological safety and quality is usually determined using 'marker' organisms to indicate the presence of given pathogens or toxin formers at specified levels (Mossel 1982, Cox *et al.* 1988).

The bacteria which present a public health risk grow best at 35–37°C, while spoilage bacteria have a lower optimum temperature for growth. A total count of bacteria in the sample when incubated at the higher temperature gives an indication of the degree of contamination with potentially harmful bacteria. Determination of the incidence of *Escherichia coli* and coliforms indicates faecal contamination, and sometimes it may be useful to investigate the presence of specific pathogens such as coagulase-positive *Staphylococcus* and *Streptococcus* spp. Elevated histamine levels are taken to indicate bacterial quality more generally and the risk of scombroid poisoning.

### Food poisoning due to pathogens found in the aquatic environment

Fish-borne bacterial food poisoning may be caused by the bacteria naturally present in the aquatic environment, derived from aquatic pollution or introduced during handling and processing. Bacteria naturally present in the aquatic environment which have been implicated in food poisoning include *Vibrio* spp. (West & Colwell 1984) and *Cl. botulinum* type E (Licciardello 1983). Twenty three of 272 samples of seafood and water taken off South-west India contained *Vibrio cholerae* non–01 (Mathew *et al.* 1988), and the pathogenicity of strains of *V. cholerae* non–01, *V. parahaemolyticus*, *V. vulnificus*, *V. mimicus* isolated in the same region has been confirmed (Malathi *et al.* 1988). Sporadic cases of tropical diarrhoea have been attributed to consumption of freshwater fish carrying *Edwardsiella tarda* and *Plesiomonas shigelloides* (Van Damme & Vandepitte 1980), with species such as *Tilapia* providing the natural habitat of these bacteria. The species involved in scombroid fish poisoning (Table 17.2) also are naturally present in the aquatic environment.

If fish contaminated with these pathogens are harvested and stored at temperatures conducive to bacterial multiplication and then consumed, gastroenteritis may result. The symptoms associated with *V. parahaemolyticus* are characterized by abdominal pain, vomiting, watery diarrhoea, fever, chills and headache. The incubation period is 12–48 h and recovery is commonly within 5 days. Usually cooking or heat processing kills *V. parahaemolyticus* but low temperature storage only reduces multiplication, and organisms have been detected after two days storage at 4°C from fish contaminated with about $10^3$ cells per g. (Venugopal & Karunasagar 1988).

*V. vulnificus* causes septicaemia, chills, fever, sometimes vomiting and diarrhoea, and cutaneous lesions and ulcers may occur at the extremities. People with impaired liver function or stomach dysfunction are particularly vulnerable. Onset of symptoms is within 24 h and about half reported cases have died (Blake *et al.* 1980).

C. *botulinum* is the causative organism of botulism, a severe form of poisoning associated with headache, vision disorders, weakness and respiratory distress. There are vomiting, abdominal pain and diarrhoea followed by neurological involvement within 1–6 days. Resulting partial paralysis may persist for months, but if the outcome is fatal this usually occurs within the first 10 days. The incidence is low. Since records were first kept in the United States of America there have been 227 cases in 100 outbreaks of seafood associated botulism, with 33% of them fatal (Bryan 1986). Most were due to *C. botulinum* type E toxin. There have been no recorded cases of botulism arising from fish in Scotland or the rest of the United Kingdom in the last 10 years (Dr J.C.M. Sharp, personal communication), the last documented case occurring in Birmingham in 1978 (Ball *et al.* 1979).

### Scombroid fish poisoning

The symptoms of scombroid fish poisoning resemble an allergic reaction, with a burning sensation in the mouth, flushing, headache, palpitations, itching and gastrointestinal disturbance. It is caused by eating scombroid fish (tuna, mackerel, bonito, etc.) and some non-scombroid fish in which bacterial metabolism has resulted in high levels of histamine being produced in the fish muscle (Taylor *et al.* 1989). Dark fleshed fish in particular contain large amounts of the free amino acid histamine which can be decarboxylated by certain bacteria, especially Enterobacteriaceae (Table 17.2), to histamine. The effect of histamine is considered central to the physiological process of poisoning although other compounds such as cadaverine may also be involved (Taylor *et al.* 1984). The incubation period and the duration of the illness is usually brief and the episode usually resolves within a day.

Histamine is not endogenous to fish muscle and its presence is an indicator of earlier microbial decomposition (Pan 1985). The United States Food and Drug Administration has set a limit of 20 mg histamine per 100 g as indicative of mishandling and 50 mg per 100 g as a health hazard (Federal Register 1982). Levels of several hundred mg per 100 g have been recorded. The bacteria involved are nearly all Gram-negative rods in the family Enterobacteriaceae, with *Proteus margonii* a major contributor. Isolates of *Vibrio* and *Clostridium* capable of forming histamine in decomposed tuna have also been reported (Frank 1985).

Between 1976 and 1986, 258 incidents of scombrotoxic food poisoning involving 638 cases were reported in the United Kingdom (Bartholomew *et al.* 1987) and this may be an under-representation resulting from a low level of public and medical awareness of this condition (Main & Yates 1990). Fresh, canned, dried and salted fish have all been implicated, and prevention of histamine formation is by rapid refrigeration after catching and a high standard of hygiene during processing.

**Bacterial contamination after harvest or catching**

During storage, processing or preparation for consumption fish may become contaminated by potential pathogens which can multiply rapidly with a favourable storage temperature. Polluted waters in fish processing plants can introduce serious diseases such as cholera and typhoid, but this is rare. More commonly food poisoning bacteria are introduced by handlers or by contact with contaminated fomites. Bacteria involved are *Salmonella* and *Shigella* spp., *Bacillus cereus*, *C. perfringens* and *Staphylococcus aureus* (Bryan 1986, Eyles 1986, Communicable Diseases Scotland Unit 1980–9).

**Control and prevention**

Fish, like poultry and dairy produce, provides an excellent growth medium for a wide range of bacteria. Because fish deteriorates relatively quickly, spoilage may occur before potential pathogens can grow to toxigenic proportions, and a public health risk is thereby avoided. The key to prevention is to maintain a high standard of hygiene through all handling processes. At an international level there are regulatory and advisory groups such as the Codex Alimentarius, International Commission on Microbiological Specifications for Food (ICMSF), etc., to ensure the microbiological safety of food. In developed countries there are national agencies to implement effectively the relevant regulations.

A study of epidemiological data has shown the factors which have contributed to outbreaks of seafood-transmitted diseases, namely eating raw fish, heat-process failure, cross contamination of cooked fish with raw fish and other improper procedures (Bryan 1986). These factors are directly related to critical control points (CCP) in ensuring food safety. A system of hazard analysis of critical control points (HACCP) has been developed to prevent and control seafood-borne infections (World Health Organisation (WHO)/ICMSF 1982, Codex Alimentarius Commission 1984). The HACCP system sets out to determine the hazards and assess severity, identify critical control points, establish control measures, monitor critical control points and take action when monitoring indicates this is necessary (Bryan 1986).

In line with stringent controls set by the United States Food and Drug Administration for home produced fish, manufacturers supplying the American market are required to comply with equally strict import regulations. In response the FAO has sponsored training on the principles and application of the HACCP system for fish producers in countries, for example, of the Indo-Pacific region (Warne 1985).

With workers trained in safe procedures for processing fishery products, public health hazards associated with contamination and outgrowth of potential human pathogens and agents of scombroid poisoning could, to a large extent, be avoided.

## Antimicrobial agents in the control of bacterial diseases in fish: implications for human health

Antimicrobial agents are used widely throughout the world to treat bacterial diseases in animals raised for human consumption. Intensively reared fish and shellfish are subject to equivalent epizootic infections and consequently to the control measures of vaccination and chemotherapy. It is essential to ensure that chemicals and chemotherapeutics used in all food production industries do not present a health hazard to the consumer. In common with agriculture, virtually all countries require that a rigorous testing programme be undertaken to demonstrate safety, quality and efficacy of a chemotherapeutic agent before it can be used in aquaculture. The range of agents available varies considerably from country to country, depending on the aquatic species cultured and the individual legal requirements of the country concerned. Safety requirements generally relate to the fish being treated, the operatives handling the material, the eventual consumer of the treated fish product and the environment. Strict quality control during the synthesis and manufacturing process ensures the constancy of the compound in terms of stability and avoids unwanted contaminants or by-products. Such control also ensures consistency between batches, so that tests of efficacy and toxicity carried out prior to marketing authorisation will be reflected in eventual field use, provided that treatment regimes are adhered to carefully.

Of particular concern to the eventual consumer of treated fish are detailed pharmacokinetic and toxicity studies, which establish patterns of metabolism and excretion of both the parent treatment compound and any excipient and any of their metabolites produced under varying conditions of temperature, salinity and life-cycle stage. Such studies are necessary in order to regulate the 'withdrawal period' or time interval between last administration of treatment compound and eventual harvesting for human consumption. Before a withdrawal period can be established, toxicological studies, including long-term mammalian studies, are necessary to establish any damaging side-effects of the compounds concerned. These studies are also necessary to establish a '0−effect' level for the compound. Using a safety factor (often × 100 for minor toxic effects but up to × 2000 for a potentially severe effect) an acceptable daily intake of the product concerned (the ADI) for humans can be established and from this figure, and a knowledge of the likely intake of fish products by the human population, and information from residue studies, a maximum residue limit (the MRL) deduced (Woodward 1991*a,b*). When combined with the pharmacokinetic and residues depletion studies mentioned earlier, the withdrawal period is then established, commonly utilizing a degree-day concept to account for temperature variation and its effect on metabolism in fish.

The establishment of such methodologies is backed up in developed countries with ever-increasing monitoring of samples of fish, both from home production and from importation. If any samples exceed the MRL, further investigation of the origin of the sample takes place and prosecution may result if abuse of the law is detected. Legislation concerning record-keeping on farms is also used to ensure rapid and effective follow-up. With the clear popular swing in the West towards regarding fish as a health-promoting product it is apposite to review current practice and to evaluate the level of risk.

## Nature of risk associated with antimicrobial agents

Antimicrobial agents have been widely used for many years in other forms of intensive stock rearing, e.g. pigs, poultry and cattle, to treat disease and as growth promoters, and the potential hazards associated with these practices have been considered by the Joint Committee on the Use of Antibiotics in Animal Husbandry and Veterinary Medicine (1969) commonly referred to as the 'Swann Committee'. This Committee produced a report (Swann Report) which identified some of these hazards. These were:

(1) increase in the antibiotic resistance of enteric bacteria of animal origin,
(2) ingestion by man of such resistant bacteria (e.g. salmonellae) with resultant human infection,
(3) intake of antibiotic residues with direct toxic or allergic consequences, and
(4) emergence of strains resistant to essential human drugs, this related particularly to the value of chloramphenicol in treating *S. typhi* in man being undermined by wider use in animals

The degree of risk associated with these hazards is generally considered to be very low.

Nevertheless strict controls are in place to limit the levels of residues in animal products used for human foodstuffs. Current European MRL values (1992) (admittedly based on toxicological rather than on antimicrobial hazard) for meat, including fish, for commonly-used antimicrobial compounds are:

| | |
|---|---|
| Amoxycillin | 50 μg/kg |
| Sulphonamides | 100 μg/kg |
| Trimethoprim | 50 μg/kg |
| Nitrofurans | 5 μg/kg* |
| Tetracyclines | 100 μg/kg* * |

\* Provisional figures for all residues with an intact 5-nitro structure — additional data required by 1 January 1993.

\* \* Provisional figures — additional data required by 1 January 1994.
In addition, similar provisional figures are provided of 600 μg/kg for kidney, 300 μg/kg for liver and 10 μg/kg for fat.

Continued monitoring demonstrates the extent to which these levels are exceeded.

Although only limited information is currently available to quantify these risks reliably in relation to fish, data are being gathered and there are reports on the levels detected. For example, samples of farmed trout examined in a field survey in the UK in 1984 revealed no residues of sulphonamides or furazolidone but oxytetracycline was detected at levels of between 0.008 and 0.04 mg/kg in seven out of 54 samples of eight to ten fish, all of which were below the current MRL level (Working Party on Veterinary Residues in Animal Products 1987).

However, enforcement of regulations is not easy in the Western World, far less in the developing countries. Few have a systematic monitoring system and there is certainly no international standardization. Consequently irregularities have been occurring and food, including seafood, has been found at market containing antibiotics at excessive levels. (e.g. Brown & Higuera-Ciapara 1992).

Consider now the extent to which the potential hazards defined by Swann have been realized and the methods available to monitor levels and set appropriate safety standards.

### Ingestion of resistant bacteria producing human disease

The extent to which resistant bacteria have been transferred from animals to man is a subject of considerable debate. Some authors suggest a clear correlation between emerging resistance in human pathogens and overuse of antimicrobial agents by the medical profession (Walton 1988). Others suggest that such use does not play a major role, for example in the case of antibiotic-resistant salmonellae infections (Holmberg *et al.* 1984). Epidemiological tracing has shown that organisms with particular plasmid profiles affecting humans could be traced back to infections in cattle, via either meat products or farm workers (Holmberg *et al.* 1984 cited by Midtvedt & Lingaas 1992, Spika *et al.* 1987).

Of particular concern is the possibility of multiple-resistant salmonellae from farm animals producing bacteraemia in the human population, with resultant difficulties in chemotherapy. Threlfall *et al.* (1992), in a study of salmonella bacteraemia in England and Wales between 1981 and 1990, concluded that it was rare (overall incidence 1.5% of non-typhoidal salmonella isolates) and even when present, only infrequently associated with multiply resistant isolates. Multiple-resistance in salmonellae isolated from man is, however, increasing and there is some evidence to suggest that this may be a reflection of an increase in multiple-resistant salmonellae in animals, at least in some phage types (Ward *et al.* 1990).

Quinolone resistance in campylobacter in the Netherlands has been shown to have increased similarly in poultry and man between 1982 and 1989, coinciding with an increasing use of fluoroquinolones in both human and veterinary medicine during this period. However, it is suggested, though not proven, that this increase in man is almost exclusively due to transmission of campylobacter from chicken to man (Endtz *et al*. 1991).

There is also the possibility of resistance to certain antibiotics used in animals conferring resistance to similar, though not identical, antibiotics used in man. A particular example is the use of apramycin in animals conferring resistance to gentamycin, an antibiotic primarily used in man (Threlfall *et al*. 1986). Any transfer of resistant bacteria from animals to man could therefore create significant problems in human chemotherapy. However, clear evidence that transfer of resistant organisms from animals to man is of frequent occurrence is lacking, and the significance of resistance in bacteria in the human population arising from animals rather than man is not apparent.

Fortunately, particularly because of their poikilothermic nature, very few organisms found in farmed fish produce human infections and so resistant bacteria in fish are extremely unlikely to produce human disease.

The extent to which these concerns are justified is not easy to quantify at present. It should not be forgotten that selection pressure for the production of antimicrobial resistant strains is usually of short duration, and that when that pressure is removed the resistant mutant then seldom has equivalent survival properties to the original wild strain. However, there is an overall increase in drug-resistant organisms in the environment (Mitsuhashi 1977) and many bacteria possessing R-plasmids do show high survival rates in aquatic environments (Kelch & Lee 1978). Such isolates can, however, be found in remote regions such as the Antarctic, suggesting a background level of R-plasmid-carrying bacteria (Yndestad 1992).

Extensive studies carried out in Japan however have shown that the R-plasmids from fish pathogens are in fact different from those of R-plasmids of bacteria affecting man and domestic animals, suggesting that direct spread of resistance from fish to man is unlikely (Aoki 1992).

Austin (1985) has reported survival of resistant bacteria in effluent water from fish farms undergoing antibiotic therapy, although this was rapidly reduced after the end of the therapy period, while Husevag *et al*. (1991) found an increase in resistant bacteria for some considerable time after cessation of antibiotic use.

**Drug hypersensitivity (allergy)**

Hypersensitivity to drugs generally develops after repeated exposure to low or moderate doses of a particular agent. Once developed, subsequent exposure may result in a variety of outcomes ranging from localized skin reactions to respiratory problems such as asthma to generalized anaphylactic shock.

Licensing of veterinary medicines takes account of the risk of hypersensitivity in a number of ways and covers occupational and consumer exposure. Local application or contamination of the allergenic material to skin surfaces constitutes by far the most common route in the development of sensitization (Schulz

1982) and drugs vary widely in their ability to produce this type of effect. The penicillins are notorious as a class of drug commonly producing this effect. For this reason, data sheets and label information for veterinary products usually recommend precautions to be taken to avoid contact, ranging from the use of protective clothing such as gloves, face masks or specific breathing apparatus if powders are being used which contain particles in the respirable range. There is thus an immediate risk to persons mixing concentrated powders with fish feed at the feed mill or fish farm and a degree of risk thereafter to the person feeding medicated diets to fish. It should be rementioned that such precautions are intended, not only to prevent sensitization and subsequent hypersensitivity reactions in people handling medicated diets, but also to prevent hypersensitivity reactions in people previously sensitized by another route of exposure, e.g. in human chemotherapy.

The other potential area of risk is exposure to drugs contained as residues in food-producing animals. Fortunately, despite extensive use of therapeutics in animals over many years, there are few published reports implicating allergic reactions resulting from intake of residues in human food (Yndestad 1992), and the few that exist are not validated (Woodward 1991*a*). Such reports that do exist have never implicated residues in fish, and indeed the recent report of the Joint FAO/WHO Expert Committee on Food Additives (JECFA 1989) concluded that hypersensitivity reactions due to the ingestion of food of animal origin containing allergic drug residues are unlikely to be of major health significance. Stringent MRLs are set to ensure that the risk is reduced as far as possible, and the constant improvement in controls to prevent unacceptable residue levels in treated animals reaching the human consumer should reduce any risk even further.

### Resistance to essential drugs

The Swann Report of 1969 expressed concern that the use in animals, of antibiotics of particular relevance to human medicine, might lead to resistant strains developing in animals and subsequently being transferred. Of particular moment was resistance of *Salmonella typhi* to chloramphenicol through its use in treating animal disease, since at that time it was one of the few effective treatments for typhoid fever. Since then there has been no evidence to suggest that transfer of resistance to chloramphenicol has occurred through R factor transfer, and indeed it has been suggested by Murray *et al.* (1985) that such R factors, even if acquired, would not persist.

Most materials authorised at the present time for use in fish are those which have been utilized over a very long period in human medicine and have been largely superseded by newer antimicrobial agents. In the case of more novel treatment compounds, the companies concerned in registration have generally developed such treatments for animals and not for man, or used compounds such as the quinolones which do not develop plasmid-mediated resistance.

There is widespread resistance of fish pathogens to many of the commonly used antibiotics, and such resistance is increasing with continued and repeated usage necessitated by the lack of a range of available compounds. The physical transfer of stocks carrying bacteria with multiple drug resistance is also thought to exacerbate the problem (Richards *et al.* 1992). There is, however, no evidence that the use of such drugs in fish is having any cumulative effect on already-existing resistance to those older compounds among the commensal and pathogenic organisms found in man.

There is, however, a perceived risk of transferable drug resistance, where resistance plasmids in fish organisms or bacteria in the aquatic environment around aquaculture sites may hypothetically be transferred to organisms of human significance such as the Enterobacteriaceae (Hedges *et al.* 1985).

**Detection methods**

The reader is referred to the extensive review on this subject by McGill & Hardy (1992).

Traditional methods used to detect residues in fish generally relied on micro-biological assessment, utilizing an organism that was particularly sensitive to the agent in question. Usually this involves the measurement of a zone of growth inhibition, within a fixed time period, around tissue extracts placed in wells in agar plates seeded with an indicator organism. Calibration curves are used to provide concentration levels. Such methods, however, are restricted, firstly by their level of sensitivity and secondly by their lack of specificity, particularly when dealing with metabolites of a parent compound. Micro-biological methods do, however, provide a relatively rapid, inexpensive and easily applied means of screening for antimicrobial compounds.

More commonly now, physicochemical methods are utilized because of their specificity, sensitivity and reproducibility. Lack of uniformity in methodology and extraction procedures does present problems and there is a pressing need for standardization if acceptance of monitoring between countries is to be established. The most common means of physicochemical analysis is high performance liquid chromatography (HPLC), although thin layer chromato-graphy (TLC) or gas chromatography (GC) have been preferred in individual cases. Such methods are generally preferred to microbiological methods and are increasingly becoming accepted as the norm for statutory requirements. Other methods are also constantly being examined, either because of their sensitivity in particular cases, or because of their ease of use and reproducibility. Recent examples include the use of a radiobioassay system (Penicillin Assays, Malden, Massachussetts, USA), in which specific microbial receptors or anti-bodies are applied to bind to antibiotics in tissue extracts or fluids in competition with a radiolabelled tracer antibiotic. The reduction of labelled antibiotic fixed in the test is proportional to the amount of antibiotic in the sample.

Bound residues present a particular problem as it is important to know if these are bioavailable, and hence able to exert any harmful effects. Moreover, it is important to differentiate between bound residues and those arising from metabolic incorporation or mineralization (e.g. to bicarbonate ion). The Joint FAO/WHO Expert Committee on Food Additives (JECFA) has recently recommended methodologies for examining bound residues (JECFA 1990).

Of general concern at the present time is the possible requirement for permitted limits to be decided by the ever more sensitive methods of detection rather than by criteria of safety. Within the EC, this is unlikely to be a problem as the Working Group on the Safety of Residues of the Committee for Veterinary Medicinal Products (CVMP) is establishing MRLs based on toxicology.

**The situation in Europe**

Though Member States of the EC have their own national legislation to ensure food safety, this is increasingly controlled by a number of Directives emanating directly from the EC (Woodward 1991*b*). European marketing authorization for veterinary products is primarily controlled through Directives 81/851/EEC and 81/852/EEC, amended from 1 January 1992 by Directive 90/676/EEC (Hankin 1992), and Directive 70/524/EEC, which applies specifically to medicated and non-medicated feed additives. Directive 87/22/EEC provides control over products derived from high technology, and from January 1992 Directive 90/672/EEC will extend controls to cover immunological products. In all cases, controls regarding safety, quality and efficacy are applied prior to marketing authorization being given.

The so-called residues Directive, 86/469/EEC, defines monitoring requirements, though this formal legislation does not currently require national surveillance plans for fish. Voluntary screening of fish for residues is in force in a number of member states in order to determine whether there is, in fact, a potential problem with residues in fish (Hankin 1992). From January 1992, MRL values for new veterinary active ingredients will be established centrally at European Community level by the Committee for Veterinary Medicinal Products by way of its Working Group on the Safety of Residues, under Regulation EEC No. 2377/90. MRLs will be established for existing drugs used in food producing animals by 1996 (Woodward 1991*c*).

Of particular significance from 1 January 1992 is the requirement to demonstrate safety to the environment prior to giving marketing authorization.

**Extra-label use in fish**

One of the principal problems facing those attempting to control disease in fish is the extremely narrow range of products currently licensed for fish use. Even when products are approved, this generally applies only to one or two species of fish. The ever escalating cost of licensing requires careful examination of the potential market size and penetration of new products to prevent the perpetuation of the small range of currently available products.

In recognition of the need for other products in the face of specific lack of available licensed materials, a new amendment to Directive 81/851/EEC is intended to make specific exemptions to the normal licensing requirements. This will be approved only if undertaken by a veterinary surgeon in respect of animals under his direct care when no licensed product is available for that species. He may then use a product fully licensed for another species, or in exceptional circumstances a product approved for use in man, or lastly he may prescribe an extemporaneous medication (Hankin 1992). In such cases a withdrawal period of at least 500 degree days must be applied and detailed records kept of such use. If used in feed, the products must be licensed as such.

In practice, the use of such extra-species application is likely to be severely restricted; first because those products authorised for in-feed animal use (the most common method of administration to fish) are generally of low concentration of active ingredients and cannot be used for surface coating pelleted feed for use in fish because of their increased bulk; second, because of the impracticability of individually treating thousands of animals by some other route; or third, often because of the high relative cost of alternatives.

### Assessment of present overall risks

Published reports of adverse health effects in humans arising from consuming antibiotic residues in meat and milk are few (e.g. Tinkelman & Bock 1984). There appears to be no published record of any incidents of fish origin, and with the legislation currently in place and anticipated, future risk is slight. In those developing countries as yet without detailed controls, future legislation and monitoring systems will be stimulated by the regulations of importing countries if export of fish products is to take place. Perhaps the most pressing current need is the development of sensitive low-cost technology to help with monitoring at the site of production.

# References

Aoki, T. (1992) Past, present and future problems concerning the development of resistance in aquaculture. In *Proceedings of OIE Symposium: Problems of Chemotherapy in Aquaculture: from theory to reality*, Paris 12–15 March 1991 (Ed. by D.J. Alderman & C. Michel), pp. 256–64. Office International des Epizooties, Paris.

Austin, B. (1985) Antibiotic pollution from fish farms — effect on aquatic microflora. *Microbiological Sciences*, **2**(4), 113–17.

Austin, B. & Austin, D.A. (1989) *Methods for the Microbiological Examination of Fish and Shellfish*. Ellis Horwood Ltd, John Wiley & Sons, New York.

Backhoff, P.H. (1976) Some chemical changes in fish silage. *Journal of Food Technology*, **11**, 353–63.

Ball, A.P., Hopkinson, R.B., Farrell, R.B., Hutchinson, J.F.P., Paul, R., Watson, R.D.S., Page, A.J.F., Parker, R.G.F., Edwards, C.W., Snow, M., Scott, D.K., Leone-Ganado, A., Hastings,

A., Ghosh, A.C., Gilbert, R.J. (1979) Human botulism caused by *Clostridium botulinum* type E: The Birmingham outbreak. *Quarterly Journal of Medicine*, **48**, 473–91.

Bartholemew, B.A., Berry, P.R., Rodhouse, J.C., Gilbert, R.J. & Murray, C.K. (1987) Scombrotoxic fish poisoning in Britain: features of over 250 suspected incidents from 1976–1986. *Epidemiology and Infection*, **99**, 775–82.

Blake, P.A., Weaver, R.E. & Hollis, D.G. (1980) Diseases of humans (other than cholera) caused by vibrios. *Annual Review of Microbiology*, **34**, 341–67.

Borgstrom, G. (1962) Fish in world nutrition. In *Fish as Food* (Ed. by G. Borgstrom), pp. 267–360. Academic Press, New York.

Brown, J.H. & Higuera-Ciapara, I. (1992) Antibiotic Residues in Farmed Shrimp – a developing problem? In *Proceedings of OIE Symposium: Problems of Chemotherapy in Aquaculture: From theory to reality*, Paris 12–15 March 1991 (Ed. by D.J. Alderman & C. Michel), pp. 394–403. Office International des Epizooties, Paris.

Browne, S. de la R. (1990) Food safety concerns and aquaculture. In Aquaculture International Congress Proceedings. September 4–7, 1990, Vancouver BC, Canada, pp. 210–12.

Bryan, F.L. (1980) Epidemiology of foodborne diseases transmitted by fish, shellfish and marine crustaceans in the United States, 1970–78. *Journal of Food Protection*, **43**, 859–76.

Bryan, F.L. (1986) Seafood-transmitted infections and intoxications in recent years. In *Seafood Quality Determination* (Ed. by D.E. Kramer & J. Liston), pp. 319–37. Elsevier Science, Amsterdam.

Buck, J.D. & Spotte, S. (1986) The occurrence of potentially pathogenic vibrios in marine animals. *Marine Mammal Science*, **2**(4), 319–24.

Codex Alimentarius Commission (1984) Report of the Twentieth Session of the Codex Committee on Food Hygiene, Alinorm 85/13A. Codex Alimentarius Commission, Rome.

Colwell, R.R. (1984) *Vibrios in the environment*. John Wiley & Sons, New York.

Communicable Diseases (Scotland) Unit (1980–1989). Annual reports of the surveillance programme for foodborne infections and intoxications, Scotland. Information and Statistics Division, Scottish Health Service, Edinburgh.

Connell, J.J. (1990) *Control of Fish Quality*, 3rd edn. Fishing News Books, Blackwell Scientific Publications Ltd, Oxford.

Cox, L.J., Keller, N. & Schothorst, M. van (1988) The use and misuse of quantitative determination of Enterobacteriaceae in food microbiology. In *Enterobacteriaceae in the environment and as pathogens* (Ed. by B.M. Lund, M. Sussman, D. Jones & M.F. Stringer) Society for Applied Bacteriology Symposium Series No. 17. Blackwell Scientific Publications, London, pp. 237–49.

Damme, L.R. van & Vandepitte, J. (1980) Frequent isolation of *Edwardsiella tarda* and *Plesiomonas shigelloides* from healthy Zairese freshwater fish: a possible source of diarrhoea. *Applied Environmental Microbiology*, **39**(3), 475–9.

Dussault, H.P. (1958) TMA test for evaluating the quality of rosefish fillets. *Fisheries Research Board of Canada Progress Report of Atlantic Coast Station*, **67**.

Endtz, H.P., Ruijs, G.J., van Klingeren, B., Jansen, W.H., van der Reyden, T. & Mouton, R.P. (1991) Quinolone resistance in campylobacter isolated from man and poultry following the introduction of fluoroquinolones in veterinary medicine. *Journal of Antimicrobial Chemotherapy*, **27**, 199–208.

Eyles, M.J. (1986) Microbiological hazards associated with fishery products. CSIRO Food Research Quarterly, **46**(1), 8–16.

FAO (1977) Microbiological specifications for foods. Report of the second joint FAO/WHO Expert Consultation, Geneva 21 Feb–2 March 1977. Food and Agriculture Organization of the United Nations, Rome.

FAO (1981) Parasites, infections and diseases of fish in Africa. CIFA Technical Paper No. 7, 216.

FAO (1988) Yearbook of fishery statistics 1988, **66**. Catches and landings.

FAO (1990) Aquaculture production (1985–1988). Fisheries Circular No. 815. Revision 2, Rome p. 136.

Federal Register (1982) US Food and Drug Administration. Federal Register 4 September 1982.

Fox, B. (1978) *Food Science – a Chemical Approach*. Hodder & Stoughton, London.

Frank, H.A. (1985) Histamine forming bacteria in tuna and other marine fish. In *Histamine in Marine Producis* (Ed. by B.S. Pan & D. James), pp. 2–3. FAO Fisheries Technical Paper 252.

Gutting, R.E. (1990) Consumer perceptions in the seafood market. In Aquaculture International Congress Proceedings, 4–7 September 1990, Vancouver BC, Canada pp. 7–10.

Hankin, R. (1992) Veterinary Medicines Regulations for Fish in the EEC. In *Proceedings of OIE Symposium. Problems of Chemotherapy in Aquaculture: From theory to reality*, Paris 12–15 March 1991 (Ed. by D.J. Alderman & C. Michel), pp. 116–21. Office International des Epizooties, Paris.

Hebard, C.E., Flick, G.J. & Martin, R.E. (1982) Occurrence and significance of trimethylamine oxide and its derivatives in fish and shellfish. In *Chemistry and Biochemistry of Marine Food Products* (Ed. by R.E. Martin, G.J. Flick, C.E. Hebard & D.R. Ward), pp. 149–304. AVI Publishing Company, Westport, Connecticut.

Hedges, R.W., Smith, P. & Brazil, G. (1985) Resistance plasmids of aeromonads. *Journal of General Microbiology*, **131**, 2091–5.

Herbert, R.A., Hendrie, M.S., Gibson, D.M. & Shewan, J.M. (1971) Bacteria active in the spoilage of certain seafoods. *Journal of Applied Bacteriology*, **34**(1), 41–51.

Higgins, B.C. & Kolbye, A.C. (1984) Risks and benefits of seafood. In *Seafood Toxins* (Ed. by E.P. Regelis), pp. 59–67. American Chemical Society Symposium Series No. 262.

Hood, M.A., Ness, G.E. & Blake, N.J. (1983) Relationship between fecal coliforms, *Escherichia coli* and *Salmonella* spp. in shellfish. *Applied Environmental Microbiology*, **45**, 122–6.

Holmberg, S.D., Wells, J.G. & Cohen, M.L. (1984) Animal-to-man transmission of antimicrobial-resistant *Salmonella*: investigations of US outbreaks 1971–1983. *Science*, **225**, 833–5.

Husevag, B., Lunestad, B.T., Johannessen, P.J., Enger, O. & Samuelsen, O.B. (1991) Simultaneous occurrence of *Vibrio salmonicida* and antibiotic resistant bacteria in sediments at abandoned aquaculture sites. *Journal of Fish Diseases*, **14**(6), 631–41.

Huss, H.H. (1983) Fersk Fisk-Kvalitet og Holdbarhed. Monograph, Technological Laboratory, Ministry of Fisheries, Technical University, Lyngby, Denmark.

Huss, H.H., Trolle, G. & Gram, L. (1986) New rapid methods in microbiological evaluation of fish quality. In *Seafood Quality Determination* (Ed. by D.E. Kramer & J. Liston), pp. 299–318. Proceedings of International Symposium, Sea Grant College Programme, Anchorage. Elsevier, Amsterdam.

ICMSF (1986) *Micro-organisms in Foods, 2. Sampling for Microbiological Analysis, Principles and Specific Applications*, 2nd edn. ICMSC, University of Toronto Press.

Janda, J.M. & Bryant, R.G. (1987) Pathogenic *Vibrio* spp.: an organism group of increasing medical significance. *Clinical Microbiology Newsletter*, **19**(7), 49–53.

JECFA (1989) Thirty fourth Report. Evaluation of certain drug residues in food. WHO, Geneva.

JECFA (1990) Evaluation of certain veterinary drug residues in food. WHO, Geneva.

Joint Committee on the use of Antibiotics in Animal Husbandry and Veterinary Medicine (1969) Report by the Secretary of State for Scotland, the Minister of Agriculture, Fisheries and Food and the Secretary of State for Wales (Chairman Prof. M.M. Swann). Command 4190. HMSO, London.

Kelch, W.J. & Lee, J.S. (1978) Antibiotic resistance pattern of gram-negative bacteria isolated from environmental sources. *Applied Environmental Microbiology*, **36**, 450–6.

Licciardello, J.L. (1983) Botulism and heat-processed seafoods. *Marine Fisheries Review*, **45**(2), 1–7.

Liston, J. (1980) Microbiology in fishery science. In *Advances in Fish Science and Technology* (Ed. by J.J. Connell), pp. 138–57. Fishing News Books Ltd, Farnham.

Liston, J. (1982) Recent advances in the chemistry of iced fish spoilage. In *Chemistry and Biochemistry of Marine Food Products* (Ed. by R.E. Martin, G.J. Flick, C.E. Hebard & D.R. Ward), pp. 27–37. AVI Publishing Company, Westport, Connecticut.

McGill, A.S. & Hardy, R. (1992) Review of the methods used in the determination of antibiotics and their metabolites in farmed fish. In Proceedings of the OIE Symposium: *Problems of Chemotherapy in Aquaculture: From theory to reality*, Paris 12–15 March 1991 (Ed. by D.J. Alderman & C. Michel), pp. 343–80. Office International des Epizooties, Paris.

Main, R. & Yates, B.D. (1990) Two cases of scombrotoxin fish poisoning. In *Surveillance Programme for Foodborne Infections and Intoxications, Scotland 1988*, Report 9 (Ed. By P.W. Collier, J.C.M. Sharp, K. Barratt & G.I. Forbes). Common Services Agency, Scottish Health Service.

Malathi, G.R., Karunasagar, I., Suseela, P.M. & Karunasagar, I. (1988) Role of hemolysins in the pathogenicity of Vibrios associated with seafoods. In *The First Indian Fisheries Forum* (Ed. by

M. Mohan Joseph), pp. 365–7. Asian Fisheries Society, Indian Branch, Mangalore.

Martin, R.E., Flick, G.J., Hebard, C.E. & Ward, D.R. (1982) *Chemistry and Biochemistry of Marine Food Products.* AVI Publishing Company, Westport, Connecticut.

Mathew, S., Karunasagar, I., Malathi, G.R. & Karunasagar, I. (1988) *Vibrio cholerae* in seafoods and environs, Mangalore, India. *Asian Fisheries Science,* **2,** 121–6.

Midtvedt, T. & Lingaas, E. (1992) Putative Public Health Risks of Antibiotic Resistance Development in Aquatic Bacteria. In *Proceedings of OIE Symposium: Problems of Chemotherapy in Aquaculture: From theory to reality,* Paris 12–15 March 1991 (Ed. by D.J. Alderman & C. Michel), pp. 304–15. Office International des Epizooties, Paris.

Mitsuhashi, S. (1977) Epidemiology of bacterial drug resistance. In *R-Factor Drug Resistance Plasmid* (Ed. by S. Mitsuhashi) University Park Press, Baltimore.

Morris, J.G. & Black, R.E. (1985) Cholera and other vibrioses in the United States. *New England Journal of Medicine,* **312,** 343–50.

Mossel, D.A.A. (1982) Marker organisms in food and drinking water. Semantics, ecology, taxonomy and enumeration. *Antonie van Leeuwenhoek International Journal of General and Molecular Microbiology,* **48,** 609–11.

Murray, B.E., Levine, M.M., Cordano, A.M., D'Ottone, K., Jananetra, P., Kapecko, D., Pan-Urae, R. & Prenzel, I. (1985) Survey of Plasmids in Salmonella typhi from Chile and Thailand. *Journal of Infectious Diseases,* **151,** 551–5.

Palumbo, S.A., Bencivengo, M.M., Delcorral, F., Williams, A.C. & Buchanan, R.L. (1989) Characterization of the *Aeromonas hydrophila* group isolated from retail foods of animal origin. *Journal of Clinical Microbiology,* **27**(5), 854–9.

Pan, B.S. (1985) Histamine formation in the canning process. In *Histamine in Marine Products* (Ed. by B.S. Pan & D. James), pp. 41–4. FAO Fisheries Technical Paper No. 252.

Richards, R.H., Inglis, V., Frerichs, G.N. & Millar, S.D. (1992) Variation in antibiotic resistance patterns of *Aeromonas salmonicida* isolated from Atlantic salmon *Salmo salar* L. in Scotland. In Proceedings of OIE Symposium: *Problems of Chemotherapy in Aquaculture: From theory to reality,* Paris 12–15 March 1991 (Ed. by D.J. Alderman & C. Michel), pp. 278–39. Office International des Epizooties, Paris.

Schulz, K.H. (1982) Allergy to chemicals: problems and perspectives. In *Allergy and Hypersensitivity to Chemicals.* WHO, Copenhagen.

Shewan, J.M. (1961) The microbiology of sea-water fish. In *Fish as Food,* Vol. 1 (Ed. by G. Borgstrom), pp. 478–560. Academic Press, New York.

Shewan, J.M. (1962) The bacteriology of fresh and spoiling fish and some related chemical changes. In *Recent Advances in Food Science,* Vol. 1 (Ed. by J. Hawthorn & J.M. Leitch), pp. 167–93. Butterworth, London.

Shewan, J.M. (1971) The microbiology of fish and fishery products – a progress report. *Journal of Applied Bacteriology,* **34**(2), 299–315.

Shewan, J.M. (1977) The bacteriology of fresh and spoiling fish and biochemical changes induced by bacterial action. In *Proceedings of the Conference on the Handling, Processing and Marketing of Tropical Fish,* pp. 51–66. London Tropical Products Institute.

Shewan, J.M., Hobbs, G. & Hodgkiss, W. (1960) The *Pseudomonas* and *Achromobacter* groups of bacteria in the spoilage of marine white fish. *Journal of Applied Bacteriology,* **23**(3), 463–8.

Spencer-Garrett, E. (1988) Microbiological standards. Guidelines and specifications and inspection of seafood products. *Food Technology,* March 1988, 90–3.

Spika, J.S., Waterman, S.H., Soo Hoo, G.W., St Louis, M.E., Pacer, R.E., James, S.M., Bissett, M.L., Mayer, L.W., Chiu, J.Y., Hall, B., Green, K., Potter, M.E., Cohen, M.L. & Blake, P.A. (1987) Chloramphenicol-resistant *Salmonella newport* traced through hamburger to dairy farms – a major persisting source of human salmonellosis in California. *New England Journal of Medicine,* **316,** 565–70.

Spreekens, K.J.A. van (1977) Characterization of some fish and shrimp spoiling bacteria. *Antonie van Leeuwenhoek International Journal of General and Molecular Microbiology,* **43,** 283–303.

Taylor, S.L., Hui, J.Y. & Lyons, D.E. (1984) Toxicology of scombroid poisoning. In *Seafood Toxins* (Ed. by E.P. Ragelis), pp. 417–30. American Chemical Society, Washington DC.

Taylor, S.L., Stratton, J.E. & Nordlee, J.A. (1989) Histamine poisoning (scombroid fish poisoning): an allergy-like intoxication. *Clinical Toxicology,* **27**(4 & 5), 225–40.

Threlfall, E.J., Rowe, B., Ferguson, J.L. & Ward, L.R. (1986) Characterization of plasmids conferring resistance to gentamycin and apramycin in strains of *Salmonella typhumurium* phage type 204c isolated in Britain. *Journal of Hygiene (Cambridge)*, **97**, 419–26.

Threlfall, E.J., Hall, M.L.M. and Rowe, B. (1992) Salmonella bacteraemia in England and Wales, 1981–1990. *Journal of Clinical Pathology*, **45**, 34–6.

Tinkelman, D.G. & Bock, S.A. (1984) Anaphylaxis presumed to be caused by beef containing streptomycin. *Annals of Allergy*, **53**, 243–4.

Todd, E.C.D. (1978) Foodborne diseases in six countries — a comparison. *Journal of Food Protection*, **41**, 559–65.

Venugopal, M.N. & Karunasagar, I. (1988) Effect of chemical preservatives on *Vibrio parahaemolyticus* in fish. In *The First Indian Fisheries Forum* (Ed. by M. Mohan Joseph), pp. 407–8. Asian Fisheries Society, Indian Branch, Mangalore.

Walton, J.R. (1988) Antibiotic resistance. An overview. *Veterinary Record*, **122**, 249–57.

Ward, L.R., Threlfall, E.J. & Rowe, B. (1990) Multiple drug resistance in salmonellae in England and Wales: a comparison between 1981 and 1988. *Journal of Clinical Pathology*, **43**, 563–6.

Warne, D. (1985) Introduction to the hazard analysis critical control point (HACCP) concept for canned fish manufacture. In Spoilage of tropical fish and product development (Ed. A. Reilly). *Symposium Proceedings of Indo-Pacific Fishery Commission, Royal Melbourne Institute of Technology*. FAO Fisheries Report No. 317, Supplement.

West, P.A. (1989) Human pathogens and public health indicator organisms in shellfish. In *Methods for the Microbiological Examination of Fish and Shellfish* (Ed. by B. Austin & D.A. Austin), pp. 273–308. Ellis Horwood, Chichester.

West, P.A. & Colwell, R.R. (1984) Identification and classification of Vibrionaceae — an overview. In Vibrios in the Environment (Ed. by R.R. Colwell), pp. 285–363. John Wiley & Son, New York.

WHO/ICMSF (1982) Report on hazard analysis. WHO, Geneva.

Wood, E.J.F. (1953) Heterotrophic bacteria in marine environments of Eastern Australia. *Australian Journal of Marine and Freshwater Research*, **4**, 160–200.

Woodward, K.N. (1991a) Hypersensitivity in humans and exposure to veterinary drugs. *Veterinary and Human Toxicology*, **33**(2), 168–72.

Woodward, K.N. (1991b) Use and regulatory control of veterinary drugs. In *Food Production in Food Contaminants, Sources and Surveillance* (Ed. by C.S. Creaser & R. Purchase), pp. 99–108. Royal Society of Chemistry, London.

Woodward, K.N. (1991c) The licensing of veterinary medicinal products in the United Kingdom — the work of the Veterinary Medicines Directorate. *Biologist*, **38**(3), 105–8.

Working Party on Veterinary Residues in Animal Products (1987) Anabolic, anthelminthic and antimicrobial agents. Twenty-second report of the Steering Group on Food Surveillance. Food Surveillance Paper, No. 22. HMSO, London.

Yndestad, M. (1992) Public Health Aspects of Residues in Animal Products — Fundamental Considerations. In *Proceedings of OIE Symposium: Problems of Chemotherapy in Aquaculture: From theory to reality*, Paris 12–15 March 1991 (Ed. by D.J. Alderman & C. Michel), pp. 494–509. Office International des Epizooties, Paris.

# Index